T0190130

Register Now for Online Access to Your Book!

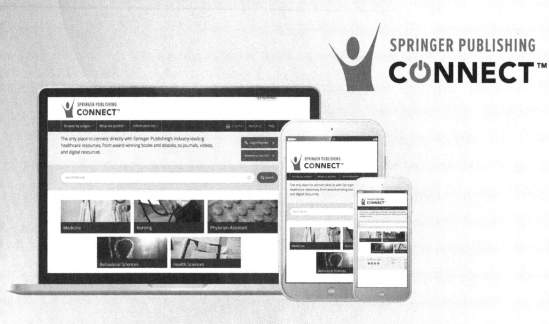

Your print purchase of *Assisted Living Administration and Management, Second Edition,* **includes online access to the contents of your book—** increasing accessibility, portability, and searchability!

Access today at:
http://connect.springerpub.com/content/book/978-0-8261-6199-4
or scan the QR code at the right with your smartphone
and enter the access code below.

51SMM006

Scan here for quick access.

If you are experiencing problems accessing the digital component of this product, please contact our customer service department at cs@springerpub.com

The online access with your print purchase is available at the publisher's discretion and may be removed at any time without notice.

Publisher's Note: New and used products purchased from third-party sellers are not guaranteed for quality, authenticity, or access to any included digital components.

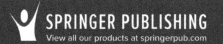

SPRINGER PUBLISHING
View all our products at springerpub.com

"Assisted living is incredibly complex, with great nationwide variability in regulation, size, services, staffing, delivery models, and financing. Out of the chaos, this book offers clarity and understanding. Considered through a multidisciplinary lens, with appreciation of state-level differences, each chapter offers a complete picture of the nuances of field.

"Chapters include perspectives on the history of assisted living; policy; organizational structure; care; staffing; safety; business; financial management; law and liability; disaster preparedness; concepts of aging; principles and models of care; facility design; ethnic, cultural, and sexual diversity; physiological and psychological changes with aging; dementia, hospice, and palliative care; and elder resident rights.

"The second edition of *Assisted Living Administration and Management: Effective Practices and Model Programs in Elder Care* should be a first stop for anyone with an interest in assisted living."

Daniel David, PhD, RN
Assistant Professor
Rory Meyers College of Nursing
New York University
New York, NY

"Propelled by the COVID-19 pandemic, society faced the daunting revelation that older adults residing in long-term care settings faced high rates of morbidity and mortality due to inadequacies in the administration and management of these facilities. In the United States, assisted living facilities are the fastest growing segment in this sector. The timely publication of this book, needed now more than ever, offers the critical knowledge about evidence-based practices and resources relevant to administrators, staff, families, gerontology students, and policy makers to address these inadequacies. Each chapter is written by one or more content experts on the topic with explicit objectives, related historical background, regulatory landscape, practical care delivery aspects, challenges, resources, and future directions. Given the lack of national standards in assisted living and the variety of regulatory approaches across the states, the contemporary tables and charts that highlight these differences by state along with links to key policy, advocacy, and consumer resources are very helpful. The second edition not only updates the award-winning content from the first edition but also adds contemporary material on ethics, ethnicity, culture, diversity, disparity, and resident rights issues. For those interested in learning about assistive living, *Assisted Living Administration and Management: Effective Practices and Model Programs in Elder Care* is a necessity!"

Diane Feeney Mahoney, PhD, GNP-ret, FGSA, FAAN
Professor Emerita, MGH Institute of Health Professions
and Senior Gerontologist, EDDEE Consulting
Boston, MA

"Assisted living facilities account for a substantial proportion of the long-term care recipient population, yet as we were reminded by the COVID-19 pandemic, these facilities are often under-resourced. This book offers a practical approach to key issues in routine and crisis management of an assisted living facility. It is especially pleasing to see the long needed collaboration between nursing and social services, and the emphasis given to the training needs of the direct-care staff. The authors have made an important update to their first edition. This work continues to be a milestone for the field of aging and assisted living administration."

Robert Newcomer, PhD
Professor Emeritus, Institute for Health & Aging
University of California
San Francisco, CA

"The second edition of *Assisted Living Administration and Management: Effective Practices and Model Programs in Elder Care,* offers a well-written and thorough overview of assisted living administration and management that can be of benefit to a broad audience. From increasing awareness of family members who are looking for a better understanding of long-term care options and information related to the unique characteristics of the assisted living environment, to long-term care administrators who desire increased insight into the multiple components of assisted living management, this book is an essential and valuable resource. The inclusion of information pertaining to common age-related changes in neuropsychological functioning, in addition to overviewing psychological conditions as they relate to adjustment and adaptation to optimal functioning for individuals within the assisted living setting, emphasizes the depth and relevance of this invaluable resource."

Lisa Lind, PhD
Licensed Psychologist
Chief of Quality Assurance
Deer Oaks Behavioral Health
San Antonio, TX
and President
Psychologists in Long-Term Care

ASSISTED LIVING ADMINISTRATION AND MANAGEMENT

Darlene Yee-Melichar, EdD, FGSA, FAGHE, is professor and coordinator of gerontology at San Francisco State University (SF State) where she also serves as director of long-term care administration. She is the recipient of numerous awards and honors for her teaching excellence and service contributions to the campus, community, and profession.

Dr. Yee-Melichar's research interests in healthy aging, long-term care administration, minority women's health, and safety research and education are reflected in the five books, 109 journal articles, book chapters, book reviews, and technical reports she has written, and the numerous professional and scholarly presentations she has made. She was active on the National Institutes of Health (NIH) Advisory Committee for Research on Women's Health, NIH Review Committee for Research Enhancement Awards Program, and Agency for Healthcare Research and Quality (AHRQ) special emphasis panels on Translating Research into Practice and Health Research Dissemination.

She chaired the U.S. Department of Health and Human Services (DHHS) Office on Minority Health (OWH) Minority Women's Health Panel of Experts, served on the U.S. DHHS–Centers for Medicare & Medicaid Services' Advisory Panel on Outreach and Education, and the U.S. DHHS–OWH Region IX Women's Health Advisory Council, cochaired the International Association of Gerontology and Geriatrics 2017 World Congress on Gerontology and Geriatrics Local Arrangements Committee and the Regional Health Equity Council for Region IX (RHEC IX).

Dr. Yee-Melichar is a charter Fellow of the Academy for Gerontology in Higher Education; Fellow of the Gerontological Society of America; Fellow of the American Alliance for Health, Physical Education, Recreation and Dance Research Consortium; and member of Sigma Xi, the national research society. She has served on the editorial boards of the *Journal of Gerontological Social Work, Journal of Health Education,* and other peer-reviewed publications. She also serves on the board of directors for the California Advocates for Nursing Home Reform (CANHR) and as an OMH Health Equity Mentor for the U.S. DHHS.

She received her BA in biology from Barnard College, MS in gerontology from the College of New Rochelle, and MS and EdD in health education focusing on gerontology from Columbia University.

Cristina Flores, PhD, RN, FGSA, has been a registered nurse for more than 30 years. Her nursing practice has included many aspects of the continuum of care such as home health care, assisted living communities, and the acute care hospital. She holds an MA in gerontology from San Francisco State University (SF State) and a PhD in nursing health policy from the University of California, San Francisco (UCSF). At present, she is the owner and licensee of three six-bed residential care facilities for the elderly in California, a lecturer in the gerontology program at SF State, and an adjunct professor for UCSF. She has published several journal articles, book chapters, and two books relative to long-term care administration and quality of care. She is a Fellow of the Gerontological Society of America and was the recipient of the 2009 Kenji Murase Distinguished Alumni Award, School of Social Work, SF State.

Andrea Renwanz Boyle, PhD, RN, FNAP, is a graduate of the University of California, San Francisco, where she received a PhD in nursing science. Dr. Boyle received her MS in nursing from Boston University and adult nurse practitioner certification from Peter Bent Brigham Hospital. Currently, Dr. Boyle is the chair and professor of nursing at Dominican University of California and a Distinguished Practice Fellow in the National Academies of Practice. Dr. Boyle is the Co-President of Sigma Theta Tau International Nursing Honor Society (Rho Alpha Chapter) and an emerita associate professor at San Francisco State University. Dr. Boyle is widely published in the areas of health-related issues in aging and assisted living, nursing education, evidence-based practice, problem-based learning, and interprofessional practice in palliative care. She has presented her work at a number of international and national scholarly research and professional conferences and currently serves as a manuscript reviewer for interprofessional, geriatric, and nursing journals. Dr. Boyle has served as a member of national and international nursing boards and organizations, including the International Council of Nurses Nurse Practitioner/Advanced Practice Nursing Network and the Regional Health Equity Council for Region IX (RHEC IX). Dr. Boyle has served as a commissioner on the California Workforce Policy Commission, been certified as a residential care facility for the elderly (RCFE) administrator, and worked in primary care settings as an adult and geriatric nurse practitioner. Dr. Boyle received the 2009 SF State Distinguished Faculty Award for Excellence in Service.

ASSISTED LIVING ADMINISTRATION AND MANAGEMENT

Effective Practices and Model Programs in Elder Care

Second Edition

Darlene Yee-Melichar, EdD, FGSA, FAGHE

Cristina Flores, PhD, RN, FGSA

Andrea Renwanz Boyle, PhD, RN, FNAP

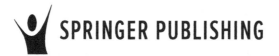 SPRINGER PUBLISHING

Springer Publishing Company, LLC
11 West 42nd Street, New York, NY 10036
www.springerpub.com
connect.springerpub.com/

Acquisitions Editor: David D'Addona
Compositor: Exeter Premedia Services Private Ltd.

ISBN: 978-0-8261-6194-9
ebook ISBN: 978-0-8261-6199-4
DOI: 10.1891/9780826161994

Qualified instructors may request supplements by emailing textbook@springerpub.com

Test Bank ISBN: 978-0-8261-6197-0 (Also available on Respondus®.)

20 21 22 23 24 / 5 4 3 2 1

The author and the publisher of this Work have made every effort to use sources believed to be reliable to provide information that is accurate and compatible with the standards generally accepted at the time of publication. The author and publisher shall not be liable for any special, consequential, or exemplary damages resulting, in whole or in part, from the readers' use of, or reliance on, the information contained in this book. The publisher has no responsibility for the persistence or accuracy of URLs for external or third-party Internet websites referred to in this publication and does not guarantee that any content on such websites is, or will remain, accurate or appropriate.

Library of Congress Cataloging-in-Publication Data

Names: Yee-Melichar, Darlene, author. | Flores, Cristina, author. |
  Boyle, Andrea Renwanz, author.
Title: Assisted living administration and management : effective practices
  and model programs in elder care / Darlene Yee-Melichar, Cristina
  Flores, Andrea Renwanz Boyle.
Description: Second edition. | New York, NY : Springer Publishing Company,
  LLC, 2020. | Includes bibliographical references and index.
Identifiers: LCCN 2020038069 (print) | LCCN 2020038070 (ebook) | ISBN
  9780826161949 (paperback) | ISBN 9780826161994 (ebook)
Subjects: MESH: Assisted Living Facilities--organization & administration |
  Homes for the Aged | Nursing Homes | Aged
Classification: LCC HV1454 (print) | LCC HV1454 (ebook) | NLM WT 27.1 |
  DDC 362.61068--dc23
LC record available at https://lccn.loc.gov/2020038069
LC ebook record available at https://lccn.loc.gov/2020038070

Contact sales@springerpub.com to receive discount rates on bulk purchases.

Publisher's Note: New and used products purchased from third-party sellers are not guaranteed for quality, authenticity, or access to any included digital components.

Printed in the United States of America.

Dedicated to the students and practitioners in health and human services who are committed to enhancing the quality of care and quality of life of older adults residing in assisted living facilities and other long-term care communities.

With love and gratitude to our families and friends for their continuing patience and moral support.

CONTENTS

PART TWO: HUMAN RESOURCES MANAGEMENT

CONTRIBUTORS

Benjamin Bongers, MA, Associate Director, Health and Science Center Inc., Lima, Pennsylvania

Edwin P. Cabigao, PhD, RN, Director of Clinical Services, Generations Healthcare, Santa Ana, California

Anthony M. Chicotel, JD, MPP, Staff Attorney, California Advocates for Nursing Home Reform, San Francisco, California

Mark J. Cimino, JD, Chief Executive Officer, CiminoCare, Citrus Heights, California

Brian de Vries, PhD, Professor Emeritus, Gerontology, San Francisco State University, San Francisco, California

David Hahklotubbe, MA, Disrupter, Red Kite Movement, Monterey, California

Joseph F. Melichar, PhD, Research Consultant, Gerontology, San Francisco State University, San Francisco, California

Pauline Mosher Shatara, MA, Deputy Director, California Advocates for Nursing Home Reform, San Francisco, California

Raymond Yee, MBA, MPH, Director of Finance and Administration, Healthdata EZ Consulting Corporation, Fair Lawn, New Jersey

FOREWORD

If you are reading this book because you are preparing for or have entered a career in long-term care, then you probably already know that the population 65 years of age and older is expected to grow dramatically from 53 million older adults today to 70 million in 2030 and 95 million by 2060. What you may not know is that if you have chosen to work with older people, your decision is comparatively rare. In spite of the fact that we have expected this growth for decades, we have not adequately prepared a healthcare workforce and have failed to recruit enough other necessary professionals, especially in long-term care settings. Today less than 3% of medical students choose electives about aging and less than 1% of nurses are certified gerontological nurses. In spite of the fact that 75% of social workers serve older adults and their families, only 4% have completed gerontological training.

There are many reasons people select particular career paths including remuneration, family expectations, talent, and opportunity. Public judgments about the desirability of various careers also influence our choices. Negative perceptions about older people and stereotypic views equating old age with disease, poverty, loneliness, and other afflictions have no doubt discouraged some from pursuing careers in gerontology.

Gerontological researchers, policymakers, educators, and advocates have attempted to dispel negative stereotypes by pointing out that the older population of the future will be more racially and ethnically diverse, more likely to be employed, less likely to live in poverty, and better educated than previous generations. Influential organizations such as the Gerontological Society of America (GSA) and the AARP launched initiatives to promote positive attitudes about aging, improve perceptions of older adults, and counter ageism. The World Health Organization (WHO) mounted the "Age-Friendly Cities" movement that reimagines living environments supporting well-being and engagement for all generations. These and other undertakings have achieved some success in changing narratives about aging in a more positive direction, but ageism and the marginalization of older adults can resurface when conditions are ripe.

While this book was being prepared for publication in the spring of 2020, the world was gripped by a global pandemic caused by a novel coronavirus. At this time, over 100,000 Americans have died, and nearly two million have been infected by COVID-19, the disease caused by the coronavirus. Around the world, infected older adults have been disproportionately more likely to experience severe disease and death. Because COVID-19 spreads readily through respiratory droplets, it spiked in living and working environments where people clustered in close proximity. America's long-term care facilities were particularly hard hit. In addition to the congregate living environment, the incidence of co-morbidities (diabetes, heart disease, compromised immune systems, etc.) rendered this population especially vulnerable. In the spring of 2020, nearly 32,000 of the 100,000 Americans who died were reported to have been residents of nursing homes. This alarming number was an undercount of the long-term care death toll since not all nursing homes had reported and assisted living residents were not included in the Centers for Medicare & Medicaid Services (CMS) data.

Governments around the world attempted to stop the spread of the virus by imposing quarantines. These policies, however, had a devastating economic impact, rivaling the Great Depression, as businesses and "nonessential" services closed down. Public debate focused on whether to maintain quarantines, thus exacerbating unemployment, business collapse, and financial hardship or to re-open businesses thus allowing the virus to spread, with especially adverse consequences for older people, in general, and those in assisted living/residential care, in particular.

In the crisis moment, expressions of ageism appeared. Seniors were encouraged to sacrifice themselves for the sake of their grandchildren. Editorials suggested that some proportion of older adults were "expendable," for the good of the economy and the "American way of life." Contrary opinions insisted that it is a false choice between saving the economy and saving older adults as, in actuality, the health of the economy depends on the productive contributions and consumer power of those over 65. It seems likely that as such crises are brought under greater control, overt expressions of ageism will recede while the underlying sentiment remains below the surface of public discourse.

These events have shown that we have much more educational work to do. This is especially true regarding residents of long-term care communities who are most likely to suffer from negative stereotyping that ignores the diversity of this population. Therefore, it is fortunate that the second edition of *Assisted Living Administration and Management: Effective Practices and Model Programs in Elder Care* is being published at this particular time.

This book is a practical resource for professionals, a textbook for students, and a study manual for those preparing for state certification exams. It locates the expanding field of long-term care within a social context and corrects many misperceptions. New chapters in this edition address topics such as inter-professional practice; home- and community-based services; information and communication technology; LGBTQ and other diverse groups; memory care; and palliative and hospice care.

Importantly, the book is based on core competencies required to operate assisted living communities, and each of its five parts focuses on a core competency (i.e., domain of practice). Thus, it is consistent with the competency movement in higher education, an evidence- and measurement-based approach to learning promoted by the Academy for Gerontology in Higher Education (AGHE), the Accreditation for Gerontology Education Council (AGEC), and the National Association for Professional Gerontologists (NAPG). Credentialing and state certification/licensure, based on demonstrated competencies, professionalizes a field by maintaining standards that improve the quality of care. Credentialed professionals positively affect the public's perceptions and expectations about standards of care. A public that expects superior services also improves the quality of care for the elderly. Public perceptions about gerontology and long-term care that hold these fields in high regard lead to more positive attitudes toward the elderly themselves and greater interest in professional training for careers that serve them.

The second edition of *Assisted Living Administration and Management: Effective Practices and Model Programs in Elder Care* makes a timely and essential contribution to professional training and is a welcome resource for those dedicated to improving long-term care services for older adults.

Donna E. Schafer, PhD, CPG
Executive Director
National Association for Professional Gerontologists

PREFACE

This second edition of *Assisted Living Administration and Management: Effective Practices and Model Programs in Elder Care* reflects the way society views the growing elderly population and the implications of this demographic trend for the field of long-term care. Long-term care continues to be the fastest growing segment of the healthcare industry; there is a critical need to educate and train a core of professional personnel with the knowledge and skills to address the complex issues in aging, health, and human services. Long-term care administration is in a period of diversification and expansion. Professional requirements vary widely depending on state and federal regulations for the specific area of administration. Long-term care administrators manage and direct the daily operations of a variety of communities and facilities.

This book aims to provide a useful reference of content information, effective practices, and model programs in elder care related to assisted living/residential care (AL/RC) administration. Similar to the first edition, this book is based on the core competencies required to operate assisted living communities. This book contains five parts; each part focuses on a core competency in assisted living administration such as organizational management, human resources management, business and financial management, environmental management, and resident care management. This book embraces chapter features such as useful learning objectives, case studies, effective practices, and model programs in elder care that are relevant to assisted living communities.

The positive responses of faculty, students, and AL/RC practitioners to the first edition suggest that we have been successful in achieving our goals for this book. Based on feedback from our readers, this second edition builds on and expands on the chapters in the first edition. This book has six new chapters (8, 15, 16, 18, 21, 22), and the other 17 have been considerably revised and updated as needed. The new chapters in this edition include: Interprofessional Practice: Issues for Assisted Living Administrators, Home- and Community-Based Services as an Alternative to Assisted Living, Information and Communication Technology in Assisted Living, LGBTQ Issues in Assisted Living, Memory Care Units in Assisted Living: Benefits and Challenges for Administrators, and Palliative and Hospice Care. We updated each original chapter as needed according to the National Center for Assisted Living (NCAL) 2019 Assisted Living State Regulatory Review, *Compendium of Residential Care and Assisted Living Regulations and Policy: 2015 Edition*; and currently available research literature.

Part I focuses on organizational management and includes three chapters. Chapter 1 introduces the reader to the assisted living concept. A historical background, nomenclature, definitions, and an overview description of the industry are included. The evolution and emergence of assisted living are discussed. Individual states are responsible for the licensing, monitoring, and oversight of assisted living. Chapter 2 summarizes basic laws and regulations regarding assisted living and discusses some of the similarities and differences across states. A description of various regulatory models is included. Chapter 3 provides an overview of the organizational models used in assisted living communities. States' staffing requirements and staff educational requirements for assisted living communities are described.

Part II focuses on human resources management and includes five chapters. The success of an assisted living community depends greatly on the hiring of appropriate staff that is based on the specific needs of the community. Chapter 4 describes the recruitment and hiring of suitable staff persons, including the administrator and direct care workers. Factors influencing recruitment, recruitment sources, and the hiring process are included. Chapter 5 describes the training processes of staff in assisted living. Concepts, such as orientation, on-the-job training, and the evaluation of training processes, are incorporated. A summary of the various state requirements regarding staff training is included. In Chapter 6, strategies for the retention of key and high-quality personnel are discussed. The needs of employees, such as economic security and job satisfaction, are considered. Strategies for empowering staff to participate in the vision of the assisted living community are described. Staff development concepts, including continuing education requirements, for personnel are discussed in Chapter 7. An overview of the various state requirements for ongoing training and continuing education for the administrator and direct care staff is included. Examples of important continuing education topics are integrated into the chapter. Chapter 8, a new chapter in this second edition, describes the important need for interprofessional practice roles in assisted living communities. Definitions of interprofessional practice, descriptions of interprofessional team member roles, and benefits and issues of interprofessional practice are presented.

Part III focuses on business and financial management and includes three chapters. Chapter 9 offers a comprehensive introduction to business, management, and marketing in assisted living communities with attention to essential management theories, management method and style, management and organizational structure, the business plan, operational plan and planning system, information and technology support services, and marketing approaches for assisted living communities. Chapter 10 presents key information on accounting systems, organization, financial reporting, account procedures, accounts records, budget preparation, ratio analysis, risk management, and accounting terms used in assisted living communities. Updates to this chapter include information about GAAP; the National Investment Center for Senior Housing; real estate aspects of assisted living communities, such as lease agreements and real estate investment trust (REITs); differences between a publicly traded company, a privately held one, and nonprofits (charity and noncharities) and the reporting obligations associated; and financial analysis using proformas for acquisitions or ground-up startups. Chapter 11 provides fundamental information on tort law and negligence, *respondeat superior,* corporate negligence, governing body, contracts, evictions, wills, trusts, conservatorships, guardianships, advance directives, living wills, and durable power of attorney.

Part IV focuses on environmental management and includes five chapters. Chapter 12 is updated to describe selected federal regulations, laws, and statutes. Accessibility, fire safety, workplace safety, and disaster preparedness issues are identified and discussed. Chapter 13 provides a discussion of care delivery philosophy in assisted living communities. An updated discussion of the medical model, Greenhouse model, and Eden Alternative is presented and includes the benefits and challenges associated with each care model. Chapter 14 provides updated descriptions of universal design and aging-in-place programs for assisted living communities. Selected elements of universal design and aging in place are discussed along with the benefits and challenges associated with each approach. Chapter 15, a new chapter in this second edition, introduces home- and community-based services (HCBS) as an alternative for consumers wishing to avoid leaving their homes to reside in assisted living. It describes the benefits of HCBS services, long-term care services, the historical evolution of HCBS, three existing HCBS programs, and the need for expansion of HCBS programs in light of the challenges experienced by consumers in accessing services. Chapter 16, another new chapter in this second edition, provides a comprehensive discussion on what information communication technologies (ICT) are, and how they can be of use in an assisted living/residential care community. ICT general terminology, history and evolution, ICT and their uses in aiding older adults, and examples of practice use in assisted living are discussed.

Part V focuses on resident care management and includes seven chapters. Chapter 17 offers an update on cultural elements and diversity issues for assisted living residents in selected groups, including but not limited to African Americans, Hispanics, Asian Americans, and Native Americans. Chapter 18 is a new chapter that is important to include in this second edition. It contains vital information regarding LGBTQ older adults in the context of assisted living. Key terms are defined, specific barriers faced by this population are discussed, and best practices and resources are addressed. Chapter 19 is an updated discussion of normal physiologic changes in aging. Updated information is presented on nutrition, sleep assessment, mobility, falls prevention, and pain management. Chapter 20 presents information on normal psychological changes associated with aging and is updated to provide strategies for memory maintenance. Issues including depression, dementia, and alcohol and substance abuse in elders are also discussed. Chapter 21 is a new chapter designed to describe the need for memory care units in assisting living communities. Definitions of neurocognitive disorders are presented along with a discussion of the regulatory requirements and selected benefits and challenges associated with assisted living memory care units. Chapter 22, another new chapter in this second edition, describes palliative and hospice care and the possible benefits this type of care can be to assisted living residents. The reader will learn how to address challenges and barriers related to implementing these programs and learn about model programs. Finally, yet very important, Chapter 23 provides an updated focus on the protection of elderly residents and resident rights in assisted living communities. Selected state statutes and federal civil rights legislation are described.

Assisted Living Administration and Management: Effective Practices and Model Programs in Elder Care, Second Edition, serves as a useful reference for professionals who are associated with AL/RC organizations. It can also function as a primary textbook for undergraduate and graduate courses in gerontology, health administration, and long-term care administration that focus on assisted living/residential care administration. *Assisted Living Administration and Management: Effective Practices and Model Programs in Elder Care,* Second Edition, is the "go-to book" if you wish to study for your state certification exam and/or review some of the chapters for hands-on information in running an assisted living community, especially when used in conjunction with your AL/RC state regulations. We have attempted to make the book practical for all readers by including useful learning objectives, case studies, effective practices, and model programs in elder care that are relevant to assisted living communities. Readers can obtain test questions for each chapter from Springer Publishing Company, LLC. Faculty can use these test questions to challenge their students on midterm or final exams; students can use these test questions to prepare themselves for the AL/RC Administrator State Certification Exam. We take this opportunity to express our gratitude to our readers who intend to use this book in their efforts to enhance the quality of care and quality of life for residents in AL/RC communities.

Darlene Yee-Melichar
Cristina Flores
Andrea Renwanz Boyle

REFERENCE

Office of the Assistant Secretary for Planning and Evaluation. (2015). *Compendium of residential care and assisted living regulations and policy: 2015 edition.* https://aspe.hhs.gov/basic-report/compendium-residential-care-and-assisted-living-regulations-and-policy-2015-edition#:~:text=Compendium%20 of%20Residential%20Care%20and%20Assisted%20Living%20Regulations,PUBLIC%20 FINANCING%20OF%20SERVICES.%20...%20More%20items...%20

Qualified instructors may obtain access to a supplemental test bank by emailing textbook@springerpub.com

ACKNOWLEDGMENTS

We are grateful to the many people who have contributed meaningfully to the successful completion of edition two of this book.

In particular, we thank David D'Addona and Jaclyn Shultz at Springer Publishing Company, who helped to extend the idea of this book and invited us to improve it. We appreciated very much the encouragement, patience, and support that our colleagues at Springer have provided during the past year in broadening and updating the manuscript.

We especially wish to thank the contributing authors who have shared their respective areas of expertise within this book. Benjamin Bongers, Edwin P. Cabigao, Anthony M. Chicotel, Mark Cimino, Brian de Vries, David Hahklotubbe, Joseph F. Melichar, Pauline Mosher Shatara, and Raymond Yee have provided informed, insightful, and invaluable contributions to this edition. You are the best!

For their capable assistance in writing test questions related to the chapters in this book, we are grateful for the proficient work of Victoria Aguila, Yadira Aldana, Mark Cimino, Mia Enriquez, Terry Ervin, Pauline Mosher Shatara, Ismael Tellez, and Connie Yuen. Thank you all for the successful teamwork.

San Francisco State University student assistants Victoria Aguila, Yadira Aldana, Christine Reyes, Cyrus Riahi, Annabelle Stein, and Elke Tekin provided helpful assistance with literature reviews and updating references. Your behind-the-scenes support was much appreciated.

Our families and friends have been a mainstay of encouragement and support throughout the preparation of the second edition of this book, and we take this opportunity to express our gratitude to all of them:

- Joseph and Helen Melichar and Yuen Hing and Raymond Yee
- Robert and Irene Benjamin, Jacqueline and Jake Angelo, and Albert Ujcic
- Robert and Bubba Boyle

We could not have done this without you—thank you all for your help and support in making the second edition of this book the best it could be.

Darlene Yee-Melichar, EdD, FGSA, FAGHE
Cristina Flores, PhD, RN, FGSA
Andrea Renwanz Boyle, PhD, RN, FNAP

LIST OF FIGURES

LIST OF TABLES

ORGANIZATIONAL MANAGEMENT

THE ASSISTED LIVING INDUSTRY: CONTEXT, HISTORY, AND OVERVIEW

LEARNING OBJECTIVES

Upon the completion of Chapter 1, the reader will be able to:

- Describe assisted living in the context of the continuum of long-term care services and supports.
- Discuss the historical evolution of assisted living.
- Cite a variety of operational definitions of assisted living.
- Describe the characteristics of assisted living residents, such as resident profiles and sources of payment.
- Discuss the challenges faced by the assisted living industry, such as quality of care and safety concerns.
- Describe quality-improvement strategies of the assisted living industry.

INTRODUCTION

The purpose of this first chapter is to introduce the reader to the assisted living industry. First, the context of long-term care services, needs, and associated costs is described. Next, the historical evolution of assisted living is included to help the reader understand the background and development of today's assisted living communities. Because there is no single nationally accepted definition of *assisted living*, multiple definitions—along with their sources—are provided. A description of common resident characteristics is incorporated, including resident profiles, length-of-stay averages, reasons residents leave assisted living communities, and common payment sources. This chapter closes with an overview of some of the challenges related to quality of care in assisted living, highlighting the important need for knowledgeable administrators in the industry.

Context

Assisted living is a prominent and significant component of long-term care for older persons in the United States. Concerns regarding nursing home quality, states' interests in containing long-term care costs, as well as consumer demand have produced a dramatic growth in the industry. The assisted living industry is often referred to as the fastest growing segment of long-term care. The number of assisted living beds doubled between 1990 and 2002 (Harrington et al., 2005). In 2007, states reported 38,373 licensed assisted living/residential care communities with 974,585 units/beds, compared to 36,218 communities with 935,364 units/beds in 2004 (Mollica et al., 2007). In a national report covering the years 2015 and 2016 prepared for the U.S. Department of Health and Human Services, Harris-Kojetin et al. (2019) reported a total of 28,900 communities with 996,100 beds. These numbers are indicative of the growth of larger sized communities.

Long-Term Care

Long-term care (LTC) has been defined "as an array of healthcare, personal care and social services generally provided over a sustained period, 90 days or more, to persons with chronic conditions and with functional limitations" (Wunderlich & Kohler, 2001). Today, the National Institute on Aging (n.d.) defines *long-term care* as "a variety of services designed to meet a person's health or personal care needs during a short or long period of time. These services help people live as independently and safely as possible when they can no longer perform everyday activities on their own."

Functional limitations include limitations with activities of daily living (ADL) and/or instrumental activities of daily living (IADL). *ADL* typically refer to basic functions that include bathing, dressing, eating, transferring in and out of bed (mobility), and toileting. *IADL* are considered additional activities that are necessary to live independently such as light housework, shopping, managing money, using the telephone, communicating verbally or in writing, preparing meals, and taking medications.

Long-term care is distinct from acute care in duration and emphasis concerning personal and social services. Services may be regular or intermittent and occur over months, years, or a lifetime. Services include personal care, rehabilitation, social services, medical care coordination, transportation, skilled and custodial care, and more. Services are delivered in a variety of settings, from individual homes to institutional environments. *Formal long-term care* refers to a variety of supportive and healthcare services provided by organizations and persons paid to provide services. *Informal long-term care* remains a more common form of long-term care, in which care is provided by family members and friends on an unpaid basis.

Traditionally, much of formal long-term care was provided in institutional settings such as large state hospitals and skilled nursing facilities. Today, the focus of long-term care has shifted to consumer-centered care. *Consumer-centered care* (also referred to as patient-centered care) is care that is aligned with the needs, wants, and preferences of the person requiring care. Developments in legislation, such as the Americans with Disabilities Act (ADA) of 1990, have supported the growth and acceptance of consumer-centered care. The Patient Self-Determination Act of 1990 requires all healthcare facilities that participate in Medicare or Medicaid to inform adult patients about advanced directives. Furthermore, the U.S. Supreme Court's 1999 landmark *Olmstead* decision concluded that confining persons with disabilities in institutions without adequate medical reasons is a form of discrimination that violates the Americans with Disabilities Act. In the *Olmstead* decision, the Supreme Court held that states cannot make institutionalization a condition for publicly funded health coverage unless it is clinically mandated. Instead, states must direct their health programs for persons with disabilities toward providing community-based care. Therefore, the growth of community-based long-term care, including assisted living communities, has been rapid.

Need for Long-Term Care

The steady increase of an aging population and an increase in life expectancy present many challenges to the formation of public policy in the United States. The population is aging, and the older adults population is growing older and living longer. The fastest growing age group in the country is 85 years and older. As the "baby boom" generation begins to age, the demand for long-term care services is expected to increase. In a report to Congress, the U.S. Department of Health and Human Services (2003) noted that by 2050, the number of individuals using paid long-term care services in any setting (e.g., at home, residential care such as assisted living, or skilled nursing facilities) will likely double from 13 million using services in 2000, to 27 million people. This estimate is influenced by growth in the population of older people in need of care.

Although people of many ages may need long-term care, older persons are the primary recipients of long-term care services because functional disability increases with advancing age. According to the Centers for Disease Control and Prevention (2013), annually 8,357,100 people receive support from the five main long-term care services: home health agencies (4,742,500), nursing homes (1,383,700), hospices (1,244,500), residential care communities/assisted living facilities (713,300), and adult day health centers (273,200). In 2018, the Administration for Community Living reported that the need for caregiving increases with age. In January to June 2018, the percentage of older adults aged 85 and over needing help with personal care (20%) was more than twice the percentage for adults ages 75 to 84 (9%) and five times the percentage for adults ages 65 to 74 (4%).

As the U.S. population ages, the number of people needing long-term care will rise. On average, 52% of people who turn 65 today will develop a severe disability that will require long-term care at some point (Favreault & Dey, 2015). The average duration of need, over a lifetime, is about two years. Unsurprisingly, women are disproportionately more likely to need long-term care than men. Women live longer and have higher rates of disability than men, so older women are more likely to need care (58% versus 47%), and on average need care for longer (2.5 years versus 1.5 years). While most people will need some long-term care, only 14% are expected to need it for 5 years or more.

Long-Term Care Providers

The majority of long-term care continues to be provided by unpaid family and friends often in the home setting. Others require care in long-term care facilities. Although the majority of public funding supports persons residing in skilled nursing facilities (commonly called nursing homes), long-term care is largely and increasingly provided outside of these institutions in community-based group residential settings, such as assisted living. According to the Congressional Budget Office (2013), in 2012, there were 1.4 million people in nursing homes nationally. Harris-Kojetin et al. (2019) reported that 811,500 people were living in assisted living in 2015 to 2016. Table 1.1 illustrates many of the long-term care provider options available today.

The Cost of Long-Term Care

Long-term care is very expensive. According to the Administration on Aging (2017), the national average costs for long-term care in the United States as of 2016 include:

- $225 a day or $6,844 per month for a semi-private room in a skilled nursing facility
- $253 a day or $7,698 per month for a private room in a skilled nursing facility

TABLE 1.1 LONG-TERM CARE PROVIDER OPTIONS

Home care	Home care can include medical care (nursing, social work, rehabilitation therapies) and also help around the home. Skilled professionals come directly to the home to provide care. Home health aides or personal care service workers can visit daily or as needed to help with activities of daily living, such as bathing and grooming. They can also assist with housekeeping, meals, and shopping.
Adult day care Adult day health care	Adult care programs are a type of long-term care that offers social interaction and meals from one to five days a week, depending on the program. Some adult care programs provide transportation to and from the care center. Activities often include exercises, games, trips, art, and music. Some adult care programs include medical services, such as help taking medications or checking blood pressure.
Senior housing	This type of housing is often rental apartments that have been adapted for seniors, including railings installed in the bathrooms and power outlets placed higher on the walls. Other services offered by senior housing communities include meals, transportation, housekeeping, and activities.
Assisted living/ community-based residential care	Assisted living communities offer room and board with provisions for assistance with ADL such as bathing, dressing, eating, grooming, continence, and eating. In addition, assistance with transportation, housekeeping, laundry, obtaining medical and social services, and the supervision of medications and other medical needs is often offered.
Skilled nursing facility Nursing Home	Skilled nursing facilities or nursing homes offer 24-hour nursing care. These services are for those who need more medical care than other long-term care options can offer, such as wound care, rehabilitative therapy, and help with respirators or ventilators.
Continuing-care retirement community	Continuing-care retirement communities offer several levels of care in one setting. They can enable persons to remain in one place for the rest of their life rather than moving each time a new level of care is needed. Typically, there are senior housing apartments, assisted living units, and skilled nursing facilities in a CCRC. A fee or endowment is often required to enter a CCRC.

ADL, activities of daily living; CCRC, continuing-care retirement community

- $119 a day or $3,628 per month for care in an assisted living facility (for a one-bedroom unit)
- $20.50 an hour for a health aide
- $20 an hour for homemaker services
- $68 per day for services in an adult day healthcare center

These costs are extremely variable throughout the country and vary considerably relative to the region, accommodations, amenities, services, and staffing availability.

There are a variety of payment sources for long-term care. Medicare generally does not pay for long-term care. Medicare also does not pay for help with activities of daily living or other care that most people can do themselves. Some examples of activities of daily living include eating, bathing, dressing, and using the bathroom. Medicare will help pay for skilled nursing or home healthcare when certain criteria are met (e.g., rehabilitation services after an acute event). If income and resources are limited, persons may qualify for Medicaid benefits. Private long-term care insurance, personal savings, and assets are other options people utilize to finance long-term care. Table 1.2 summarizes some of the public and private funding sources frequently utilized for the payment of long-term care services.

TABLE 1.2 LONG-TERM CARE PAYMENT SOURCES

Medicare	A federal health insurance program for people 65 and older and younger people with disabilities. Medicare will pay part of the cost for skilled nursing and rehabilitative services in a skilled nursing home (up to 100 days) following a recent related stay in a hospital. Medicare will pay for some home healthcare such as skilled nursing services or therapy through a Medicare-certified home health agency if ordered by a physician. In addition, Medicare will also pay for medical and support services from a Medicare-approved hospice agency for the terminally ill. Many seniors believe that the federal Medicare program will pay for long-term care costs, such as costs for a nursing home or assisted living, but this is not true.
Medicaid	A federal- and state-funded program run by states that helps certain low-income individuals and families pay for some or all of their medical bills. People must meet eligibility criteria set by federal and state law. Medicaid may help pay for nursing home care and sometimes services at home. People whose income is higher, but who have high medical or long-term care bills, can also become eligible for Medicaid. Certain income and assets rules apply. Some states have home- and community-based waiver programs for which Medicaid can help pay some costs associated with assisted living—the programs are limited and differ by state policy.
Veterans Affairs	Provides long-term care for service-related disabilities or for certain eligible veterans. Veterans who do not have service-related disabilities, but who are unable to afford to pay for long-term care, are also eligible for assistance.
Long-term care insurance	Some, but few persons, purchase private long-term care insurance. It is specifically designed to cover the costs of long-term care services. Depending on the policy, long-term care insurance may pay for care in nursing homes, assisted living communities, and/or at home. The cost of long-term care insurance depends on what type of coverage you buy and at what age you buy it. Coverage is variable and often quite expensive to purchase.
Personal savings and investments	Personal savings and investments are how most people who are not on Medicaid pay for long-term care services.

HISTORICAL EVOLUTION OF ASSISTED LIVING

Assisted living is not a new phenomenon in long-term care. Historically, some form of residential and community-based care arrangements or supportive housing has long been available. Residential settings for older people with health problems, ranging from ordinary boarding homes to philanthropically funded organizations often called *homes for the aged*, typically predate the 1965 enactment of Medicare and Medicaid (Cohen, 1974). After 1965, some homes for the aged converted into nursing facilities with encouragement from state governments. These facilities received matching federal money to help state and local governments finance long-term care services. Some residential care facilities did not convert into nursing facilities, either because they did not want to become medical facilities or because they could not meet the regulatory standards. These types of facilities are known by more than 30 different names across the country, including residential care, community care, personal care, domiciliary care, supervisory care, sheltered care, adult foster care, board and care, and family, group, and boarding homes (Newcomer & Grant, 1990). Even as the demand for nursing facility beds grew, the residential care industry continued to develop and expand.

An overlapping type of residential care, termed assisted living, has become increasingly popular in the past two decades. Most states now have a licensing category or statute that uses the term *assisted living* (Carder et al., 2015).

It is difficult to identify the exact beginnings of assisted living. Keren Brown Wilson (2007) explored the historical evolution of assisted living. She wrote,

> To my knowledge, the first written use of the term (and my first such use of it) was in a 1985 proposal to the State of Oregon to fund a pilot study whereby the services for 20 nursing-home-level Medicaid recipients would be covered in a new residential setting. By 1988, assisted living was being used in presentations at professional meetings and in early trade publication articles. By 1991, when Hawes, Wildfire, & Lux (1991) published a national study of board and care homes, many residential care facilities that offered or arranged care were calling themselves assisted living, and the study included assisted living as an explicit subset of residential care.

In this book, the term *assisted living* is used to describe all types of group residential care settings for elder persons, because many states use the term *assisted living* generically to cover every type of group residential care on the continuum between home care and nursing homes (Mollica et al., 2007). We also acknowledge that for some stakeholders the term *assisted living* represents a unique model of residential care that differs significantly from traditional types of residential care. We include a discussion of the distinct assisted living philosophy that is included in some states' regulations in Chapter 2.

DEFINING *ASSISTED LIVING*

The setting for the delivery and receipt of long-term care is often discussed as a continuum, with one's own home at one end and the nursing home at the other. These end points also are used to symbolize the continuum from personal independence to institutionalization. Assisted living is typically considered to fall somewhere in between these extreme ends where personalized care and supervision can be provided outside of an institutionalized environment, with an emphasis on optimizing physical and psychological independence.

In general, assisted living communities offer room and board with provisions for assistance with ADL such as bathing, dressing, eating, grooming, continence, and eating. In addition, assistance with transportation, housekeeping, laundry, obtaining medical and social services, the supervision of medications, as well as other medical needs is often offered.

It is noted that the exact definition of assisted living remains a question, and that the ambiguity surrounding the various definitions and regulatory models used throughout the country make for great confusion for clinicians, consumers, and researchers. Some see this as a unique mix of services and privacy, while others view it as a new term for the type of care and assistance that has been available historically.

There has never been a single nationally accepted definition of an assisted living facility. Instead, states that have the responsibility for regulating the supportive housing industry have each developed their own definitions and guidelines. While there is much in common among the states, there are also differences in the terms used to label various housing types and levels of care, and variation in the standards and restrictions for which these operations are held accountable. Provider and trade associations, formal associations, and governmental agencies, as well as academic researchers, have developed a vast variety of definitions designed to capture both the definition and essence of assisted living communities and suit their own needs and purposes. In 1992, Lewin-VHI, Inc. (1996) conducted a literature review and policy synthesis for the Office of the Assistant Secretary for Planning and Evaluation, Administration on Aging, and the U.S. Department of Health and Human Services. They determined that overall, assisted living was used to refer to housing for the older adults with supportive services in a homelike environment; the term was used interchangeably throughout the states with other common labels, such as residential care and board and care. However, it was also determined that proponents of assisted living often assert that assisted living offers a special philosophy that includes maximizing functional capability and autonomy and utilizing the environment as an aid for independence and socialization that makes assisted living distinguishable from other types of supportive housing for the older adults. Over time, additional definitions have been suggested. Table 1.3 illustrates some selected definitions for *assisted living* and *residential care*.

These selected definitions illustrate that the definitions and concepts of assisted living are not uniform. Depending on one's perspective, different dimensions and descriptions are included or excluded. Commonly, stressing the importance of privacy, dignity, and autonomy are seen in these definitions. Privacy is often addressed, and in some cases private rooms and baths are required to fit the definition. Lists of services that must be available are also included, with some distinct statements regarding response to residents' needs around the clock. Although some assisted living communities may offer high-quality care in settings that afford maximum privacy and dignity, others lack adequately trained staff and sufficient levels of care and supervision. This gap is most obvious when philosophy aims to combine privacy, such as locking doors and providing individual kitchens, with high service levels regardless of changes in health, physical, or cognitive functioning.

TABLE 1.3 SELECTED DEFINITIONS OF ASSISTED LIVING

ASSOCIATION OR RESEARCHER	DEFINITION
Argentum (formerly Assisted Living Federation of American) (n.d.)	A special combination of housing, personalized supportive services, and healthcare designed to meet the needs—both scheduled and unscheduled—of those who need help with activities of daily living.
Assisted Living Workgroup (ALW; 2003)	Assisted living is a state-regulated and monitored residential long-term care option. Assisted living provides or coordinates oversight and services to meet the residents' individualized scheduled needs, based on the residents' assessments and service plans and their unscheduled needs as they arise. Services that are required by state law and regulation to be provided or coordinated must include but are not limited to: • 24-hour awake staff to provide oversight and meet scheduled and unscheduled needs • Provision and oversight of personal and supportive services (assistance with activities of daily living and instrumental activities of daily living) • Health-related services (e.g., medication management services) • Social services • Recreational activities • Meals • Housekeeping and laundry • Transportation A resident has the right to make choices and receive services in a way that will promote the resident's dignity, autonomy, independence, and quality of life. These services are disclosed and agreed to in the contract between the clinician and resident. Assisted living does not generally provide ongoing, 24-hour skilled nursing.

(continued)

TABLE 1.3 SELECTED DEFINITIONS OF ASSISTED LIVING (*CONTINUED*)

ASSOCIATION OR RESEARCHER	DEFINITION
American Seniors Housing Association (n.d.)	These communities are a popular option for adults who need a little extra help with the tasks of daily living. The physical environment may resemble a condominium or upscale apartment where residents feel at home. Seniors who choose an assisted living community do so knowing they will be able to maintain their independence in a private apartment while having around-the-clock support from nearby caregivers. The most commonly needed services in an assisted living community are medication reminders and personal care (bathing, grooming, dressing). Housekeeping, meals, laundry and life enrichment programs are included. Some form of transportation service is usually offered.
Centers for Medicare & Medicaid Services (n.d.)	Assisted living is a type of living arrangement in which personal care services such as meals, housekeeping, transportation, and assistance with activities of daily living are available as needed to people who still live on their own in a residential facility. In most cases, the "assisted living" residents pay a regular monthly rent. Then, they typically pay additional fees for the services they get.
Kane and Wilson (1993)	Assisted living is any group residential program that is not licensed as a nursing home that provides personal care to persons with need for assistance in the activities of daily living and that can respond to unscheduled need for assistance that might arise.
National Center for Assisted Living (n.d.)	Assisted living is part of a continuum of long-term care services that provides a combination of housing, personal care services, and healthcare designed to respond to individuals who need assistance with normal daily activities in a way that promotes maximum independence. Assisted living services can be provided in freestanding communities, near or integrated with skilled nursing homes or hospitals, as components of continuing care retirement communities, or at independent housing complexes. Assisted living communities offer a multi-faceted residential setting that provides personal care services, 24-hour supervision and assistance, activities, and health-related services, designed to: Minimize the need to relocate. Accommodate individual residents' changing needs and preferences. Maximize residents' dignity, autonomy, privacy, independence, choice, and safety. Encourage family and community involvement.
U.S. Department of Housing and Urban Development (n.d.)	ALFs are designed to accommodate frail elderly people and people with disabilities who can live independently but need assistance with activities of daily living (e.g., assistance with eating, bathing, grooming, dressing, and home management activities). ALFs must provide support services such as personal care, transportation, meals, housekeeping, and laundry.
Wilson (1990)	Offered a paradigm to describe what she called *AL* in which: • AL is a setting where a person can create his/her own place. • AL is responsive to the needs of individuals at different levels of physical and mental abilities. • AL encourages sharing the responsibility with residents and their family members. • AL provides autonomy and independence to residents.

AL, assisted living; ALFs, assisted living facilities.

RESIDENT CHARACTERISTICS

In order to address quality and safety in assisted living communities, it is important to know the population of residents residing in and being served within these settings. The research in this area (although limited by methodology) has begun to suggest that residents residing in these communities are becoming increasingly dependent and frail, which makes issues of quality and safety more critical. Residents enter assisted living communities from a variety of places, including (a) the community, (b) other assisted living communities, (c) skilled nursing facilities, (d nursing homes, and (e) hospitals.

General Resident Profile

In their report for the Centers for Disease Control and Prevention, Caffrey et al. (2012) noted that:

- The majority of residents living in residential care facilities in 2010 were non-Hispanic, White, and female. More than half of all residents were aged 85 and over.
- Nearly two in 10 residents were Medicaid beneficiaries, and almost six in 10 residents under age 65 had Medicaid.
- Almost four in 10 residents received assistance with three or more activities of daily living, of which bathing and dressing were the most common.
- More than three fourths of residents have had at least two of the 10 most common chronic conditions; high blood pressure, Alzheimer's disease, and other dementias were the most prevalent.

These findings suggest a vulnerable population with a high burden of functional and cognitive impairment. The percentage of residents needing assistance with ADL is illustrated in Table 1.4.

Length of Stay and Reasons for Leaving

The median stay in an assisted living facility is 22 months (National Center for Assisted Living, 2018). About 60% of residents in assisted living transitioned to a skilled nursing facility. Reasons for residents leaving assisted living include:

- Need for higher level of care (voluntary relocation or involuntary eviction),
- Locations closer to loved ones,
- Dissatisfaction,
- Financial concerns/running out of money.

TABLE 1.4 ASSISTED LIVING RESIDENTS' NEEDS FOR ASSISTANCE

Assistance with bathing	72%
Assistance with dressing	52%
Assistance with bathroom needs	36%
Assistance with transferring and mobility	25%
Assistance with eating	22%

Source: From Caffrey, C., Sengupta, M., Park-Lee, E., Moss, A., Rosenoff, E., & Harris-Kojetin. (2012). *Residents living in residential care facilities: United States, 2010.* NCHS data brief, no 91. National Center for Health Statistics. https://www.cdc.gov/nchs/data/databriefs/db91.pdf

Sources of Payment in Assisted Living

Although Medicaid coverage for assisted living services has increased gradually, assisted living remains a primarily private-pay segment of long-term care. Therefore, the majority of assisted living residents pay with their own funds. Others receive some support from family members and some have private long-term care insurance. The lack of public subsidies and frequent high costs of assisted living often make it unaffordable for persons with low to moderate incomes.

CHALLENGES IN THE ASSISTED LIVING FIELD

The concept of assisted living, as illustrated by the varying definitions, is far less uniform than most realize. In addition, today's assisted living communities are caring for more physically frail and cognitively impaired residents than ever before. For example, it is not uncommon for assisted living communities to care for residents with advanced dementia or hospice care needs.

Quality of Care and Safety Concerns

As the interest in assisted living has increased, so have concerns about the quality of care and safety that can be provided to these residents that require special care, staffing, and physical and social environments. In contrast to nursing homes, no federal quality standards exist for assisted living. In addition, states vary significantly in their licensing requirements, quality standards, monitoring, and enforcement activities (see Chapter 2).

Research, media, and reports generated throughout the country dating back to 1999 (U.S. General Accounting Office, 1999) have identified quality of care and consumer protection issues relative to the quality of care in residential care settings. Older persons receiving necessary care and services in a homelike and residential setting dedicated to preserving dignity and autonomy are attractive and appealing. These concerns continue today. The determination of what makes assisted living "good" remains an important question.

Quality-Improvement Efforts

One effort to address problems of quality was the establishment of the Assisted Living Workgroup (ALW). Formed at the request of the U.S. Senate Special Committee on Aging, the ALW was a national effort of approximately 50 organizations representing consumers, clinicians, long-term care and healthcare professionals, and regulators. In 2003, the ALW issued a report with recommendations for improving quality in assisted living. Included in their recommendations were the following components (www.theceal.org/ALW-report.php):

1. Introduction,
2. Definitions and core principals,
3. Accountability and oversight,
4. Affordability,
5. Direct-care services,
6. Medication management,
7. Operations,
8. Resident rights,
9. Staffing.

To continue and expand the work of the ALW, 11 organizations that participated in the ALW have formed an organizing committee to develop a Center for Excellence in Assisted Living (CEAL). The CEAL has continued to support and foster high quality, affordable assisted living by disseminating research and information, and providing technical assistance. Today, the CEAL (n.d.) is a unique collaborative of nine diverse organizations:

1. Alzheimer's Association,
2. American Assisted Living Nurses Association,
3. American Seniors Housing Association,
4. Argentum,
5. National Association of States United for Aging and Disability,
6. The Society for Post-Acute and Long-Term Care Medicine,
7. Leading Age,
8. National Center for Assisted Living,
9. Pioneer Network.

Furthermore, in an effort to promote improved quality in assisted living, there are many local, state, and federal professional provider associations, as well as advocacy groups, that provide education and support to providers of assisted living (see Chapter 7 for more information on continuing education for administrators and providers).

CONCLUSIONS

This chapter provides the reader with the context, history, and overview of assisted living communities. Although assisted living has promised to be a consumer-centered alternative to institutionalized settings for long-term care, quality-of-care concerns have become increasingly apparent. This chapter illustrates the need for today's assisted living administrators to be well informed and well prepared in the effort to provide high-quality long-term services to older adults persons in a challenging and evolving environment.

REFERENCES

Administration on Aging. (2017). *Costs of care.* https://longtermcare.acl.gov/costs-how-to-pay/costs-of-care.html

Administration for Community Living. (2018). *2018 profile of older Americans.* https://acl.gov/sites/default/files/Aging%20and%20Disability%20in%20America/2018OlderAmericansProfile.pdf

American Seniors Housing Association. (n.d.). *Where you live matters: Maximize your living.* https://www.whereyoulivematters.org

Argentum. (n.d.). *Argentum definition of assisted living.* https://quizlet.com/155093319/argentum-assisted-living-exam-flash-cards

Assisted Living Workgroup. (2003). *Assuring quality in assisted living: Guidelines for federal and state policy, state regulations, and operations.* U.S. Government Printing Office. https://www.huduser.gov/portal/publications/Assuring-Quality-in-Assisted-Living-Guidelines.html

Caffrey, C., Sengupta, M., Park-Lee, E., Moss, A., Rosenoff, E., & Harris-Kojetin. (2012). *Residents living in residential care facilities: United States, 2010.* NCHS data brief, no 91. National Center for Health Statistics. https://www.cdc.gov/nchs/data/databriefs/db91.pdf

Carder, P., O'Keeffe, J., & O'Keeffe, C. (2015). *Compendium of residential care and assisted living regulations and policy: 2015 edition.* U.S. Department of Health and Human Services, Office of the Assistant Secretary for Planning and Evaluation, Office of Disability, Aging and Long-Term Care Policy and Research

Triangle Institute. https://aspe.hhs.gov/basic-report/compendium-residential-care-and-assisted-living-regulations-and-policy-2015-edition

Center for Excellence in Assisted Living. (n.d.). *Who CEAL is.* https://www.theceal.org

Centers for Disease Control and Prevention. (2013). *Long-term care services in the United States: 2013 overview.* https://www.cdc.gov/nchs/data/nsltcp/long_term_care_services_2013.pdf

Centers for Medicare & Medicaid Services. (n.d.). *Glossary.* https://www.cms.gov/apps/glossary/default .asp?Letter=ALL

Cohen, E. (1974). An overview of long-term care facilities. In E. M. Brody (Ed.), *Social work guide for long-term care facilities* (pp. 11–26). U.S. Government Printing Office.

Congressional Budget Office. (2013). *Rising demand for long-term services and supports for elderly people.* https://www.cbo.gov/sites/default/files/113th-congress-2013-2014/reports/44363-ltc.pdf

Favreault, M., & Dey, J. (2015). *Long-term services and supports for older Americans: Risks and financing research brief.* U.S. Department of Health and Human Services. https://aspe.hhs.gov/basic-report/long-term-services-and-supports-older-americans-risks-and-financing-research-brief

Harrington, C., Chapman, S., Miller, E., Miller, N., & Newcomer, R. (2005). Trends in the supply of long-term care facilities and beds in the United States. *Journal of Applied Gerontology, 20,* 1–19.

Harris-Kojetin, L., Sengupta, M., Lendon, J. P., Rome, V., Valverde, R., & Caffrey C. (2019). *Long-term care providers and services users in the United States, 2015–2016.* National Center for Health Statistics. https://www.cdc.gov/nchs/data/series/sr_03/sr03_43-508.pdf

Kane, R., & Wilson, K. (1993). *Assisted living in the United States: A new paradigm for residential care for frail older persons?* American Association of Retired Persons.

Lewin-VHI, Inc. (1996). *National study of assisted living for the frail elderly: Literature review update.* Research Triangle Institute.

Mollica, R., Sims-Kastelein, K., & O'Keeffe, J. (2007). *Residential care and assisted living compendium, 2007.* U.S. Department of Health and Human Services, Office of the Assistant Secretary for Planning and Evaluation, Office of Disability, Aging and Long-Term Care Policy and Research Triangle Institute. https://aspe.hhs.gov/report/residential-care-and-assisted-living-compendium-2007

National Center for Assisted Living. (n.d.). *What is assisted livin*g? https://www.ahcancal.org/ncal/about/ assistedliving/Pages/What-is-Assisted-Living.aspx

National Center for Assisted Living. (2018). *Residents.* https://www.ahcancal.org/ncal/facts/Pages/Residents .aspx

National Institute on Aging. (n.d.). *What is long-term care?* https://www.nia.nih.gov/health/what-long-term-care

Newcomer, R., & Grant, L. (1990). Residential care facilities: Understanding their role and improving their effectiveness. In D. Tilson (Ed.), *Aging in place: Supporting the frail elderly in residential environments.* Scott Foresman.

Wilson, K. (1990). *Assisted living: The merger of housing and long-term care services. Long-term care advances.* Duke University Center for the Study of Aging and Human Development.

Wilson, K. (2007). Historical evolution of assisted living in the United States: 1979 to the present. *The Gerontologist, 47,* 8–22.

Wunderlich, G., & Kohler, P. (Eds.). (2001). *Improving the quality of long-term care.* National Academies Press.

U.S. Department of Health and Human Services and U.S. Department of Labor. (2003). *The future supply of long-term care workers in relation to the aging baby boom generation: Report to Congress.* Office of the Assistant Secretary for Planning and Evaluation. https://aspe.hhs.gov/basic-report/future-supply-long-term-care-workers-relation-aging-baby-boom-generation

U.S. Department of Housing and Urban Development. (n.d.). *Assisted Living Conversion Program.* https://www.hud.gov/program_offices/housing/mfh/progdesc/alcp

U.S. General Accounting Office. (1999). *Assisted living: Quality of care and consumer protection issues* (GAO/T-HEHS-99-111).

POLICY, LICENSING, AND REGULATIONS

Upon the completion of Chapter 2, the reader will be able to:

- Explain the challenges in generically describing assisted living policy, licensing, and regulations.
- Cite examples of current changes to state regulation and policy.
- Describe state policy related to Medicaid reimbursement for assisted living.
- Describe policy and regulations related to assisted living labels, licensure, and philosophy.
- Recognize a variety of state regulatory models in assisted living.
- Understand the variability of policy and regulations related to assisted living communities.
- Describe federal statutes that impact assisted living.

INTRODUCTION

This chapter addresses key issues in assisted living policy, licensing, and regulations. Because states are primarily responsible for the monitoring and oversight of assisted living, this chapter provides a broad overview of the models and regulations used by individual states. An assisted living administrator is required to thoroughly understand the regulations and requirements specific to their individual state, which is beyond the scope of this book. This section addresses regulatory models and similarities and variations in policy and regulations across states. Key concepts typically covered by state regulations are discussed, including but not limited to assisted living philosophy, resident agreements and disclosure requirements, admission and retention criteria, and resident rights. Finally, a summary of federal laws that may pertain to the assisted living industry is included.

The Challenge

Although there are some similarities across states in the licensing, regulations, and policy relative to assisted living communities, these concepts are challenging to describe genericall for several reasons. Similar to the assisted living nomenclature and definitions, state regulations and policy are variable and continually changing. Assisted living is a broad and general licensing category in some states and a detailed model in others. Some states (as well as providers) utilize the term *assisted living* interchangeably with other terms, such as *residential care*, whereas others have different licensing categories based on size, services, and/or philosophy of care. For example, in California, the label "assisted living" is not used in the state regulations, but it is frequently used by clinicians. Furthermore, some states have additional licensure requirements that allow for higher levels of care to be provided, such as limited nursing care, specialized dementia care, and hospice care for the terminally ill.

The most comprehensive work in tracking state policy and regulation has been conducted by Dr. Robert Mollica and his colleagues. Paula Carder and her colleagues have continued to provide periodic updates to this work (Carder et al., 2015). Additional sources of information utilized for this chapter include the National Center for Assisted Living and recognized experts in the field. Furthermore, because there are no specific federal regulations for assisted living communities, the recommendations of the Assisted Living Workgroup from their report, *Assuring Quality in Assisted Living: Guidelines for Federal and State Policy, State Regulations, and Operations*, are included on important topics such as resident agreements, disclosure medication management, resident rights, and staff training requirements (Assisted Living Workgroup, 2003). The Assisted Living Workgroup was an initiative of approximately 50 national organizations, including clinicians, consumers, long-term care and healthcare professionals, and regulators that came together at the request of the U.S. Senate Special Committee on Aging to develop recommendations for federal guidelines for assisted living.

STATE POLICY AND REGULATION

State policy regarding regulations for assisted living communities continues to evolve. Every year some changes are made, so it is important for the assisted living administrator to be aware of current law, pending legislation, and newly developed or revised regulations. The National Center for Assisted Living (2019), in the report *2019 Assisted Living State Regulatory Review*, provided summary information and examples of the current changes in state policy across the country. Some examples are:

- More than half of states reported changes between June 2018 and June 2019 that will affect assisted living communities. Specifically, 27 states and the District of Columbia reported changes to a variety of requirements, either to the licensing requirements or to other regulations that also apply to assisted living providers (e.g., nursing scope of practice or life safety).

- Minnesota passed a bill finalizing comprehensive changes affecting assisted living providers. Effective in 2021 and subject to the rule-making process, the state will have two new levels of licensure: assisted living and assisted living with dementia care.

- States continue efforts to enhance protections for residents, which were the majority of changes. Specifically, the most common changes were to disclosure or notification requirements, efforts to prevent or address alleged abuse or neglect, staff training, emergency preparedness, and life safety.

- The most frequent change over the past year was an update to disclosure and notification requirements. Four states (Colorado, Minnesota, Oregon, and Virginia) and the District of Columbia passed laws requiring new types of notification either to the resident or to the state.

- Efforts to protect against elder abuse and neglect was another common change. Continuing last year's trend regarding state background checks, two states (Utah and West Virginia) reported updates for background checks of employees.

- Both Minnesota and North Dakota passed legislation allowing a resident or the resident's representative to conduct electronic monitoring in the resident's room in specified circumstances.

- Twenty-three states reported no finalized legislative or regulatory changes between June 2018 and June 2019 affecting assisted living communities.

Medicaid Reimbursement

Although very limited in availability, many (42) states now have several options for using Medicaid to fund services in assisted living communities (Carder et al., 2015). As seen in Table 2.1, the majority of states currently utilize Home- and Community-Based Services waivers (also called *1915(c) waivers*), others utilize state plans, and some utilize both. States' ability to expand the availability of home and community services to Medicaid is an ongoing challenge and often limited by resources.

Labels

The number of states utilizing the label *assisted living* has increased over time. Most states now have a licensing category or statute that uses the term *assisted living*. Some names used are *assisted living, assisted living facility, assisted living residence,* and *assisted living community.* Another common label is *residential care,* which includes terminology such as *residential care facility, residential care home,* or *residential care facility for the elderly.* In addition, some states continue to use traditional names such as *board and care homes, homes for the aged,* and *personal care homes.* Some states utilize more than one label for various types or levels of assisted living and residential care.

TABLE 2.1 STATES UTILIZING MEDICAID REIMBURSEMENT FOR ASSISTED LIVING

HCBS WAIVER		STATE PLAN	HCBS WAIVERS AND STATE PLAN
Alaska	Nebraska	Michigan	Arkansas
Arizona	Nevada	Missouri	Florida
California	New Hampshire	North Carolina	Idaho
Colorado	New Jersey	South Carolina	Maine
Connecticut	New Mexico		Massachusetts
Delaware	Ohio		New York
District of Columbia	Oklahoma		North Dakota
Georgia	Oregon		Vermont
Hawaii	Rhode Island		Washington
Illinois	South Dakota		Wisconsin
Indiana	Tennessee		
Iowa	Texas		
Kansas	Utah		
Maryland	Wyoming		
Mississippi			
Minnesota			
Montana			

HCBS, home- and community-based services.

Source: From Carder, P., O'Keeffe, J., & O'Keeffe, C. (2015). *Compendium of residential care and assisted living regulations and policy: 2015 Edition.* U.S. Department of Health and Human Services, Office of the Assistant Secretary for Planning and Evaluation, Office of Disability, Aging and Long-Term Care Policy and Research Triangle Institute. https://aspe.hhs.gov/pdf-report/compendium-residential-care-and-assisted-living-regulations-and-policy-2015-edition

Licensure

Although there are some federal laws that impact assisted living communities, the main public oversight is through the enforcement of state regulations. This generally occurs in the form of the initial licensure of communities, periodic license renewal surveys (inspection visits), and visits in response to consumer complaints or other administrative follow-up. All states have some kind of policy, regulations, or requirements for assisted living communities.

Philosophy

More than half of the states and the District of Columbia report that provisions regarding assisted living concepts such as privacy, autonomy, and decision-making are included in their assisted living regulations (Mollica et al., 2007). Overall, this philosophy represents a consumer-focused model where the delivery of care is centered on the resident. How the philosophy of assisted living is incorporated into state laws is highly variable. For example, regulations may state the importance of privacy and may require private unit residence while some states have mixed requirements, allowing bedrooms in some settings and individual apartments in others. Other states allow sharing (apartments or bedrooms) by resident choice. Two examples of how states incorporate the assisted living philosophy into their regulations come from Florida and Oregon (Mollica et al., 2007):

1. **Florida's** statute describes the purpose of assisted living as "to promote availability of appropriate services for elderly and disabled persons in the least restrictive and most home-like environment, to encourage the development of facilities which promote the dignity, privacy, and decision-making ability" of residents. Florida law also states that facilities should be operated and regulated as residential environments, not as medical or nursing facilities. Regulations require facilities to develop policies maximizing independence, dignity, choice, and decision-making.

2. **Oregon**, the first state to adopt a specific philosophy for assisted living, states that: assisted living is a program that promotes resident self-direction and participation in decisions that emphasize choice, dignity, privacy, individuality, independence, and home-like surroundings.

Regulatory Models

One way to consider state regulatory models is to consider the levels of care. Eric Carlson (2005) reviewed laws and regulations of all 50 states in his work with the National Senior Citizens Law Center. To understand the variation in state regulatory models, Carlson (2005) described two regulatory systems utilized by states:

1. *Single-level system*
   In the single-level system, a state licensing agency licenses only one type of residential care/assisted living. In this model, any residential care/assisted living facility is licensed to accept or retain any resident, as long as the resident does not have a condition that disqualifies the resident from residential care/assisted living generally.

2. *Multilevel system*
   In a multilevel system, residential care/assisted living facilities are licensed to care for residents only up to a particular care need. In this model, a resident typically may not be admitted or retained if they need a level of care that exceeds the specific level at which the facility is licensed.

Many states recognize more than one level of care. For example, Florida allows communities to be licensed for standard assisted living services, limited nursing services, some mental health services, and extended congregate care. Arizona and Montana allow for multiple levels of care with each level allowing for a higher level of care to be delivered at the assisted living communities. Carlson (2005) made the important point that even states with "single level" systems (e.g., California) often allow for exceptions within state regulations for specific residents or communities.

Unit Requirements

The newer models of assisted living communities became popular with older persons in large part because of the privacy and ability to retain control over personal activities, such as bathing, dressing, eating, and sleeping. The older, more traditional homes offered shared rooms and bathrooms. Some stakeholders believe that private rooms must be made available to adhere to true assisted living philosophy, while others accept the use of shared rooms as a cost-effective alternative. Consequently, there are many types of occupancy styles in assisted living. This is controlled by both consumer demand and state regulations.

To describe the various models relative to facility size and unit types, Zimmerman and Sloane (2007) describe a three-part typology to understand the multiple classifications of assisted living facilities across various states:

1. Facilities with fewer than 16 beds,
2. Larger homes of the traditional board-and-care type,
3. New-model facilities with 16 beds or more—this new-model facility is described as (a) built in or after 1987 and (b) having two or more private-pay rates, at least 20% of residents who required assistance in transfer, at least 25% of residents who were incontinent, or a registered nurse or licensed practical nurse on duty at all times.

States set occupancy requirements in a variety of ways (Carder et al., 2015). Some states use the label assisted living for homes that only provide private rooms while other states allow for shared rooms to be offered. Some states have different licensing categories, allowing shared rooms in some settings and requiring private rooms in others.

Resident Agreements/Contracts

Dating back to 1999, the U.S. Government Accounting Office (GAO) reported that most assisted living communities provide information about services offered, but do not routinely provide information regarding discharge criteria, staff training and qualifications, services not available from the facility, grievance procedures, and medication policies. The majority of the 721 communities that responded to the GAO survey stated that they generally provide prospective residents with written information about many of their services and costs before they apply for admission. However, only about half indicated that they provide information on the circumstances under which the cost of services may change their policy on medication assistance, or their practice for monitoring residents' needs. Furthermore, less than half said they provide written information in advance about discharge criteria, staff training and qualifications, or services not covered or available from the facility. The report concluded that the provision of adequate information to prospective and current residents is a major issue that requires additional oversight. This issue has become a key topic in assisted living today, with consumer advocates expressing ongoing concern regarding the quality of resident agreements.

To address these historic concerns, states now have more regulations and requirements relating to the resident agreement. According to Carder et al. (2015):

■ Nearly all states require a residency agreement and describe the type of information that it must include. Some states also require clinicians to furnish a separate document to inform prospective residents about services and rates, typically called a Disclosure Statement.

■ Most states specify that residency agreements must include information about basic services and fees, optional services if any, admission and discharge criteria, limits on the scope of services that may be provided, resident rights and responsibilities, and information for reporting grievances and complaints.

■ Most states require the resident (or a representative, if there is one) to sign the contract, though the timing for doing so varies.

■ Ten states require that the residency agreement include information about medication services and policies.

The Assisted Living Workgroup (2003) included the following recommendations regarding resident agreements/contracts within the resident rights component of their report, *Assuring Quality in Assisted Living: Guidelines for Federal and State Policy, State Regulations, and Operations*:

1. *Consistency in contracts and marketing*
   All information conveyed by an assisted living residence to prospective residents (e.g., marketing materials, sales presentations, and tours) should be consistent with the contract.

2. *Contracts and agreements: Consistency with applicable law*
   All contract provisions shall be consistent with applicable law. The parties may agree to modify the contract as long as all parties agree to the modification and signify their agreement. Such modification will be consistent with applicable law.

3. *Contracts and agreements: Readability and pre-signing review*
   Contracts shall be written in simple language and be understandable. Prior to signinge, the prospective resident has the right to review a contract and/or have the contract reviewed by a third party. Prior to the execution of the contract, a representative of the assisted living residence shall offer to read and explain the contract and answer any questions.

4. *Contracts and agreements: Required elements*
   Contracts/agreements should include at a minimum the following information:
   a. The term of the contract,
   b. A comprehensive description of the assisted living residence's billing and payment policies and procedures,
   c. A comprehensive description of services provided for a basic fee,
   d. A comprehensive description of the fee schedule for services provided on an á la carte basis or as part of a tiered pricing system that are not included in a basic fee,
   e. The policy for changing the amount of fees,
   f. The amount of advance notice the assisted living residence will give before the changing of fees (e.g., 30 days, 60 days); notices should be readable and understandable by the resident,
   g. Whether the assisted living residence requires an entrance fee, security deposit, and/or other fee(s) at entry, the amount of those fees and/or deposits, the policies

for whether or not fees and deposits are refundable, and procedures for refunding those fees and/or deposits,

h. A description of the circumstances under which residents may receive a refund of any prepaid amount such as monthly rent,

i. A description of the assisted living residence's policy during a resident's temporary absence,

j. The process for initial and subsequent assessments and the development of the service plan based on these assessments, including notification that the resident has the right to participate in the development of the service plan,

k. A description of all requirements for assessments or physical examinations, including the frequency and assignment of financial responsibility for such assessments and/or examinations,

l. An explanation of the use of third-party services (including all health services), how they may be arranged, accessed, and monitored (whether by the resident, family, or the assisted living residence), whether transportation is available if the services are not provided on-site, any restrictions on third-party services, and who is financially responsible for the third-party services and transportation costs,

m. A description of all circumstances and conditions under which the assisted living residence may require the resident to be involuntarily transferred, discharged, or evicted, an explanation of the resident's right to notice, the process by which a resident may appeal of the assisted living residence's decision, and a description of the relocation assistance (if available) offered by the assisted living residence,

n. A description of the assisted living residence's process for resolving complaints or disputes, including any appeal rights, and a list of the appropriate consumer/regulatory agencies (if applicable; e.g., appropriate state/local long-term care ombudsman program, the state regulatory agency, the local legal services program, and other advocacy bodies/agencies),

o. A description of the procedures the resident or assisted living residence shall follow to terminate the agreement,

p. A list of residents' rights as detailed in the statute or regulations governing assisted living residences, incorporated by reference and attached.

5. *Contracts and agreements: Prohibition on waiver of right to sue*
The contract should not require the resident to waive the right to sue the assisted living residence under applicable law. The contract may disclose but not require options for alternative dispute resolution available to the resident or assisted living residence.

6. *Contracts and agreements: Third-party responsibility*
The contract shall disclose clearly that a signature by a third party (such as a "responsible party") does not indicate acceptance of any personal financial responsibility for fees, costs, or charges incurred by the resident, and does not make the third party a guarantor, unless the third party has signed a separate agreement indicating such. The separate agreement shall include, at a minimum, the following information:

a. Third party voluntarily agrees to be financially liable for paying the residents' expenses as agreed.

b. Third party has the right to have this agreement reviewed by an attorney or other person.

c. Third party has the right to revoke the separate agreement with 30 days' notice.

Preadmission Disclosures

The Assisted Living Workgroup (2003) included the following recommendations regarding preadmission disclosure within the resident rights component of their report:

1. *Preadmission disclosure for specialized programs of care*
   Assisted living residences that represent in any way that they provide special care programs for persons with Alzheimer's disease or other dementias, or any other specific health conditions, shall disclose how the program and its services are different from the basic services. At a minimum, the assisted living residence shall disclose the following information to each prospective resident prior to admission:

   a. The assisted living residence's philosophy of the special care program,

   b. The process and criteria for placement in, and transfer or discharge from, any specialized unit and/or the assisted living residence,

   c. The process for assessing residents and establishing individualized service plans,

   d. Additional services provided and the costs of those services relevant to the special care program,

   e. Specialized (condition-specific) staff training and continuing education practices relevant to the special care program,

   f. How the physical environment and design features are appropriate to support the functioning and safety of residents with the specific condition(s),

   g. The frequency and types of activities offered to residents,

   h. Options for family involvement and the availability of family support programs.

2. *Preadmission disclosure on advance directives*
   Assisted living residences shall provide residents with information about their rights under state law to make decisions about medical care, including their right to accept or refuse health-related services, the right to formulate advance medical directives, such as a living will, a directive to physicians, or durable power of attorney for healthcare. The assisted living residence information should disclose its philosophy and policies about implementation of advance medical directives, including, but not limited to, implementation of Do Not Resuscitate orders (DNRs) and medical directives that require limitations on delivery of medical services, food, or hydration, and situations in which the assisted living residence is required to summon emergency medical services.

3. *Preadmission disclosure on end-of-life care*
   Assisted living residences shall clearly disclose information to residents about applicable state laws and about the assisted living residence's philosophy and policies regarding delivery of end-of-life care, including delivery of hospice and palliative care services. Disclosure shall include the circumstances, if any, under which a resident with terminal illness or in the process of dying may be required to leave.

Admission and Retention

In general, states often utilize specific criteria that determine whether or not a person can be admitted to or retained in an assisted living community. Typically, these include the general condition of the resident, health-related conditions, functional conditions, physical function, cognitive function, behavioral problems, and health needs that may require the need for nursing care. A primary purpose of regulating admission and retention is to ensure that providers are able to meet the needs of the population they serve (Carder et al., 2015). The goal is to ensure that communities will be able to meet their residents' needs.

Resident Rights

Regulations regarding resident rights are included in many states. Resident rights include such concepts as personal rights, disclosure of information regarding services and fees, and marketing practices. A further exploration of the significant challenges related to resident rights in assisted living communities is found in Chapter 23. The Assisted Living Workgroup (2003) included the following recommendations regarding resident rights in their report to the U.S. Senate Special Committee on Aging, *Assuring Quality in Assisted Living: Guidelines for Federal and State Policy, State Regulations, and Operations* to the U.S. Senate Special Committee on Aging:

1. ***Resident rights***
   Within the boundaries set by law, residents have the right to:

   a. Be shown consideration and respect;

   b. Be treated with dignity;

   c. Exercise autonomy;

   d. Exercise civil and religious rights and liberties;

   e. Be free from chemical and physical restraints;

   f. Be free from physical, mental, fiduciary, sexual and verbal abuse, and neglect;

   g. Have free reciprocal communication with and access to the long-term care Ombudsmen program;

   h. Voice concerns and complaints to the assisted living residence orally and in writing without reprisal;

   i. Review and obtain copies of their own records that the assisted living residence maintains;

   j. Receive and send mail promptly and unopened;

   k. Private unrestricted communication with others;

   l. Privacy for phone calls and access to a phone;

   m. Privacy for couples and for visitors;

   n. Privacy in treatment and caring for personal needs;

   o. Manage their own financial affairs;

   p. Confidentiality concerning financial, medical, and personal affairs;

   q. Guide the development and implementation of their service plans;

   r. Participate in and appeal the discharge (move-out) planning process;

   s. Involve family members in making decisions about services;

   t. Arrange for third-party services at their own expense;

   u. Accept or refuse services;

   v. Choose their own physicians, dentists, pharmacists, and other health professionals;

   w. Choose to execute advance directives;

   x. Exercise choice about end of life care;

   y. Participate or refuse to participate in social, spiritual, or community activities;

   z. Arise and retire at times of their own choosing;

   aa. Form and participate in resident councils;

   ab. Furnish their own rooms, and use and retain personal clothing and possessions;

ac. Exercise choice and lifestyle as long as it does not interfere with other residents' rights;

ad. Unrestricted contact with visitors and others as long as that does not infringe on other residents' rights;

ae. Have the rights that one would enjoy in one's own home, such as coming and going;

af. Residents' family members have the right to form and participate in family councils.

2. *Provider responsibilities*

The provider will:

a. Promote an environment of civility, good manners, and mutual consideration by requiring staff, and encouraging residents, to speak to one another in a respectful manner.

b. Provide all services for the resident or the resident's family that have been contracted for by the resident and the provider, as well as those services that are required by law.

c. Obtain accurate information from residents that is sufficient to make an informed decision regarding admission and the services to be provided.

d. Maintain an environment free of illegal weapons and drugs.

e. Obtain notification from residents of any third party services they are receiving, and to establish reasonable policies and procedures related to third-party services.

f. Report information regarding resident welfare to state agencies or other authorities as required by law.

g. Establish reasonable house rules in coordination with the resident council.

h. Involve staff and other providers in the development of resident service plans.

i. Maintain an environment that is free from physical, mental, fiduciary, sexual and verbal abuse, and neglect;.

j. Require that providers of third-party services ensure that they and their employees have passed criminal background checks, are free from communicable diseases, and are qualified to perform the duties they are hired to perform.

Services

Services offereded in assisted living communities vary both by state admission and retention criteria, and by individual assisted living providers. Typically services that may be offered by assisted living communities include:

1. Twenty-four-hour care and supervision,

2. Oversight of personal and supportive services (assistance with activities of daily living and instrumental activities of daily living),

3. Health-related services (e.g., medication management services, hospice care),

4. Social services,

5. Recreational activities,

6. Meals and snacks,

7. Housekeeping and laundry,

8. Transportation.

Many states now seek to allow communities to facilitate aging-in-place and to offer consumers a full range of long-term care options. However, in some cases, most states specify the range of allowable services and a minimum that must be provided, but do not require communities to provide the full range of allowable services. There are varying opinions on what services assisted living communities should be expected to provide. Some believe that assisted living should remain a social model, and communities should not be expected to provide services to persons with medically complex conditions or high levels of disabilities. On the other hand, some believe that assisted living communities should provide additional services to residents as care needs increase in an effort to minimize the need to relocate to a skilled nursing facility or nursing home.

Training Requirements

State regulations generally specify initial training requirements for assisted living administrators, as well as direct-care staff. However, some states stipulate general requirements, and others include specific topics, such as the number of hours required (see Chapter 5 for more information on direct-care staff training requirements).

Administrator Requirements

Administrator requirements also vary by state. Each state requires assisted living settings to employ a manager, director, or an administrator who is responsible for daily operations, including staffing, oversight, and complying with regulatory requirements (Carder et al., 2015). Generally, the administrator is expected to be employed full-time, but states may permit smaller settings with a licensed resident capacity under a specified number to employ a part-time administrator. Initial and ongoing training requirements for administrators are typically required.

Direct Staff Requirements

Assisted living communities employ direct-care workers to provide personal care and related daily services to residents. States use a variety of terms to describe these staff, including *personal care assistant*, *attendant*, and *caregiver* (Carder et al., 2015). Most often, these direct-care staff are unlicensed, though states may require training and/or certification, as seen in Chapter 5.

Carlson (2005) makes the important notation that direct-care standards for assisted living communities are far less stringent than those that apply to nursing home staff members, where under the terms of the federal Nursing Home Reform Law, direct-care staff must complete at least 75 hours of initial training under the supervision of a registered nurse with a minimum of 2 years' experience and at least 1 year of nursing experience in long-term care.

Dementia Care

States continue to adopt more regulations with regard to residents with dementia in assisted living (Carder et al., 2015). Two examples of the various additional requirements for communities serving dementia residents include:

1. *Disclosure*
   Most states require that facilities disclose their dementia care-specific services. These facilities are required to describe in writing how they are different from other facilities. This may include philosophy of care, admission/discharge criteria, the process for arranging a discharge, services covered and the cost of care, and special activities that are available.

2. *Staffing and training*
    Most states now have requirements for dementia training and staffing for facilities
    serving people with Alzheimer's disease and other dementias, which may include
    additional training hours or staffing ratios.

Medication Administration

Medication management and administration is a key issue for assisted living communities that offers many challenges. In their report, *Assisted Living: Quality of Care and Consumer Protection Issues*, the U.S. General Accounting Office (1999, p. 3) found "not providing residents with appropriate medications and not storing medications properly" to be a common problem in assisted living facilities. Regulators have also cited medication administration and assistance with self-medication as a major concern (Mollica et al., 2007).

There is much variability in how states address medication issues within their regulations in assisted living communities. However, several states now report that they are paying closer attention to medication issues, including the tracking of medication problems as the acuity level of residents served increases. Some states allow for trained aides to administer medications, while others allow only trained aides to administer medications or to assist with self-administration of medications. Some states require communities to have a consulting pharmacist, and several states require licensed nurses to review medication records on a regular basis. Some states are now requiring additional training for direct-care staff who administer or assist with self-administration of medications (e.g., California).

The Assisted Living Workgroup (2003, p. 170) included the following recommendation with regards to medication management in their report, *Assuring Quality in Assisted Living: Guidelines for Federal and State Policy, State Regulations, and Operations*, to the U.S. Senate Special Committee on Aging:

The assisted living residence will have and implement policies and procedures for the safe and effective distribution, storage, access, security, and use of medications, related equipment, and services of the residence by trained and supervised staff.

Policies and procedures of the residence should address the following issues:

1. Medication orders, including telephone orders;
2. Pharmacy services;
3. Medication packaging;
4. Medication ordering and receipt;
5. Medication storage;
6. Disposal of medications and medication-related equipment;
7. Medication self-administration by the resident;
8. Medication reminders by the residence;
9. Medication administration by the residence;
10. Medication administration—specific procedures;
11. Documentation of medication administration;
12. Medication error detection and reporting;
13. Quality-improvement system, including medication error prevention and reduction;

14. Medication monitoring and reporting of adverse drug effects to the prescriber;

15. Review of medications (e.g., duplicate drug therapy, drug interactions, monitoring for adverse drug interactions);

16. Storage and accountability of controlled drugs;

17. Training, qualifications, and supervision of staff involved in medication management.

Quality-Assurance Efforts

As the interest in assisted living has increased, so have concerns about quality of care and safety that can be provided to those residents who require special care, staffing, and physical and social environments. These concerns have been described in media reports throughout the country and in a 1999 report from the U.S. General Accounting Office (U.S. GAO; 1999). In 2004, the U.S. GAO issued another report, *Assisted Living: Examples of State Efforts to Implement Consumer Protections*, which describes the quality-assurance initiatives in Florida, Georgia, Massachusetts, Texas, and Washington.

Quality-assurance strategies by states described in the U.S. GAO report (2004) include:

1. Provide technical assistance and follow-up.

2. Act within 10 days on complaints.

3. Have clear lines of communication and definition of duties for survey staff.

4. Develop clear enforcement procedures that are well understood by state staff meeting with providers to discuss issues.

5. Provide training.

6. Conduct follow-up visits.

7. Maintain a consumer perspective that focuses on improving care, not just punishing past failures.

In addition, states described a number of initiatives to improve quality:

1. Provide training for providers.

2. Implement new training requirements for medication aides.

3. Revise the survey process.

4. Develop a more formalized consultation program.

5. Provide more technical assistance.

6. Conduct forums for providers to discuss quality issues.

7. Implement quality-assurance and quality-of-care initiatives.

Furthermore, additional strategies focused on conducting regulatory reviews to bring facilities up to national standards and to tighten standards for assessment, training, and level of care:

1. Work with providers to develop minimal standards for assessments, service plans, negotiated risk agreements, and disclosure requirements.

2. Add disclosure requirements for dementia care providers.

3. Increase staff training requirements.

4. Establish specific staffing requirements for special care units.

5. Increase requirements for a comprehensive resident assessment.

Quality assurance and quality improvement continue to be key issues addressed by researchers, educators, industry professionals, and advocacy groups.

FEDERAL STATUTES THAT IMPACT ASSISTED LIVING

Although states are primarily responsible for the licensing and oversight of assisted living communities, federal statues also impact the operations of assisted living. Some examples of federal statutes that are important for the assisted living administrator to have knowledge of are offered by the Assisted Living Federation of America (2008):

Americans With Disabilities Act

The Americans With Disabilities Act (ADA) affects assisted living operators in two primary ways: first, as employers under Title I of that law; and second, as "public accommodations" under Title III of that law. Title I of the ADA covers all employers with 15 or more employees, although religious organizations may require all employees, including those with disabilities, to conform to their religious tenets. The principal obligation of employers under Title I of the ADA is to provide "reasonable accommodations" to employees with disabilities, which are defined as physical or mental impairments that substantially limit "major life activities"—such as walking, breathing, and working—in order to allow them to perform the "essential functions" of a job. In addition, under Title I of the ADA, assisted living employers must refrain from making adverse decisions based on an individual's having a record of a physical or mental impairment, as well as from erroneously regarding an individual as disabled and treating him or her differently on that basis. Finally, the ADA prohibits employers from inquiring whether an applicant has a medical condition or disability prior to extending a conditional offer of employment. Alcoholism is a protected disability under the ADA, although current drug users (as opposed to the rehabilitated) are not covered under the Act, and the Act does not affect the ability of assisted living employers to test employees for drug use.

Title III of the ADA prohibits discrimination on the basis of disability by "commercial facilities" and "places of public accommodation' —such as "social service center establishments" and offices of "service establishments," regardless of size. Title III's prohibitions, however, do not apply to "religious organizations or entities controlled by religious organizations."

Under Title III of the ADA, "commercial facilities" are specifically defined to exclude residential facilities and facilities otherwise covered by or exempted from the requirements of the Fair Housing Act of 1968 as amended by the Fair Housing Amendments Act (FHAA) of 1988. Because the term *dwelling"* under the FHAA has been interpreted broadly, the coverage of assisted living facilities as "commercial facilities" under Title III of the ADA may be correspondingly narrow. However, as certain physically public parts of assisted living facilities, such as lobbies, hallways, sales and management offices, and parking lots, may separately qualify as "places of public accommodation" under Title III of the ADA, assisted living operators can expect the coverage of Title III of the ADA and the FHAA to overlap with respect to such areas. In any event, under either law, assisted living operators will generally be required to make those architectural modifications to facilities that do not constitute "undue hardships."

Moreover, to the extent an assisted living operator offers social services such as dining, counseling, and transportation to its residents, the public areas of an entire facility may independently be deemed a covered "place of public accommodation." As such, if a resident or guest meets the definition of "disabled" under the ADA, the resident will be entitled to reasonable accommodations that will allow the resident to access the facility and its services on a nondiscriminatory basis. Assisted living operations must ensure that their delivery of services does not result in any of the types of discrimination prohibited under Title III of the ADA. This generally will mean making reasonable accommodations to ensure that facilities and programs give the disabled equal opportunities to participate and benefit in the most appropriate integrated setting.

Civil Rights Act of 1991

The Civil Rights Act of 1991 consisted primarily of amendments to Title VII of the Civil Rights Act of 1964, which, like the ADA, covers assisted living operators employing 15 or more employees. It also affects the prohibition on intentional racial discrimination contained in the Reconstruction Civil Rights Act of 1866 (42 U.S.C. Sec. 1981), which covers assisted living operators regardless of the number of workers they employ.

Prior to the Civil Rights Act of 1991, Title VII of the Civil Rights Act of 1964 had been designed primarily to promote informal resolution of employment discrimination claims, and remedies were generally limited to declaratory judgments, injunctions, orders of reinstatements and/or backpay, and attorney's fees. The most dramatic change caused by the 1991 Act was the replacement of this system with a tort-like compensation scheme for intentional employment discrimination, including compensatory damages for emotional pain and suffering, punitive damages, and jury trials. Though it expanded the range of remedies available under Title VII, Congress also capped damages, however, at levels rising in three increments from $50,000 to $100,000, $200,000, and $300,000, for employers with up to 100, 200, 500, and over employees, respectively. These caps notwithstanding, the 1991 Act still significantly raised the financial stakes and risks for assisted living operators litigating federal employment discrimination claims.

In addition, the 1991 Act specifically overruled several Supreme Court decisions that had narrowed the scope of the Reconstruction Civil Rights Act and Title VII. In particular, Congress reversed a 1989 Supreme Court decision that had limited the reach of the Reconstruction Civil Rights Act, and expanded the kinds of acts prohibited by that law to encompass intentional discrimination in virtually any aspect of the employment relationship. Second, Congress adopted the broad interpretation of "adverse impact" discrimination announced by the Supreme Court in a landmark 1971 case—*Griggs v. Duke Power Co.*—thereby legislatively reversing another 1989 Supreme Court decision that briefly appeared to make it more difficult for plaintiffs to prevail in challenges to employment practices with disproportionate negative effects on classes of employees protected under Title VII. Finally, the 1991 Act also helped plaintiffs by partially reversing another 1989 decision of the Supreme Court—*Price Waterhouse v. Hopkins*—and newly allowing plaintiffs to "prevail" and receive declaratory judgments, injunctions, and attorney's fees even if an employer could establish that a decision adverse to an employee would have been made for legitimate reasons, any actual discriminatory motivation notwithstanding.

Rehabilitation Act of 1973

Section 504 of the Rehabilitation Act of 1973 applies to assisted living operators who receive federal financial assistance, and Section 503 of that Act applies to the rare operator who contracts with the federal government for more than $10,000 in personal property or "nonpersonal" services annually. Generally speaking, if a facility directly or indirectly receives Medicaid funds, it will likely be deemed the "recipient" of federal financial "assistance."

If an assisted living operator is covered by Section 504, the operator will effectively have no more obligations than they already had under Titles I and III of the ADA. Thus, for all practical purposes, unless the operator is exempt from the ADA for some reason, Section 504 of the Rehabilitation Act will not impact its operation. If an assisted living operator also becomes covered under Section 503 of the Rehabilitation Act, however, wholly apart from any obligations the operator may have under Titles I or III of the ADA, they will also have an obligation to take affirmative action to employ the disabled.

Family and Medical Leave Act

The Family and Medical Leave Act (FMLA) requires assisted living operators with 50 or more employees to provide up to 12 weeks of unpaid leave for family and medical reasons to employees who have worked for them for at least 12 months and a total of 1,250 hours during the previous 12-month period. Employers must maintain employees' preexisting group health insurance benefits while they are on FMLA leave, and must restore employees to the same or equivalent positions when their leave ends.

Employees can take FMLA leave for the birth of a child; adoption of a child; placement of a foster child; to care for a spouse, child, or parent with a "serious health condition"; or to care for a minor child who is unable to care for himself or herself due to a physical or mental disability as defined under the ADA. The statute also provides for leave for employees with "serious health conditions," defined as an "illness, injury, impairment or physical or mental condition that results in: (1) an overnight inpatient stay at a hospital, hospice, or residential medical care facility; (2) absence from work or other regular daily activities and continuing treatment for more than 3 days; or (3) continuing treatment for a chronic or long-term condition that if not treated would incapacitate the family member for more than 3 days" (The Family and Medical Leave Act of 1993, as amended).

An employee may take FMLA leave on a continuous or intermittent basis if medically necessary—such as when the employee or the employee's family member has an episodic illness. Though the law requires the employee give the employer 30 days' notice of needed FMLA leave when possible, fundamentally, the employee must simply make a reasonable attempt to schedule leave so as to minimize the disruption of the employer's operation. Moreover, employers may choose to designate paid leave as concurrent FMLA leave when taken by an employee qualifying for FMLA leave.

Fair Housing Amendments Act

The Fair Housing Amendments Act of 1988 altered Title VIII of the Fair Housing Act of 1968 in two main ways: First, it expanded the prohibitions contained in the Fair Housing Act to include discrimination in the sale or rental of "dwellings" on the basis of disability; and second, it enhanced the procedural enforcement options available for private litigants, as well as the Department of Housing and Urban Development (or its designated equivalent state or local agency, such as the City of Dallas), as they pursue relief under the Fair Housing Act.

Many of the residents of assisted living facilities qualify as "disabled" within the meaning of FHAA. Thus, the expansion of the Fair Housing Act to cover the disabled is having a complex effect on the assisted living industry. For example, on the one hand, the FHAA has put a new arrow in the quiver of assisted living operators faced with state and local regulations—uch as zoning restrictions—that can interfere with or prevent the construction of new (or expansion of operation of existing) facilities. On the other hand, however, the FHAA may result in new architectural burdens with respect to interior residential facilities, and may also create new potential liability for operators attempting to comply with state regulations that govern, for example, the placement of patients in assisted living (as opposed to long-term care) facilities.

The changes in the enforcement procedures contained in the FHAA also significantly increase the financial risk faced by assisted living operators sued under the Fair Housing Act. In particular, in addition to lengthening the period of time during which complaints of discrimination can be brought, in stark contrast with the prior $1,000 cap on punitive damages under the former law, the FHAA newly allows plaintiffs to recover unlimited punitive damages, and increases the ability of plaintiffs to recover attorney's fees in suits brought under the Fair Housing Act. Finally, the FHAA significantly enhances the ability of the federal government or its state or local agents to enforce the provisions of the Fair Housing Act in administrative proceedings and to recover fines for violations.

Fair Labor Standards Act

The Fair Labor Standards Act of 1938 (FLSA) is the primary federal law setting the minimum wage, overtime pay, equal pay, record keeping, and child labor standards for employers in the assisted living industry. An assisted living employer will qualify as an "enterprise" covered under the FLSA—and its non-exempt employees will be covered—if it has a gross annual sales volume of $500,000 or more, and two or more of its employees "handle," "sell," or "work on" goods or materials that have been "moved in or produced for commerce by any person." Depending on the precise nature of the services they provide, however, some assisted living operators may qualify for special exemptions from certain of the FLSA's requirements. These include, for example, exemptions related to individuals employed to provide companionship to the aged, "live-in" domestics, and workers residing on-site at their workplace.

As of July 24, 2009, the federal minimum wage is $7.25 per hour. Employers with unionized employees may not negotiate agreements that waive employees' statutory rights under the FLSA. Thus, collective bargaining agreements may only contain provisions that are more beneficial to employees than what such employees would otherwise receive under the FLSA.

Many of the questions and complexities that arise under the FLSA derive from the rules governing what constitutes compensable "hours worked" under that law, and employer errors in interpreting these rules may be particularly significant because (especially where full-time employees are concerned) they can result in unpaid overtime liability. Waiting time, on-call time, breaks, sleep time, meal periods, training, and travel time are all governed by detailed rules requiring separate analyses based on the facts and circumstances of employment.

In addition, with certain limitations, the FLSA allows assisted living employers to institute certain "alternative" work schedules. For example, under 29 U.S.C. Sec. 270(j), employers "engaged in the operation of . . . establishment[s] . . . primary engaged in the care of the . . . aged" can adopt a so-called "8–80" payroll system whereby employees are scheduled to work 80 hours on a 14-day basis rather than 40 hours on a 7-day basis.

Occupational Safety and Health Act

The Occupational Safety and Health Act of 1970 (OSHA) sets a national minimum standard for workplace safety. Section 18 of OSHA encourages states to develop and operate their own job safety and health programs, and OSHA approves and monitors state plans and provides up to 50% of an approved plan's operating costs. Some states, however, including Texas, do not maintain their own plans, and enforcement and the applicable statutes and regulations in such states are federal.

Employers of assisted living facilities have two general duties under OSHA: First, to furnish employees with employment (and a place of employment) that is free from recognized hazards that are likely to cause death or serious physical harm; and second, to comply with the detailed occupational safety and health standards promulgated under OSHA. Moreover, assisted living employers with 11 or more employees during the previous calendar year must keep records of occupational injuries and illness in the form of an OHSA Log 200.

OSHA compliance officers are authorized to inspect and investigate (at reasonable times and in a reasonable manner) places of employment for compliance with OSHA regulations, and are empowered to obtain injunctions, issue citations, and assess penalties for noncompliance through administrative proceedings.

CONCLUSIONS

This chapter provides the reader with an overview of state policy, licensing, and regulations for the assisted living industry. It is quite apparent that the states vary tremendously in regard to the licensing and monitoring of assisted living facilities. Although federal regulations do not currently exist, the reader is offered national guidelines and recommendations stemming from the work of prominent national organizations. Examples of federal statutes that impact assisted living facilities are described. This chapter illustrates the need for today's assisted living administrators to be well informed with regard to individual state laws and regulations and to remain updated as requirements are commonly changed and frequently modified.

REFERENCES

Assisted Living Federation of America. (2008). *Federal statutes that impact assisted living.* http://www.alfa .org/i4a/pages/index.cfm?pageid=3516

Assisted Living Workgroup. (2003). *Assuring quality in assisted living: Guidelines for federal and state policy, state regulations, and operations.* U.S. Government Printing Office. https://www.huduser.gov/portal/ publications/Assuring-Quality-in-Assisted-Living-Guidelines.html

Carder, P., O'Keeffe, J., & O'Keeffe, C. (2015). *Compendium of residential care and assisted living regulations and policy: 2015 edition.* U.S. Department of Health and Human Services, Office of the Assistant Secretary for Planning and Evaluation, Office of Disability, Aging and Long-Term Care Policy and Research Triangle Institute. https://aspe.hhs.gov/pdf-report/compendium-residential-care-and-assisted-living-regulations-and-policy-2015-edition

Carlson, E. (2005). *Critical issues in assisted living: Who's in, who's out and who's providing the care.* National Senior Citizen's Law Center.

Mollica, R., Sims-Kastelein, K., & O'Keeffe, J. (2007). *Residential care and assisted living compendium, 2007.* U.S. Department of Health and Human Services, Office of the Assistant Secretary for Planning and Evaluation, Office of Disability, Aging and Long-Term Care Policy and Research Triangle Institute. https://aspe.hhs.gov/system/files/pdf/75316/07alcom.pdf

National Center for Assisted Living. (2019). *2019 Assisted living state regulatory review.* National Center for Assisted Living. https://www.ahcancal.org/ncal/advocacy/regs/Documents/2019_reg_review.pdf

U.S. General Accounting Office. (1999). *Assisted living: Quality of care and consumer protection issues* (GAO/ T-HEHS-99-111).

U.S. General Accounting Office. (2004). *Assisted living: Examples of state efforts to implement consumer protections* (GAO-04-684). https://www.gao.gov/assets/250/242237.pdf

Zimmerman, S., & Sloane, P. (2007). Definitions and classification of assisted living. *The Gerontologist, 47,* 33–39.

3

ORGANIZATIONAL OVERVIEW

LEARNING OBJECTIVES

Upon the completion of Chapter 3, the reader will be able to:

- Understand the concept of aging in place in the context of assisted living.
- Describe the variation in assisted living according to the size of the community and services provided.
- Explain the differences between multiple service models in assisted living.
- Describe organizational patterns in assisted living.
- Understand the various business models in assisted living.
- Learn about assisted living communities that cater to the needs of special populations.

INTRODUCTION

This chapter considers key issues related to organizational management in the assisted living industry. First, the concept of *aging in place* is discussed in the context of models of care and levels of services within assisted living. Community size (i.e., number of beds) is highly variable among assisted living communities. Some common size variations are outlined, and how these size variations affect the organizational structure is also considered. An overview of common organizational models and patterns is described. Modern organizational designs, such as those with specific affiliation, are also included. Overall, this chapter provides the reader with an overview of common organizational considerations for assisted living communities.

AGING IN PLACE—A CONSIDERATION

"Aging in place" is a subject of much dialogue and debate among various assisted living stakeholders. As assisted living continues to evolve, questions, such as who is an appropriate resident for a certain community and how long a resident can remain, have become complicated. Should residents be allowed to remain in assisted living regardless of their care needs? Should they be allowed to die there? The concept of aging in place is a key concern for assisted living administrators as models of care and levels of services are discussed. *Aging in place* is a term used by many in the rapidly evolving senior housing industry, which includes assisted living.

"Growing older without having to move" is frequently offered as a definition of aging in place. In comparison, the definition of aging in place offered by of M. Powell Lawton (1990), a leader in aging research, described aging in place as a multiidimensional phenomenon for seniors: "Aging in place represents a transaction between an aging individual and his or her residential environment that is characterized by changes in both person and environment over time with the physical location of the person's being the only constant." In Lawton's definition there is a dynamic between the person and the environment. Lawton further explains that three types of changes occur as aging in place progresses. First, there are the psychological changes of aging. Second, there is change to the physical environment due to natural physical wear and the behaviors of other people. Third, there are changes that occur during the process of aging in place based upon alterations made to the environment to create a more supportive and private atmosphere.

In addition, Catherine Lysack (2010) expands on the idea that many elderly do not want to move from their homes as they get older. Baby boomers hope they can "live where they presently live until the end of life." However, many seniors move because of their physical limitations or the state of their house. Though many older adults are reluctant to move to an assisted living community, these communities can be beneficial in a variety of ways.

The assisted living ideal allows the physical place to stay the same and implies that necessary services to meet an older person's needs be brought to the person. Older persons usually move into supportive environments with the hope of avoiding other subsequent moves, and that the community will be able to provide for their changing needs over time. The community's ability to do this is an important aspect of security for older people. Aging in place is limited by several things in assisted living, including state regulations and community discretion. The models of care, in regard to admission and retention criteria, discharge triggers, and the availability of hospice/end-of-life care, are all important to consider.

In 2001, Jacquelyn Frank described the difficulties faced by providers of assisted living. These challenges still exist today, and perhaps even more so as older adults are living longer. She offered the following questions for consideration. *Who are suitable candidates for assisted living? When is it time for a resident to leave?* These are important questions for the assisted living administrator to consider. Although minimizing the need to move and providing prolonged residence are frequent goals of an assisted living community, "never having to move" is a promise that should not be made.

Size

Nationally, according to The National Center for Assisted Living (2016), the average assisted living community has approximately 33 licensed beds. However, assisted living community size varies greatly and communities may be much smaller or larger. In some states, different-size communities follow varying regulations and go by various names, as explained in Chapter 2, Policy, Licensing, and Regulations.

Services

As noted in previous chapters, assisted living communities typically offer services, including personal care and assistance with activities of daily living, social and recreational activities, meals, medication management, housekeeping, laundry, and transportation services. Some communities offer additional health services, such as intermittent nursing care oversight. Physical therapy as well as occupational therapy are also common services available among communities nationwide (National Center for Health Statistics, 2010). These services may be offered directly or through a third-party contractor. Under the direct services model, services are provided by the in-house staff. Under the contracted service model, outside agencies provide services to residents. Examples of contracted services include home healthcare and hospice services.

SERVICE MODELS

There is no standardized service model in assisted living. There are advantages to this, such as flexibility for industry and consumers, a wide span of services (at community's option), and a wide range of structures (site-based and imported services, bundled and unbundled charges and services). There are also disadvantages to this variety. For example, there is less clarity. A consumer's ability to plan is reduced and the accountability of the community can be unclear, creating regulatory oversight complexities. More extensive information on assisted living models of care is found in Chapter 13. Below four common examples of service models in assisted living are offered to illustrate the variety. These examples were chosen because they illustrate common models, but the reader should be aware that other models exist.

Board and Care

Small group homes that provide care for seniors and frail elders go by names. Depending on location, they may be called *board and care homes, assisted living, residential care homes for the elderly, personal care, adult foster care, adult group homes, adult family homes,* or *boarding care homes.* These residences characteristically offer room and board in a small environment, typically housing 10 persons or fewer. These homes are commonly located in residential neighborhoods and offer a less institutional alternative. A home like environment is of high priority. Although these facilities sometimes offer somewhat less independence and privacy, they often house persons with more cognitive impairments, chronic health conditions, and impairments with activities of daily living as opposed to larger models. Home healthcare and hospice services are sometimes available from third-party vendors. The ability of a resident to age in place in a board and care home is variable, depending on regulations and individual operator philosophies. Because of the smaller number of residents, these homes often have very few staff. For example, an owner or administrator may also be a direct caregiver and have only one or two additional employees.

Hospitality Model

Some assisted living facilities offer apartment-style living and hotel-type services with limited personal care assistance. These facilities offer meals, housekeeping, transportation, and security. Personal care services, such as toileting, getting up from a chair, or assistance with eating, are limited. Residents have a high degree of independence, but may not be able to stay at the facility if their care needs worsen. Hospitality-model assisted living facilities can be very appealing to consumers because of the high level of privacy that can be provided. Private units with private bathrooms and kitchenettes are common amenities. Facilities following this type of model may experience higher resident turnover rates, because of the lower level of care provided. Depending on facility size, staff size for this type of community varies. Hawes et al. (2003) classified an assisted living community as having low service status if it did not have an RN on staff and did not provide its own nursing care staff, but did provide the following:

- Twenty-four-hour staff oversight,
- Housekeeping,
- At least two meals a day,
- Personal assistance, defined as help with at least two of the following: medications, bathing, or dressing.

Larger Model

Larger or new-model assisted living facilities have typically more than 60 beds. In 2004, Hawes, Phillips, and Rose first described the newer model facilities as "high service and high privacy" (p. 11). These models have continued to evolve. The criteria for being a high-service community requires at least the following are provided:

■ Twenty-four-hour staff oversight,

■ Housekeeping,

■ At least two meals a day,

■ Personal assistance, defined as help with at least two of the following: medications, bathing, or dressing,

■ At least one full-time RN on staff,

■ Nursing care (monitoring or services) performed by its own staff.

In the report, *High Service or High Privacy Assisted Living Facilities, Their Residents and Staff: Results from a National Survey* (2000), Hawes and colleagues made several conclusions regarding high-service assisted living facilities (ALFs) nationwide: (a) the high-privacy or high-service ALFs provide this care in a setting that has many components valued by consumers, particularly in terms of privacy and environmental autonomy; (b) most high-service or high-privacy ALFs offer a wide array of services; (c) the issue of whether such services can meet residents' unscheduled needs is more complex; (d) the degree to which such facilities enable residents to age in place is clearly mixed unless one limits the concept to one of *aging in place without significant decline in physical or cognitive functioning*; and (e) assisted living is still a largely private-pay sector and, among the high-service or high-privacy ALFs, one that is largely unaffordable for most moderate and low-income older persons unless they spend down (i.e., the process of reducing the value of assets to qualify for Medicaid) their assets or receive help from relatives.

Specialized Dementia Care Model

A growing specialty area in assisted living facilities is dementia care (commonly referred to as *memory care*). The market demand for dementia care has continued to grow. Specialized facilities exist, as do specialized units within assisted living facilities. According to Rick Weisberg (2016) in *Many Different Models of Assisted Living*, an assisted living community with a special memory care unit is the most common model for people with Alzheimer's or dementia. Special care units may promote a physical environment, activities, staff training, and program philosophy that address the special care needs of individuals with memory loss and related behavioral problems. Activities, such as art and music therapy, are offered in units like these to aid with memory issues. Specialized dementia units often have a secure environment and a specialized physical design layout. To enhance the quality of life of persons with dementia, these specialty units often include additional interventions and philosophies such as:

■ Holistic assessment;

■ Regular formal assessments;

■ Referral to other professionals as appropriate;

■ Care planning involving resident, family, and staff;

■ Person-centered care;

■ Opportunities for residents to express themselves;

- Medication and nonpharmacological treatment;
- Training and management of staff;
- A positive and safe environment.

ORGANIZATIONAL PATTERNS BY SIZE AND MODEL

Assisted living communities generally have traditional departments, including :
- Marketing
- Admissions
- Direct care
- Nutritional services
- Laundry
- Housekeeping
- Maintenance

However, depending on the size and model of the community, staffing levels and organizational patterns vary greatly. Figure 3.1 illustrates a sample organizational pattern for a smaller, board-and-care type of community. Figure 3.2 illustrates a sample organizational pattern for a midsized, or hospitality-model community, and Figure 3.3 illustrates a sample organizational pattern for a larger, or new-model community.

BUSINESS MODELS

For-Profit Versus Nonprofit

Both for-profit and nonprofit investors want to see a well-managed operation. For-profit investors look for low costs, which means more profit for the organization. Nonprofit investors, on the

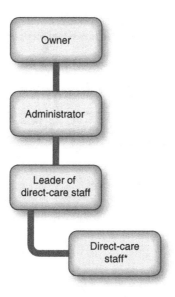

FIGURE 3.1 Sample organizational pattern for a smaller community (board and care).
*Number of direct-care staff varies based on number and needs of residents.

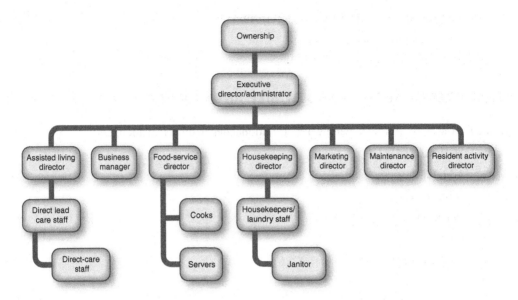

FIGURE 3.2 Sample organizational pattern for a midsize, or hospitality, community.

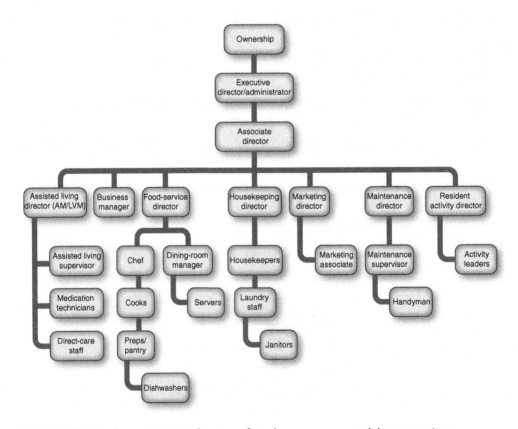

FIGURE 3.3 Sample organizational pattern for a large, or new-model, community.

other hand, are actually investing in a cause, so they want to see as much money as possible go toward that cause, not toward overhead. As an administrator, you should keep in mind that any plan you put together should build the case that you can operate the community well and deliver what you claim to offer.

For-Profit Investors

For-profit investors want to see a profitable business that offers a safe, high return on their money. You will need to demonstrate that there is a market for your product or service that is willing to pay for it out of their own pockets. If you are starting a community, for example, investors want assurance that in your location, there is enough demand at the price you charge to make a good business. Furthermore, as for-profit investors want to get their money back, the business must either generate a lot of cash or be a good candidate for acquisition. The emphasis is on profit, so much so that in some cases, companies may change their line of business in order to reach their goals.

Nonprofit Investors

Nonprofit investors are usually funded by foundations or people who want to see the organization provide a community service. They are concerned about what you will accomplish and how you'll get the results they want in the community. In a nonprofit plan, what you do is concentrate on the deed. Rarely will you find nonprofits that change their mission once they're underway. The cash-raising process for a nonprofit differs from profit fundraising as well. Foundations and donors often have their own requirements for what goes into a nonprofit proposal, and you may find that with nonprofit status, you spend a lot of time figuring out how to satisfy each organization's requirements.

For-Profit Versus Nonnprofit Board of Directors

Some differences exist among for-profit versus nonprofit boards of directors. Some knowledge of these differences may be useful to the assisted living administrator. These are summarized in Table 3.1.

Administrator's Objective

The objectives in either plan are the same: to meet the funding source's needs by laying out a plan for an organization that will get the job done better than other organizations. In for-profit, it is the bottom line that counts, and your community's plan will be geared around that. In nonprofits, it is what you do that matters, so you should set a business plan to meet that need.

SPECIFIC AFFILIATIONS

Assisted living facilities may sometimes cater to the specific needs of special populations. Although these communities do not discriminate against any person and still must comply with state regulations, they may offer services that are designed to benefit a distinct population where common values, language, food, and customs are promoted. Examples include affiliations, such as religious, ethnic, or LGBTQ groups, for example, the Catholic Health Services of the Archdiocese of

TABLE 3.1 FOR-PROFITS VS. NONPROFITS, AND BOARDS OF DIRECTORS

	FOR-PROFIT	**NONPROFIT**
Overarching goal/mission:	Generate profits for owners	Serve the needs of the public
Size:	Relatively small (3–7 residents)	Can be quite large (11–35 residents)
Membership:	Major owners and other business people	Come from business, professional, and volunteer sectors
Term of office:	Often no term limits	Increasingly, nonprofits are adopting term limits
Employees on the board:	Usually the case, often more than one	Typically, only the CEO and usually ex officio members (nonvoting)
"Owners":	Shareholders	Members of the public, , association members, donors, churches, etc.
Primary beneficiaries:	Owners	The community
Elections:	Shareholders vote according to number of shares owned	Varies: May be open to all members, trustees only, or various other arrangements
Compensation:	Often paid per meeting	Few nonprofit directors are paid for being on the board
Public accountability:	Discloses only what is required by law	High transparency: tax returns available online

CEO, chief executive officer.

Miami (www.catholichealthservices.org); Kokoro Assisted Living, established by members of the Japanese American community in San Francisco (www.kokoroassistedliving.org); and Stonewall Gardens, for LGBTQ residents (http://www.stonewallgardens.com).

FUTURE LANDSCAPE

Looking forward to the future, the Green House Project continues to be one example of an innovative model of assisted living that is being adopted and integrated by assisted living communities across the nation (www.thegreenhouseproject.org).

CONCLUSIONS

This chapter provides the reader with an overview of organizational patterns and models in the assisted living industry. Great variety exists among organizations due to varying facility sizes and service models used. Typical organizational patterns for common models are illustrated. Examples of specific affiliation models show that assisted living is emerging and advancing to serve a diverse population with varying needs. This chapter illustrates the need for today's assisted living administrators to be well informed and to remain attuned to the evolving needs, practices, and models in the industry.

REFERENCES

Frank, J. (2001). How long can I stay? The dilemma of aging in place in assisted living. *Journal of Housing for the Elderly, 15*, 5–30. https://doi.org/10.1300/j081v15n01_02

Hawes, C., Phillips, C., & Rose, M. (2000). *High service or high privacy assisted living facilities, their residents and staff: Results from a national survey.* U.S. Department of Health and Human Services.

Hawes, C., Phillips, C., Rose, M., Holan, S., & Sherman, M. (2003). A national study of assisted living facilities. *The Gerontologist, 43*, 875–882. https://doi.org/10.1093/geront/43.6.875

Lawton, M. P. (1990). Knowledge resources and gaps in housing for the aged. In D. Tilson (Ed.), *Aging in place: Supporting the frail elderly in residential environments*. Scott, Foresman.

Lysack, C. (2010). Household and neighborhood safety, mobility. In P. Lichtenberg (Ed.), *Handbook of assessment in clinical gerontology* (pp. 619–646). Elsevier.

National Center for Assisted Living. (2016). *Communities*. www.ahcancal.org/ncal/facts/Pages/Communities.aspx

National Center for Health Statistics. (2010). *National Survey of Residential Care Facilities*. https://www.cdc.gov/nchs/nsrcf/index.htm

Weisberg, R. (2016). *Many different models of assisted living*. http://assistedlivingnationwide.com/many-different-models-assisted-living

FURTHER READING

Catholic Health Services. (2019). *Assisted living facilities*. https://www.catholichealthservices.org/assisted-living

Kokoro Assisted Living. (2019). *An assisted living community*. https://kokoroassistedliving.org/about-us

NCB Capitol Impact. (2019). *The Greenhouse replication initiative*. http://www.socialimpactexchange.org/organization/ncb-capital-impact

Stonewall Gardens. (2019). *Stonewall gardens*. http://www.stonewallgardens.com/index.php

II

HUMAN RESOURCES
MANAGEMENT

4

RECRUITING AND HIRING STAFF

LEARNING OBJECTIVES

Upon the completion of Chapter 4, the reader will be able to:

- Describe the assisted living workforce.
- Discuss the challenges of workforce recruitment in assisted living.
- Understand a variety of factors that influence workforce recruitment in long-term care.
- Identify the steps in the recruitment and hiring process.
- Recognize the importance of written job requirements and job descriptions.
- Identify the legal issues surrounding recruitment and hiring.
- Consider best practices for finding and keeping direct-care workers in long-term care.

INTRODUCTION

This chapter addresses critical issues in the recruitment and hiring of personnel for an assisted living community. Background information is included, such as a description of the assisted living workforce and the challenges of workforce recruitment. Factors that influence workforce recruitment are discussed. For example, issues, such as the economy, pay and benefits, working conditions, education, and training, are discussed to provide an understanding of the complexity of today's long-term care workforce. The five steps of the recruitment process (i.e., planning, searching, screening, selection and hiring, and maintaining an applicant pool) are then described in detail with examples provided to assist the reader in understanding the included concepts.

The Assisted Living Workforce

Providing formalized long-term care in an assisted living community requires an adequate, skilled, and diverse workforce. Paraprofessionals (i.e., unlicensed, direct-care staff) represent the largest component of personnel in long-term care and will likely make up the majority of an assisted living community's staff. Today, estimates report the direct workforce comprises 4.5 million home health aides, personal care aides, and nursing assistants employed across a range of home and community-based settings (Scales, 2018). Direct-care workers help clients with essential daily tasks, such as dressing and bathing. All communities employ a licensed or certified administrator and many larger communities also employ licensed nurses (i.e., registered nurses, licensed vocational nurses). Other employed or typical personnel include those who work in various support departments such as business (e.g., accounting, marketing), nutritional services (e.g., cooks, dieticians), personal support (e.g., activities, social services), laundry, housekeeping, and maintenance. Other professionals necessary for the provision of long-term care include physicians, social workers, therapists, pharmacists, podiatrists, dentists, and mental health providers. These other professionals are typically third-party contractors who provide services to the residents and are not employed by the assisted living community. Developing a successful recruitment and retention strategy tasks time and effort, but even a small investment can pay off.

Challenges of Workforce Recruitment

The recruitment and hiring of quality personnel is a growing challenge for assisted living communities. Staffing challenges are not entirely unique to the organization—they are shaped by trends affecting long-term care employers across the country. This is especially true for paraprofessionals (i.e., direct-care staff) due to low wages and benefits, hard working conditions, and work that is stigmatized by society (Stone & Weiner, 2001).

In a 2013 report to Congress, the Commission on Long-Term Care described several issues relative to today's long-term care workforce:

1. Family caregivers today provide the majority of long-term care. Those who take on this unpaid role risk the stress, physical strain, competing demands, and financial hardship of caregiving, and thus are vulnerable themselves. Due to declining birthrates, which will result in fewer available family caregivers than in years past, there may be a larger caregiver responsibility for fewer family caregivers, and the availability and quality of paid caregivers will become increasingly important.

2. Direct-care workers, whether working in residential settings or in a person's home, are often most familiar with the individual and the individual's service needs and are best able to provide services and support in a person-centered way. Individuals with high levels of disability and complex health conditions increasingly receive long-term care in home and community-based settings, increasing the skill demands both for family caregivers and paid workers.

3. Many home-care workers are employed by home-care agencies, and many others are employed directly by individuals and their families, as personal care attendants under a Medicaid consumer-directed services program or as private household employees. Rarely do any of these workers receive adequate training to meet the demands of providing long-term care in a home setting, resulting in high rates of injury and high rates of turnover, reducing continuity of service. Low wages and few, if any, benefits with little opportunity for advancement compound to make it more difficult to retain a trained workforce. Growth of the older adult population and increasing integration of medical services with long-term care for all populations with cognitive or functional limitations will require more professional and direct-care workers in long-term care settings, care planning, and participation in teams providing direct care.

4. Efforts to improve the availability and quality of paid and unpaid caregivers need to be framed in the context of the fiscal and economic pressures facing this country and the challenge of ensuring access to quality healthcare and long-term care for an aging population.

Paraprofessional workers or direct-care staff make up the majority of the long-term care workforce (Paraprofessional Healthcare Institute, 2013). As with many caregiving jobs, the majority of direct-care staff are women. There is a significant geographic variation in the race and ethnicity profile of direct-care workers. In some areas, more minority workers are available and willing to work in long-term care. Direct-care workers most often have some economic disadvantages, such as low levels of education and low household earnings. These "frontline" workers engage in very demanding and important work, but the occupation itself is relatively low paying.

FACTORS INFLUENCING WORKFORCE RECRUITMENT

The Economy

The current state of the economy as well as labor market influence directly impact the ability of assisted living communities to recruit and hire staff. In a stronger economy, many workers move to other industries that offer better job quality, whether higher wages, more stable hours, safer working conditions, opportunities for advancement, or other advantages.

Pay and Benefits

Pay and benefit considerations are critical for attracting personnel. This is especially problematic with the paraprofessional workforce in long-term care because wages and benefits are typically quite low considering the level of responsibility expected, difficult workloads, and high injury rates. The actual level at which salaries would have to be set to attract adequate personnel for assisted living communities is unknown. A living wage and better benefits are two essential elements for boosting recruitment and retention in direct care.

Working Conditions

The way in which an assisted living workplace is organized and managed affects the working conditions. The utilization of mentoring, recognition, coaching, and collective involvement of staff in decision-making is a way to create positive working conditions. Nurses and aides often complain about managers who lack respect for the knowledge and skills they bring to the job and refuse to share information.

Image of the Industry

Workforce recruitment in long-term care is often difficult because of the image of the industry. Ageism in society coupled with media reports of poor care quality, scandals, and elder abuse can bias the view of the public. Frontline worker jobs in long-term care are sometimes viewed by the public as unpleasant and poor paying.

Education and Training

The professional and paraprofessional workforce often lacks the necessary training to address the special health and medical care needs of the frail elderly. Standards for direct-care staff training are often minimal and not specific. Few nurses or physicians specialize in geriatrics. Long-term care is not a traditional component of a nursing curriculum. Administrator requirements vary by state but are often inadequate.

Transportation

The ease with which potential employees can commute to work may affect the geographic area from which employees can be recruited. The availability of an efficient public transportation system improves access to employees who do not drive. This may be especially true with regard to direct-care staff.

THE RECRUITMENT PROCESS

Recruitment is the process of sourcing, screening, and selecting people for a job or vacancy within an organization. Box 4.1 lists the main components of the recruitment process, which are then discussed in detail.

Planning

Planning recruitment efforts begin with forecasting employment needs. The assisted living administrator is responsible for projecting the needs (e.g., number of residents, levels of care) of the community, and identifying the personnel requirements necessary to meet those needs. Advanced planning for employment needs is critical to the success of the community.

Projections

Advanced knowledge of trends in the industry can assist in the planning of recruiting employees. As noted earlier, consider the factors that influence workforce availability (i.e., labor market and economy, wages and benefits, education and training, image of the industry, transportation). The U.S. Department of Labor (DOL) and the Employment Security Commission (within individual states) may also be sources of information to consider in the planning phase.

Job Requirements

Defining job requirements is a necessary and essential step in the planning of recruitment. In assisted living communities, some job requirements are mandated by state regulation (e.g., criminal background checks, education, and experience). Job requirements for direct-care staff are minimal, and training is often completed on the job (see Chapter 5 for training requirements for direct-care staff). Requirements for the administrator are specific to each state. A summary of current state requirements is available from the National Center for Assisted Living (2019). Remember, state requirements represent only minimal standards, and assisted living communities may consider higher standards regarding job requirements for personnel.

When defining job requirements, the assisted living administrator must understand the responsibilities involved with the job, the tasks involved with the job, and the background (i.e., education and experience) necessary to complete the job. In addition, it is important to consider the personal characteristics that may be required (e.g., interpersonal skills, decision-making skills, motivation), the culture of the community, and managerial style of the administrator.

BOX 4.1: STEPS IN THE RECRUITMENT PROCESS

1. Planning
2. Searching
3. Screening
4. Selection and hiring
5. Maintaining applicant pool

Job Descriptions

Well-developed job descriptions are imperative to the planning phase of recruitment. Job descriptions are often utilized to establish salary ranges, define performance expectations, and evaluate performance, but they can also be very useful in a successful recruitment plan. Job descriptions contain detailed information on the skills, knowledge, abilities, and experience that a candidate should possess for a specific job. Keep in mind that state regulations sometimes include specifics on what must be included in the job descriptions of assisted living personnel. Box 4.2 offers a list of information typically included in a job description.

Searching

The search process will vary depending on the type of position being filled. For example, strategies that may be appropriate for the recruitment of an administrator may be very different from the recruiting of direct-care staff. Recruitment plans should be developed accordingly, and incorporate strategies that have worked in the past, as well as allow for new ideas. If a community has a very limited candidate pool, the development of a continuous recruitment plan may be appropriate. There are both internal and external sources for recruitment. Of course, the community should choose the method that is likely to produce the best results.

Internal Sources

Recruitment of individuals from within an organization can be beneficial for several reasons. Internal recruitment often allows for internal growth opportunities and may also result in greater retention, as well as improved staff morale and loyalty. Internal recruitment may be less expensive, less time consuming, and less disruptive to a community. Internal recruitment may be facilitated by posting notices of a job opening within the organization prior to the information being published outside of the organization. Box 4.3 lists some ideas for internal recruitment. For example, postings may be distributed by memorandum email, voice mail, newsletters, bulletin boards, or

---

BOX 4.2:   INFORMATION TO BE INCLUDED IN JOB DESCRIPTION

1. Position title, name of the specific unit (if indicated), and name of the facility
2. Duties, essential job functions, and responsibilities of the position
3. Education, training experience, and licensure requirements
4. Knowledge, skills, and abilities necessary to perform assigned duties
5. Reporting relationships (i.e., hiring manager, reporting manager)
6. Hours and location of work
7. Pay grade and salary ranges (optional)
8. Background characteristics required
9. Personal characteristics required
10. Continuing education and training required to maintain competence
11. Other specifications of the position, such as legal requirements

---

BOX 4.3:   INTERNAL SOURCES FOR RECRUITMENT

1. Bulletin board notices

2. Staff meeting announcements

3. Internal email

4. Development of career ladders

---

announcements at staff meetings. The development of internal career ladders (i.e., a path in which an employee may hope to progress within a community) may also be an important internal source of recruitment.

External Sources

External recruitment sources expand the number of potential candidates. This can be beneficial because it decreases the reliance on seniority as a primary basis for promotion, and brings new talent and experience to the community. Potential methods for recruiting candidates from external sources are listed in Box 4.4.

Screening

Applicant screening involves the elimination of unqualified applicants from the recruitment pool. Screening every applicant to ensure a good fit is the easiest way to eliminate those with valid reasons for exclusion such as inadequate education or experience, or failure to pass a criminal background check. Reviewing job applications, resumes, and reference checks are common ways to learn about applicants. It is important to consider professionalism, experience, enthusiasm, and a desire to work with elderly persons when reviewing applications.

If multiple applicants are identified as candidates, consider an initial screening interview. This interview can be briefly conducted to assess the suitability of a candidate for a position. A telephone interview may be appropriate especially if the candidate lives far from the community, or to save time.

BOX 4.4:   EXTERNAL SOURCES FOR RECRUITMENT

1. Advertisements in professional journals, newspapers, professional newsletters, and internet postings

2. Personnel placement service provided by national or state agencies

3. Events, such as educational sessions or community outreach programs

4. Community job fairs

5. Educational Institutions; consider recruitment visits to colleges and universities, as well as possible internships for qualified students

6. Referrals from employees, residents, families, assisted living facilities, and provider organizations

Selection and Hiring

The key to hiring well-qualified staff is to recruit the right individuals from the start—those who are most likely to succeed in the role. For example, you will need to consider the legal aspects of hiring, the interview process, and background verification. In addition, deciding to hire and then offering the job is a part of this process.

Legal Aspects

There are a number of federal laws that employers must consider and follow when hiring employees (DOL, 2019). In general, these laws prohibit discrimination in employment decisions based on race, color, religion, gender, age, ethnic/national origin, disability, or veteran status. The DOL administers and enforces laws affecting the hiring of employees under the age of 18, veterans, and certain foreign workers. The DOL is also responsible for laws that ensure that federal contractors and grantees provide equal employment opportunities to applicants and employees. Four important examples of legal concerns (DOL, 2019) that may affect the hiring process include:

1. Equal employment opportunity (EEO): EEO laws prohibit specific types of employment discrimination. These laws prohibit discrimination on the basis of race, color, religion, sex, age, national origin, or status as an individual with a disability, or protected veteran.

2. Hiring people with disabilities: The DOL enforces laws prohibiting discrimination against individuals with disabilities, and allowing payment of special minimum-wage rates to certain individuals with disabilities.

3. Hiring foreign workers: The DOL responsibilities regarding foreign workers include certification of positions for temporary and permanent employment of aliens, as well as hiring and wage issues. Foreign labor certification programs permit U.S. employers to hire foreign workers on a temporary or permanent basis to fill jobs essential to the U.S. economy. These programs are generally designed to ensure that the admission of foreign workers into the United States on a permanent or temporary basis will not adversely affect the job opportunities, wages, and working conditions of U.S. workers.

4. Wages and the Fair Labor Standards Act (FLSA). The FLSA establishes minimum wage, overtime pay, record-keeping, and youth employment standards affecting employees in the private sector and in federal, state, and local governments.

Keep in mind that there are many other legal aspects of employment law that you must follow both in hiring and maintaining personnel. A full description is beyond the scope of this book, but as an administrator, you must become familiar with all applicable state, federal, and local laws.

Interviews

The goal of the interview process is to successfully match the best available candidate to a specific position. A successful interview should allow one to predict the future performance of candidates.

The individual interview is the most common type of interview. Individual interviews are simple, easier to schedule, and allow for a consistent perspective. They may be less intimidating to the candidate, and therefore makes it easier to evaluate the applicant more accurately, as well as allow the applicant an opportunity to ask questions.

Another type of interview is a group interview during which members of a team interview the candidate individually and then pool results, or interview the candidate as a group. This is more commonly utilized when attempting to hire a nurse or administrator than with direct-care personnel. The team approach can be advantageous because it can offer multiple perspectives. Group interviews are much more time consuming and may be more intimidating for a candidate. However, group interviews can foster an ideal of teamwork and a shared sense of responsibility.

A successful interview is an effective interview. Characteristics of an effective interview process are given in Box 4.5.

Interview methods are variable. Some interviews are more structured, whereas others are non-directive, and allow the candidate more freedom to both answer and ask questions. Although a structured interview may have very specific questions, less structured interviews may ask broader, open-ended questions, and allow for more engagement with the candidate. Box 4.6 gives some examples of interview questions.

Understanding unlawful questions and inquiries is critical to the interview process. Box 4.7 lists subjects that are inappropriate for interviews.

BOX 4.5: CHARACTERISTICS OF AN EFFECTIVE INTERVIEW PROCESS

1. Interviewers should provide information to the candidate about the facility, the agenda for the interview, and the job description.

2. The interview should be carefully planned. Allow adequate time for each part of the process.

3. Interviewers should be prepared. Information previously submitted by the candidate should be reviewed in advance of the interview.

4. Carefully planned questions should be developed in advance. Open-ended questions allow for more dialogue and a better understanding of the applicant's suitability. Take special care to maintain compliance with laws and regulations regarding suitable questions.

5. In order to create a means of comparison, a core group of questions should be established that will be asked of all candidates.

6. The interviewer should maintain focus on the criteria for the position and the qualifications of the candidates. Remember, the goal is to match the best candidate with the open position.

7. The interviewer should give the candidate a realistic perspective of the job, including favorable and unfavorable information.

8. Standards for performance and methods of evaluation should be carefully explained to the candidate. A discussion of professional growth should be included.

9. The interviewer should provide the candidate with a description of employee benefits associated with the job. For example, health insurance, vacation leave, and retirement benefits.

10. The interview should include a discussion of both initial salary and salary ranges.

11. A description of the likely work schedule should be reviewed with the candidate. Expectations regarding weekends and holidays are especially important in a long-term care facility.

12. If possible, include a tour of the facility.

13. A follow-up letter should be sent regardless of whether the candidate is hired or not. Thank the applicant and indicate any next steps. Well-organized communication improves the recruitment process.

BOX 4.6:   EXAMPLE INTERVIEW QUESTIONS

1. Personal traits/motivations:
   a. What motivates you to do your best work?
   b. Provide an example of when you went "out of your way" to get a job done.
   c. What do you think the advantages of this type of work are?
   d. What do you think the disadvantages of this type of work are?
   e. How do you define doing a good job?
   f.   What makes a job enjoyable for you?
   g. Under what conditions do you work best?

2. Goals:
   h.   Tell me what success means to you.
   i.   Do you consider yourself successful?
   j   Do you set goals for yourself and how do you do that?
   k.   Tell me your 5 year goals.

3. Communication:
   l.   Tell me how you best communicate.
   m. Tell me about a work situation you had that required excellent communication skills.
   n.   How would you grade your ability to communicate with management, customers, and peers?

4. Flexibility:
   o.   How important is communication and interaction with others in your job?
   p.   How many departments do you deal with?
   q.   What problems have occurred?
   r.   In what areas do you typically have the least amount of patience at work?

5. Stress:
   s.   You have worked in a fast-paced environment. How did you like the environment?
   t.   What kinds of decisions are most difficult for you?
   u.   What is the most difficult work situation you have faced?

6. Skill level:
   v.   What are your present job responsibilities?
   w. What are your greatest strengths on the job?
   x.   What areas need improvement?
   y.   Provide me with an example of an on-the-job problem you were able to solve.
   z.   How would you describe your professional competence?

BOX 4.7: INAPPROPRIATE INTERVIEW SUBJECTS

1. Age
2. National origin
3. Religion
4. Race
5. Marital or family status
6. Childcare arrangements or childbearing plans
7. Arrest records (although criminal background checks are required)
8. Financial information
9. Military discharge status
10. Any general information that would point out handicaps or health problems unrelated to job performance

---

Background Verification

If a candidate is under serious consideration for a position, the accuracy of all information provided by the candidate should be verified. It is important to obtain a signed request for references so that information may be obtained, especially from previous employers. In addition, the following are important sources of background verification:

1. Criminal background checks are often required by state regulation and should be completed on all staff working in an assisted living community. State and federal clearances are typically obtained through a fingerprint process.

2. Credit ratings are sometimes obtained, especially if the job requires financial responsibility. The employer must advise applicants that a credit report will be requested. If the candidate is rejected based upon the credit report, the name and address of the credit reporting agency must be given to the candidate in writing.

3. Physical examinations are required for assisted living community personnel. Tests for communicable diseases, such as tuberculosis, are included. Pre-employment physicals should be done after a job offer has been made to avoid any issues with discriminations. The physical examination will establish the physical capability of the applicant to perform the job. Recently, tests for illicit drugs are sometimes included in the physical examination.

Deciding to Hire

The decision to hire is complex. Once the candidates have been interviewed, the administrators must make an objective evaluation of each candidate. Review the important aspects, such as education and training, previous experience, job accomplishments, skills and knowledge, and personal attributes. The development of a rating system is sometimes a useful way to make objective hiring decisions. Despite efforts to maintain objectivity, evaluating candidates can still be subjective. Avoid being overly impressed with experience or maturity, or allowing personal biases to influence your assessment. Each candidate should be reviewed on a case-by-case basis to decide whether their skills and qualifications meet your community's needs.

Offering the Job

Once the decision to hire has been made, the candidate should be informed. All information, such as proposed salary, job title, description, and start date should be clearly communicated verbally and in writing. If possible, a personnel handbook should be included that describes the community's personnel policies. The process involved in the community's hiring procedures, such as work eligibility forms, tax withholding forms, and other required paperwork must then be completed.

Maintaining Applicant Pool

Maintaining an applicant pool can be useful for future needs of the community. If immediate selection is not anticipated, but the applicant is desirable, keep a file of applications and resumes. Keep applicants informed of their status indicating that they have not been selected for a current interview, but that their application will be kept on file for future needs.

CONSIDERING BEST PRACTICES

Paraprofessional Healthcare Institute (PHI), a national organization, works to transform elder-care and disability services. Their mission is to foster dignity, respect, and independence—for all who receive care and all who provide it. As the nation's leading authority on the direct-care workforce, PHI promotes quality direct-care jobs as the foundation for quality care. They offer the following strategies for success growing a strong direct-care workforce (Scales, 2018):

1. Recruit the right saff.
2. Improve the hiring process.
3. Strengthen entry-level training.
4. Provide employment supports.
5. Promote peer support.
6. Ensure efective supervision.
7. Develop advancement opportunities.
8. Invite participation.
9. Recognize and reward staff.
10. Measure progress.

CONCLUSIONS

A critical issue for today's assisted living communities is the recruitment and hiring of capable staff who understand the needs of elderly residents. The administrator of the community is responsible for identifying personnel who are committed to high-quality long-term care. This chapter identifies some of the challenges that the administrator faces relative to workforce recruitment and hiring. A five-point recruitment process is described in detail, including planning, searching, screening, selection and hiring, and maintaining an applicant pool. Possible approaches and examples are given to assist the reader in the hiring process.

REFERENCES

Commission on Long-Term Care. (2013). *Report to the Congress.* Commission on Long-Term Care. https://www.govinfo.gov/content/pkg/GPO-LTCCOMMISSION/pdf/GPO-LTCCOMMISSION.pdf

National Center for Assisted Living. (2019). *2019 Assisted living state regulatory review.* National Center for Assisted Living. https://www.ahcancal.org/ncal/advocacy/regs/Documents/2019_reg_review.pdf

Paraprofessional Healthcare Institute. (2013). *America's direct-care workforce.* PHI. https://phinational.org/wp-content/uploads/legacy/phi-facts-3.pdf

Scales, K. (2018). *Growing a strong direct workforce: A recruitment and retention guide for employers.* PHI. https://phinational.org/wp-content/uploads/2018/05/RRGuide-PHI-2018.pdf

Stone, R., & Weiner, J. (2001). *Who will care for us? Addressing the long-term care workforce crisis.* The Urban Institute and the American Association of Homes and Services for the Aging. http://aspe.hhs.gov/daltcp/reports/ltcwf.pdf

U. S. Department of Labor. (2019). *Hiring issues.* U.S. Department of Labor. https://www.dol.gov/WHD/flsa

TRAINING STAFF

Upon the completion of Chapter 5, the reader will be able to:

- Understand the importance of staff training in assisted living.
- Describe the value of orientation for assisted living employees.
- Recognize select best practices in the training of assisted living employees.
- Explain the training requirements of direct-care staff in assisted living.
- Describe the use of learning circles as a model of training.

INTRODUCTION

This chapter addresses critical factors in the training of staff in assisted living communities. Administrators are responsible to ensure that all staff are adequately trained. This chapter begins with a discussion of the importance of staff training and addresses concerns regarding training in assisted living communities. Recommendations from experts on the orientation for all assisted living staff are included. States vary in the training requirements for direct-care staff and these variations are described for the reader. Sample training components are included. The chapter concludes with a description of "The Learning Circle," a group training process that may be useful for assisted living administrators.

The Importance of Staff Training

The importance of staff training in long-term care communities is often emphasized. There is a common misconception that long-term care requires fewer skills and knowledge than acute care. However, long-term care is complex and specialized, requiring distinct skills and knowledge.

Knowledgeable and skilled employees are the greatest asset to the assisted living community, but training employees is challenging due to the costs and increased staff time, as well as the workload involved in training new employees. Pressures to contain costs may sometimes reduce training budgets. At the same time, employees are faced with increasing resident acuity, changing demands, and regulatory requirements. As a result, staff may lack the experience, knowledge, or skills to complete tasks expected of them. In general, long-term care employees recognize the importance of maintaining and developing critical skills and expertise and will turn to their employers for appropriate resources, guidance, and assistance. If these resources are not provided, frustration grows, and the consequence is often lower quality of care and increased turnover.

Training requirements are an important aspect component of quality assurance and quality improvement. For decades, government agencies and advocates have identified undertrained staff in assisted living as a concern. The U.S. General Accounting Office (1999) identified insufficient and undertrained staff, low pay rates, and high staff turnover as major contributors to quality-of-care problems in residential care/assisted living. Carlson (2005) raised concerns regarding the experience and training of direct-care staff. Although state laws and regulations consistently require certain minimum training to be provided to direct-care staff, the specifics of the training are often left to the individual communities. He cited numerous reports of the consequences of this inadequacy in training, including staff failing to administer prescribed emergency medication for a diabetic and failure of facility staff to recognize signs of acute infection, resulting in the death of a resident (Carlson, 2005). In 2014, in an article written for the American Society on Aging, Patricia McGinnis wrote *"Few states devote adequate resources to enforcement and oversight of assisted living facilities, and nearly all states have inadequate staffing and staff training requirements."*

It is critical that assisted living staff be trained in a wide variety of areas to help them fulfill their job responsibilities. However, because assisted living communities may serve different populations, providers do need a certain amount of flexibility in determining the training needs of their staff. Currently, there are no nationally accepted standards for staff training in assisted living. Argentum (n.d.), formerly known as the *Assisted Living Federation of America*, is currently working to establish voluntary, consensus-based standards for a variety of quality issues in long-term care.

ORIENTATION FOR ASSISTED LIVING EMPLOYEES

The Assisted Living Workgroup (2003) provided the following recommendations based upon practice and research in long-term care facilities regarding orientation for all assisted living employees in their report to the U.S. Senate Special Committee on Aging, *Assuring Quality in Assisted Living: Guidelines for Federal and State Policy, State Regulations, and Operations*:

1. Within 14 days of employment, all assisted living staff shall successfully complete an orientation program designed by the facility to provide information on:

    a. The care philosophy of the assisted living facility,

    b. The understanding of dementia,

    c. The understanding of the common characteristics and conditions of the resident population served,

    d. Appropriate interaction with residents and family members,

    e. Customer service policies, including resident rights and recognizing and reporting of signs of abuse and neglect,

    f. Fire and life safety, emergency disaster plans, and emergency call systems,

    g. The use of facility equipment required for job performance,

    h. The facility's employment/human resource policies and procedures.

2. All staff shall have specific orientation relevant to their specific job assignments and responsibilities.

3. Contract staff should receive orientation on topics relevant to their job tasks, including orientation of the facility's fire, life safety, emergency disaster plans, and emergency call systems.

DIRECT-CARE STAFF

Direct-Care Staff Training: General Requirements

Historically, there have been concerns regarding staff training requirements. In the report for the U.S. Department of Health and Human Services, Hawes et al. (1999), found that the types of training and orientation required for direct-care staff varied across assisted living communities, but overall, relatively little training was required. Of the unlicensed personnel, 75% were required to attend some kind of pre-service training. For those that did require training, the most common amount of required training was between 1 and 16 hours. In addition, only 11% of the staff who took the required training completed it before the start of work. Staff also reported that they did receive training on the philosophy of assisted living. Seventy-five percent of staff had participated in continuing education activities. Overall, Hawes et al. (1999) noted that staff were not well informed about normal aging processes and dementia care. Carlson (2005) noted that direct-care standards for assisted living are far less stringent that those that apply to nursing home staff members.

States have responded to identified concerns with legislative changes over the years. Still, although most states' regulations specify initial and ongoing training requirements for staff, the level of specificity varies (Carder et al., 2015; National Center for Assisted Living, 2019). Although some states specify only general requirements, others specify topics to be covered, the number of training hours required, the completion of approved courses, or some combination of topics, hours, and courses. The latest staff training requirements for each state are available from the National Center for Assisted Living (2019 Assisted living state regulatory review; https://www .ahcancal.org/ncal/advocacy/regs/Documents/2019_reg_review.pdf; see Chapter 4 for requirements for administrators). Administrators must keep in mind that policies and regulations are continuously evolving (see Chapter 2), so it is important to be aware of all current and pending legislation in your specific state.

Direct-Care Staff Training: Dementia Requirements

More and more states now have dementia-specific training requirements for direct-care staff. Forty-four states and the District of Columbia were found to have laws requiring dementia training for staff of assisted living communities, including those with Alzheimer's special care units (Burke & Orlowski, 2015). These requirements have, over time, become more specific and comprehensive. For example, Washington State requires outcome-based training for staff working with residents with dementia and includes competency tests.

Direct-Care Staff Training: Medication Requirements

Although all states require staff who assist with or administer medications to be trained, they vary in how they address who is authorized to administer medications or assist with the self-administration of medications (Carder et al., 2015). *The Compendium of Residential Care and Assisted Living Regulations and Policy: 2015* reports two primary approaches to training requirements for direct-care staff regarding medication (Table 5.1):

- Unlicensed staff who will administer medications must receive classroom-based training that some states use to certify individuals as medication aides or technicians.

TABLE 5.1 STATE TRAINING REQUIREMENTS FOR UNLICENSED STAFF WHO ASSIST WITH OR ADMINISTER MEDICATIONS

STATES THAT REQUIRE UNLICENSED STAFF TO COMPLETE AN APPROVED COURSE	STATES THAT REQUIRE UNLICENSED STAFF TO BE TRAINED BY A HEALTHCARE PROFESSIONAL AT THE FACILITY
California	Alaska
Colorado	Arizona
Connecticut	Arkansas
Delaware	Hawaii
District of Columbia	Iowa
Georgia	Louisiana
Idaho	Michigan
Indiana	Minnesota
Kansas	Montana
Maine	New Hampshire
Maryland	Oregon
Missouri	South Carolina
Nebraska	South Dakota
Nevada	Texas
New Jersey	Utah
New Mexico	Vermont
North Carolina	Washington
North Dakota	Wisconsin
Ohio	Wyoming
Oklahoma	
Pennsylvania	
Rhode Island	
Virginia	
West Virginia	

Source: From Carder, P., O'Keeffe, J., & O'Keeffe, C. (2015). *Compendium of residential care and assisted living regulations and policy: 2015 edition.* U.S. Department of Health and Human Services, Office of the Assistant Secretary for Planning and Evaluation, Office of Disability, Aging and Long-Term Care Policy and Research Triangle Institute. https://aspe.hhs.gov/basic-report/compendium-residential-care-and-assisted-living-regulations-and-policy-2015-edition

■ Unlicensed staff are taught how to assist with or administer medications by a licensed nurse and this nurse formally delegates the responsibility of medication administration to specific trained staff. *Delegation* refers to the transfer of a selected nursing task in a selected situation to a competent (unlicensed) individual, as described in the state's Nurse Practice Act.

Training Direct-Care Staff

The assisted living facility will develop a direct-care staff training program that satisfies the specific state regulatory requirements and suits the needs of the environment and residents served. The following are examples of topics that are important to include in direct-care staff training:

Direct-Care Issues

■ Principles of assisted living

■ Personal/direct-care skills

■ Meeting the needs of consumers/residents

■ Appropriate, related tasks/duties

- Hygiene
- Housekeeping/sanitation
- Nutrition/food preparation/diets
- Social/recreation activities
- Dementia/Alzheimer's care
- Mental health/emotional/behavioral needs
- Restraints

Health-Related Issues

- Basic nursing skills
- Prevention/restorative skills
- Medication administration/assistance

Knowledge Areas

- Resident rights
- Aging process/gerontology
- Working with the needs of elderly
- Death and dying
- Psychosocial needs
- Assessment skills
- Care plan development
- Communication skills
- Knowledge of community services

Safety and Emergency Issues

- CPR
- First aid
- Fire, safety, emergency procedures
- Infection prevention/control

Process Issues

- Agency/facility policies
- Regulations/law
- Reporting abuse/neglect
- Complaint procedures
- Record keeping
- Confidentiality
- Legal/ethical issues
- Survey process

BEST PRACTICES IN STAFF TRAINING

Long-Term Care Community Coalition

The Long-Term Care Community Coalition (LTCCC) is a nonprofit organization dedicated to improving quality of care, quality of life, and dignity for elderly and disabled people in nursing homes, assisted living, and other residential settings. In its 2018 comprehensive report titled *Assisted Living: Promising Policies and Practices for Improving Resident Health, Quality of Life, and Safety*, the LTCCC identified six key practices and recommendations for staff training:

1. **Require training across multiple subject areas.**
   - Ensure that training equips staff with skills in and knowledge of a range of subject areas critical to resident safety and well-being, including emergency preparedness, Alzheimer's and other dementia care, residents' rights, detecting abuse and neglect, communication skills, and (as appropriate) assisting with medication.
   - All staff who are in contact with residents and/or their records should also receive appropriate training in dignity, autonomy, and privacy.
   - Training should address social needs and understanding of the characteristics of the populations served in assisted living facilities.

2. **Specify when training must occur and how much time is required.**
   - Require that training be completed within the first 30 days of hire.
   - Unsupervised resident contact should be prohibited prior to the completion of training.

3. **Establish licensing/certification requirements as appropriate.**
   - For nonlicensed care staff, specify that staff training must be done using a personal care aide training program (or its equivalent) approved by the state.

4. **Allow for alternative training methods.**
   - Provide for use of online training programs, but for no more than half of the total required hours.

5. **Specify types of training.**
   - Categorize training requirements depending on staff type (i.e., administrator, staff working with residents who have dementia, staff assisted residents with activities of daily living.
   - Provide for a minimum of 20 to 40 hours of annual training.
   - Eight of the total hours required for administrator training must be devoted to care for residents who have Alzheimer's and/or dementia.
   - First-aid and CPR training should be required of all care staff as well as any individuals responsible for monitoring facility buildings or units overnight.

6. **Require training assessments.**
   - Staff: Conduct training assessments to ensure that staff members recall what they learned during training and are implementing this knowledge appropriately while providing care.
   - Facilities: Require modification of training programs for facilities that are cited for repeated deficiencies.

Justice in Aging

Justice in Aging, a national advocacy organization begun in 1972, identified Washington as one state with strong and comprehensive models of dementia training requirements (Burke & Orlowski, 2015). They identified five specific characteristics that should be considered when developing dementia training requirements. These include:

1.   Use of a comprehensive approach encompassing many settings and provider types, and including managerial staff.

2.   Direct state involvement in development of training content and design of competency evaluations.

3.   Use of highly detailed training objectives.

4.   Use of an outcome-based curriculum with examinations requiring demonstration that competencies have been mastered.

5.   Use of requirements for continuing education in addition to pre-service training.

FACILITATING STAFF TRAINING THROUGH LEARNING CIRCLES: A MODEL FOR TRAINING

The Learning Circle Model is used in facilities nationwide and is changing the way management, staff, and residents communicate with one another. The purpose of the learning circle is to create an environment in which people feel free to share their ideas and opinions without being criticized or reprimanded. This helps build trust among the participants, which serves to strengthen relationships. Organizations that have been successful in implementing culture change attest to the value of learning circles. For example, Meadowlark Hills Retirement Community in Manhattan, Kansas, holds learning circles daily to address concerns and work through problems, and at White Community Hospital in Aurora, Minnesota, learning circles are used between departments to strengthen relationships. Learning circles can be utilized in various ways, such as part of education and in-service training. A practice at Meadowood, in Worchester, Pennsylvania, offers a way for residents, caregivers, and available family members to determine the day's activities, as done at Northern Pines Community in Big Fork, Minnesota (Norton, 2003). The following text describes a learning circle.

The learning circle is a leveling technique that encourages quiet people to speak, talkative people to listen, and everyone to share in making decisions (Box 5.1). Participants observe, interpret, and experience not only their own feelings about an issue, but also broaden their perspective by considering the many viewpoints of others around them. Learning circles are most effective when they become a way of life in the long-term care community, and when everyone takes a turn facilitating.

Because this technique helps foster a sense of trust and connection among participants, it would also be a useful intervention to promote a more cohesive community. There are too many examples of cases in which family members sued an assisted living facility, and the underlying reason was their impression that the organization does not care or is not being honest. Techniques such as learning circles can be employed at family council meetings, resident council meetings, or community meetings involving residents, staff, and family members (Norton, 2003).

BOX 5.1: PROCEDURE FOR LEARNING CIRCLE

1. Participants sit in a circle without tables or other obstructions blocking their view of one another. Participants can include any combination of workers, residents, families, and other community members.

2. The ideal number of participants is 10 to 15. If the facilitator believes the discussion will provoke strong feelings of sadness, depression, grief, or anger, it is helpful to limit the number to five to 10.

3. One person is chosen to be the facilitator. This person poses the question or topic to the circle, gives encouragement, and keeps the circle moving in an orderly fashion.

4. The process begins when the facilitator poses the question or issue.

5. A volunteer in the circle responds with a thought about the topic.

6. The person sitting to the right or left of the respondent speaks next, moving one by one around the circle until everyone has spoken on the subject without interruption. Participants may choose to pass rather than speak. After everyone else in the circle has taken a turn, the facilitator goes back to those who passed, and allows each another opportunity to respond. Only after everyone has had a chance to speak is the floor open for general discussion.

CONCLUSIONS

This chapter addresses the important topic of staff training in assisted living communities. A variety of topics are covered to assist the administrator in understanding the importance of staff training, its context within the industry, and recommendations from national stakeholders. Best practices and a training model are included that may be useful for the administrator while staff training programs are developed.

REFERENCES

Argentum. (n.d.). *Standards for senior living*. https://www.argentum.org/research-and-initiatives/standards-for-senior-living

Assisted Living Workgroup. (2003). *Assuring quality in assisted living: Guidelines for federal and state policy, state regulations, and operations*. U.S. Government Printing Office.

Burke, G., & Orlowski, G. (2015). *Training to serve people with dementia: Is our health care system ready? Paper 2: A review of dementia training standards across health care settings*. Justice in Aging. https://www.justiceinaging.org/wp-content/uploads/2015/08/Training-to-serve-people-with-dementia-Alz2FINAL.pdf

Carder, P., O'Keeffe, J., & O'Keeffe, C. (2015). *Compendium of residential care and assisted living regulations and policy: 2015 edition*. U.S. Department of Health and Human Services, Office of the Assistant Secretary for Planning and Evaluation, Office of Disability, Aging and Long-Term Care Policy and Research Triangle Institute. https://aspe.hhs.gov/basic-report/compendium-residential-care-and-assisted-living-regulations-and-policy-2015-edition

Carlson, E. (2005). *Critical issues in assisted living: Who's in, who's out and who's providing the care*. National Senior Citizen's Law Center.

Hawes, C., Phillips, C., & Rose, M. (1999). *A national study of assisted living for the frail elderly: Results of a national survey of facilities*. U.S. Department of Health and Human Services.

Long-Term Care Community Coalition. (2018). *LTCCC Report: Assisted living: Promising policies and practices.* https://nursinghome411.org/ltccc-report-assisted-living-promising-policies-and-practices

McGinnis, P. (2014). Assisted living: A crisis in care. *American Society on Aging: Aging Today.* https://www.asaging.org/blog/assisted-living-crisis-care

National Center for Assisted Living. (2019). *2019 Assisted living state regulatory review.* https://www.ahcancal.org/ncal/advocacy/regs/Documents/2019_reg_review.pdf

Norton, L. (2003). The power of circles: Using a familiar technique to promote culture change. In A. Weiner & J. Ronch (Eds.), *Culture change in long-term care* (pp. 285–292). Hawthorne Press.

U.S. General Accounting Office. (1999). *Assisted living: Quality of care and consumer protection issues* (GAO/T-HEHS-99-111). U.S. Government Accountability Office. https://www.gao.gov/products/T-HEHS-99-111

RETAINING EMPLOYEES AND EMPOWERMENT

WITH CONTRIBUTING AUTHOR DAVID HAHKLOTUBBE

LEARNING OBJECTIVES

Upon the completion of Chapter 6, the reader will be able to:

- Discuss workforce retention as a critical issue in assisted living.
- Define *staff turnover*.
- Recognize the consequences and risks associated with staff turnover.
- Understand how to calculate staff turnover rates.
- Describe the factors associated with staff turnover and retention.
- Identify staff retention strategies.

INTRODUCTION

This chapter addresses the critical issue of workforce retention in the assisted living industry. The current trends and an increasing need for quality workforce retention in long-term care set the tone for the chapter. First, staff turnover is described and defined. The reader will also learn the consequences of staff turnover and the factors that influence this turnover and retention. The remainder of the chapter is organized into subsets of specific retention strategies: wages and benefits, working conditions, staff recognition, scheduling options, opportunities for growth, and staff empowerment. Examples and ideas are presented as possibilities for the assisted living administrator to incorporate to create both a unique and useful retention strategy.

Workforce Retention in Assisted Living: A Critical Issue

In a January 2019 publication, the Hospital and Healthcare Compensation Service reported that overall turnover in assisted living was down in 2018 compared to 2017, but the rate was up for some positions. Turnover across all positions declined from 34.96% to 31.71%. Turnover of resident assistants and personal-care aides was 36.63% in 2017 and 33% in 2018, whereas dining-service employee turnover increased from 35.74% to 36.91% during those same years. It is clear that improving retention rates is vital to better quality outcomes in assisted living.

Paraprofessionals (i.e., direct-care staff) are those providing hands-on care directly to the residents in assisted living communities. They are by far the most important people in the organization and should be treated as such. However, they are also identified as one of the most difficult staff to retain due to a variety of factors, including notoriously low wages/benefits, challenging working conditions, heavy workloads, job ambiguity, lack of perceived support by management/coworkers, and a job that has been stigmatized by society. Especially in a stronger economy, many workers move to other industries that offer better job quality: higher wages, more stable hours, safer working conditions, opportunities for advancement, or other advantages (Paraprofessional Healthcare Institute, 2019). Direct-care staff are often referred to as the "eyes and ears" of the care system (Stone & Dawson, 2008).

STAFF TURNOVER

Defining *Staff Turnover*

Turnover refers to the number of staff who leave employment at the community for any reason. *Retention* refers to keeping valued employees. To understand the community's retention challenges, the administrator should review turnover daily with all managers and department heads. All communities will experience turnover, but the extent of the turnover can be minimized with effective retention strategies. Turnover itself, depending on type, may be negative or positive. *Negative turnover* is the loss of qualified employees, whereas *positive turnover* is the result of strong employees being promoted within the community or less desirable employees leaving. The administrator's strategies should aim to minimize negative turnover and promote and maintain positive turnover.

Direct-care staff retention should be a primary focus in assisted living. Conscious effort needs to be placed not just on how to attract employees, but also on how to empower and retain staff to ensure resident quality of life. This also reduces the already high level of potential liability the operator faces daily. The challenges of retention tend to be ongoing for many assisted living operators who do not place the correct amount of value upon it (e.g., budgeted dollars and company cultural shifts through reinforcement programs). Staying ahead of the game by creating a positive and nurturing culture toward all employees appears to be a panacea to not losing valued and well-trained personnel to competitors and alternative industries.

STAFF RECRUITMENT

Purposeful Hiring

The process starts simply by engaging in a conscious and well-planned recruitment effort that seeks to find the right fit rather than filling a spot on a schedule. By hiring poorly, the whole system breaks down and the consequence is often more turnover. It is often the case that hiring managers will panic when faced with staffing shortages and in an effort to decrease overtime, avoid having to work the shifts themselves, or worse, as a result of not filling the vacant spots and burning out the team, they make desperate hires to simply patch the leak in the schedule. Clearly, this is not a winning strategy, but is an alarmingly common one.

Consequences of Staff Turnover

Consequences of staff turnover have been recognized for decades and include increased facility costs, lower job satisfaction, and lower resident quality of care in long-term care facilities (Castle &

Engberg, 2005). The exact cost of staff turnover in assisted living communities is unknown; however, the costs are substantial when considering recruitment, hiring, and training costs. Because staff turnover interrupts continuity of resident care, workload increases, and resentment of staff may build when additional responsibilities must be met. The most serious negative consequence of high staff turnover rates is the potential for negative health outcomes relative to poor quality of care. Research has long identified this concern in nursing homes, and staff turnover has been associated with quality of care in assisted living facilities as well. For example, a 2011 study, using longitudinal analysis, was able to show that favorable staffing improves quality of care (Castle & Anderson, 2011). Projections show the industry will experience an overall shortage of staff available to enter the pipeline and fill future direct-care worker positions. Because of the instability of relying on economic cycles and the upcoming shortfall of potential workers, the underlying problems associated with direct-care jobs must be addressed in order to ensure a stable, committed workforce (Institute for the Future of Aging Services and the American Association of Homes and Services for the Aging, 2010). Keep in mind that unlike most other industries, the "product" or "output" of the hands-on staff is the quality of life of human beings. In other industries, if there is a shortfall of staffing, the immediate consequence is lowered production, resulting in a decrease of revenue. It should be agreed upon that loss of revenue cannot be compared to loss of quality or quantity of life. Further, as a dovetail, large losses to the community's bottom line often come directly from either short staffing or poor staffing by way of lawsuits after an incident caused by lack of supervision. In this event, the community's financial loss through restitution far eclipses any dollars it should have spent to properly attract and retain quality personnel.

Calculating Turnover Rates

It is imperative to calculate and track turnover rates. When creating a budget, this is a line item that should get a heavy focus and should be reviewed literally every day with managers and department heads. In fact, it should be incentivized. Any bonuses given to managers and department heads who arrive under budgeted turnover quarterly will pale in comparison to the money saved, yet it will be well received and is a very effective motivator. This, of course, is only a secondary gain to the lack of headaches the managers will be enduring and the increased quality of life of everyone in the system. One common way to define and calculate staff turnover rates is to determine an annual turnover rate. Annual turnover rates are calculated by dividing the difference between the number of individuals (e.g., direct-care staff) employed during a fiscal year, and the number employed at the end of the year; this number, multiplied by 100, produces a rate. Box 6.1 illustrates how to calculate annual staff turnover. Terminations include all reasons for leaving the community such as resignation, retirement, or firing. This percentage should be calculated for each position, each unit, as well as the entire community.

Once you have calculated turnover rate for each position in your community, consider the problem areas. Are there large differences between units? Are certain positions more vulnerable to turnover? If one unit has consistent long-term staff and another does not, what issues may be affecting that particular unit? For example, is there a difference in the care levels of the residents?

BOX 6.1:   HOW TO CALCULATE TURNOVER RATES

Sum of terminations in 1 year / the sum of established positions × 100
Example: 16/50 × 100 = 32%

Asking these types of questions may assist you in identifying issues and challenges that will influence your retention strategy. In addition, when pleading your case during budget season to the parent company, you will have numerical evidence as to why you are asking for a staffing increase, or, on some occasions, a decrease in other departments.

It is important to remember that annual turnover rates are not always accurate due to the high number of staff who leave employment in long-term care communities within the first 180 days of employment. One-hundred percent turnover does not necessarily mean that every single employee leaves employment in the course of 1 year. It may mean that for every employee who stays the full year, for example, two or more came and one left a similar job at the same community. Castle (2006), well known for research in nursing home staff turnover, has offered an alternative definition of *turnover* as the total number of staff (measured in full-time equivalents) who leave employment during a 6-month period divided by the total number of staff (measured in full-time equivalents) who were employed during this period. This calculation should include all shifts, part-time staff, and voluntary and involuntary turnover.

Identifying Risk of Staff Turnover

The administrator should pay close attention to the number of employees who are at risk for leaving employment. Sometimes, staff seek new opportunities because the community cannot adequately meet their personal needs. On occasion, appropriate intervention can result in retention of a valued employee. Several warning signs of potential staff turnover are seen in Box 6.2.

If you do not know your employees well, you may have difficulty noticing these types of warning signs. Get to know your staff and elicit assistance from direct supervisors. They are important resources for identifying quality employees who are considering leaving. And, paradoxically, managers who do not know their employees well may be one of the reasons why staff are leaving.

Factors Associated With Turnover and Retention of Direct-Care Staff

To better address workforce retention, an understanding of the factors associated with staff turnover is essential. Although many factors associated with staff turnover and retention may be beyond the direct control of the assisted living community, the understanding of both *intrinsic*

BOX 6.2:   WARNING SIGNS OF POTENTIAL TURNOVER

1. Visible unhappiness

2. Complaints about workload or peers

3. Life events (e.g., childbirth, death in family, divorce, returning to school)

4. Unexplained absences

5. Increased use of sick time

6. Rejection of promotion or wage increase

7. Reduced interest in job

8. Change in job performance

9. Favorite peers or mentors leave employment

BOX 6.3:   INTRINSIC FACTORS ASSOCIATED WITH TURNOVER AND RETENTION

1. *Age:* Younger workers are less likely to remain on the job, whereas workers over the age of 30 are more likely to stay (Parsons et al., 2003; Riggs, 2001).

2. *Education:* Workers with more than a high school education are more likely to turn over (Parsons et al., 2003; Riggs, 2001). More educated workers may choose to leave their job to pursue additional education.

3. *Marital status:* Workers who are the sole source of income for themselves and dependents are less likely to turn over (Parsons et al., 2003).

4. *Social support:* Workers with reliable social support systems, such as transportation and childcare, are less likely to turn over (Riggs, 2001).

5. *Lack of job preparation:* Workers with a lack of hands-on training and inadequate skills are more likely to turn over (Lescoe-Long, 2000).

6. *Employment tenure:* Workers with a history of shorter term prior job tenure may be more likely to turn over (Parsons et al., 2003).

7. *Values and attitudes:* Workers who value being needed and who demonstrate a positive effect toward older adults are more likely to stay on the job. On the other hand, those who are more oriented to rewards, such as salary, are more likely to turn over (Lescoe-Long, 2000; Parsons et al., 2003; Riggs, 2001).

---

factors (i.e., those factors specific to the individual employee) and *extrinsic factors* (i.e., those factors not specific to the individual employee) associated with staff turnover will aid the administrator in developing strategies to improve retention over time (see Boxes 6.3, 6.4, and 6.5). These factors greatly impact job satisfaction, a primary factor in staff turnover.

RETENTION STRATEGIES

No two communities are identical. The unique cultures that exist in each specific community, with all its diverse dynamics, make it impossible to create a universal strategy to retain personnel. It is

---

BOX 6.4:   EXTRINSIC FACTORS ASSOCIATED WITH TURNOVER

1. Multiple employment opportunities
2. Inadequate job training
3. Excessive workload
4. Poor continuity of care
5. Lack of respect
6. Wages and benefits

BOX 6.5:   EXTRINSIC FACTORS ASSOCIATED WITH RETENTION

1. Clean, safe work environments
2. Higher staff ratios
3. Union contracts for workers
4. Low rates of professional staff turnover
5. Positive relationships with residents, peers, and supervisors
6. Employee recognition

---

imperative to capitalize on the uniqueness of a community and to develop a plan that incorporates not only your management team, but empowers your entire team to have an influence in development. Remember that your direct-care staff are the most important staff in your buildings and their opinions are largely discounted even though they have knowledge that would assist in operations outside of direct care. In other words, they are commonly an untapped source of valuable information. Boxes 6.3 through 6.5 suggest what to consider, as a team, when constructing a retention strategy.

Wages and Benefits

Wages

Using data from the 2004 National Nursing Assistant Survey, satisfaction with wages had the second strongest association with intrinsic job satisfaction and overall job satisfaction (Decker et al., 2009). Remember, as an administrator, if working for a large corporation you will face your most difficult challenge in advocating for wage increases for your team. Remember to advocate during budget season or your team may suffer for the entire next fiscal year. Perform due diligence in not only gathering data from competition (e.g., wage analysis surveys), but also be sure to include competing industries—for dining- room servers, for example, compare wages to restaurants and factor in that restaurants allow tipping and assisted living does not, compare hotels for housekeepers, as hotels often offer higher wages, unique perks, and less contact with bodily fluids. Be creative and stay vigilant.

Benefits

Provide health, dental, vision, and life insurance. Consider developing a pension plan and/or profit sharing for all employees. Consider sponsoring a 401k plan with an employer contribution. Assist staff with payroll deduction options. It is no secret that staff will not just be searching for intrinsic satisfaction and wages, they will be looking at benefits. It is also no secret that communities that offer higher quality and a wider variety of benefits have less turnover. Again, the money you put forward to do the right thing will come back to you in the absence of turnover dollars. Although this equation is so simple, it is routinely ignored.

Sick Time

Allow for a specified number of paid sick days per year. For employees who use no sick time, allow for a paid wellness day. Consider offering a bonus or wage increase for employees with no absences. Although most states do not have provisions for collecting sick time as you would vacation time, PTO, or paid time off, is a rare and wildly popular alternative.

Working Conditions
Attendance Policies

It is imperative to enforce attendance policies to be fair to all staff and residents. That said, it must be done in an empowering and supportive way versus one that is autocratic and punitive. Consider incentivizing being on time and not having any absences by offering a quarterly bonus to those who qualify. When staff are chronically late or have excessive absences, coach rather than punish, and aim to discover the cause rather than making assumptions. And, of course, if there is a lack of response to the coaching and write-ups, show your team respect and move to terminate rather than make an exception. The worst thing you can do is to set a precedent because termination makes you feel uncomfortable. This is a common mistake made by new administrators.

Respect

Gaining respect and commanding respect are two concepts that are polar opposites, but are often confused by first-time or misguided managers. Establishing mutual respect starts by the management team making the first gesture. Leading by example, never asking of the team anything you wouldn't or haven't done yourself and occasionally rolling up sleeves to pitch-in, even when there isn't a staffing crisis are high-profile ways of gaining respect. Respect is the cornerstone of trust and trust is the glue that binds everything in the care field. Action is what matters most and going above and beyond can mean the organization's survival.

Morale

Morale is the illusive energy that fuels productivity. If morale is high, productivity is high and the quality of the output soars. In this case, the output is quality and quantity of life of seniors, their families, and your team. You cannot tease apart morale and productivity. If morale is low, productivity will suffer. However, morale is easily shifted. To completely understand how to shift morale would take an entire book. When creating mechanisms to boost morale, the biggest mistake that is made, even with the best of intentions, is assumption. It is wise not to waste a lot of money, time, and energy developing a morale-boosting program without first inquiring of your team what that would look like from their perspective. Just engaging them and showing interest in starting a program will immediately boost morale. It is unwise to start a morale-boosting program unless you intend on maintaining it. You will effectively bring morale through the floor if you fail to maintain the program. It is better to have no program than to start one and not see it through. As obvious as this sounds, these mistakes are made routinely. The saddest thing is that the managers often mean well and genuinely want to please the team.

Performance Objectives

To avoid one of the biggest contributors to turnover, job ambiguity, performance objectives should be clear and measurable and included in each job description. When conducting performance evaluations, utilize the job description as a reference point and provide regular feedback on performance. Consider peer performance evaluations as well. Administrators should have weekly one-on-one meetings with department heads or managers and, depending upon the size of the manager's teams, they should also have a similar practice. These meetings can be as short as 10 minutes and contain some level of personal discourse prior to digging in on agendas. The managers should announce that the one-on-one meeting is the employee's meeting and that it should be tailored to whatever the employee wants in whatever format they prefer.

Consistency

Policies and procedures should be written. Establish a comprehensive system of corrective actions that are enforced consistently across disciplines and shifts. Flexibility is important in special circumstances but any deviation from the policy in its enforcement is grounds for one of the most common claims by disgruntled former employees and common cause for the labor board to get involved—perceived favoritism, which lends itself to claims of discrimination.

Supplies/Equipment

Ensure adequate supplies for the entire community. Safety and assistive equipment is important to keep up to date and in working condition. Provide personal protective equipment and ergonomic equipment as necessary. Consider new technologies that may aid staff in providing high-quality care. Always be open to suggestions by staff, perhaps a particular brand of cleaner is not as effective as another or has a better scent; a few pennies more may make a world of difference and allowing staff to have an influence in operations is worth it.

Orientation Programs

Develop excellent and efficient training programs. Consider implementing a mentoring program and pairing staff to promote teamwork. Be sure to include introductions to all staff by name and job title. See Chapter 5 for further information on training.

Shift Differential

Weekend, evening, and night shift differential should be established. Offer bonuses for covering extra shifts and incentivize taking on extra shifts when understaffed or being "on-call."

Recognition

Recognize the Value of Each Employee

Know your staff and call them by name. Let the staff see you daily on the unit and thank them for their work, yes, this means get out of your office. While it sounds obvious, it is one of the most common mistakes of an administrator to the degree that there are clinics on how to manage your day to be able to visit each department for each shift. Promote the value of the staff to all employees, residents, and families. Listen to the concerns of the staff. Involve staff with interview processes. There tends to be a segregation between departments; you will discover this at your first all-staff meeting. The housekeepers sit with the housekeepers, caregivers with caregivers, culinary with culinary, and so on. Be proactive by acknowledging this and encouraging staff to interact with each other. Provide opportunity for cross-over and shadowing in different departments; this is a brilliant strategy to decrease overtime if part-time staff especially are cross-trained.

Special Recognition/Appreciation

A staff recognition program is not optional, it is essential and the foundation of creating morale. A strong word of caution: This looks easy but even the best have made catastrophic mistakes by inadvertently alienating certain members of a team, such as the NOC (i.e., night) shift. Establish an internal committee comprised of managers and line-level staff from each department to assist in creating the recognition program. It should be multi-faceted and be on an even playing field. Keep in mind that the goal is to reinforce quality and create coaching opportunities to boost performance. Above all, when defining the reward system, it must be clear to the degree of no misinterpretation as to how to earn rewards; any ambiguity will destroy and upset your team. Fine-tuning is an inevitability and creativity is key. You need not spend a lot of money, and in fact, throwing good money after bad is the quickest way to insult your team. As was said earlier, gestures go much further than monetary tokens. Your team will have big hearts; this is your opportunity to show them yours. Never underestimate the power of saying "thank you." And although the break room should be a sanctuary, if invited, share a meal with your team. These gestures cost nothing and are personal and valuable.

Employee of the Month

Establish an official "employee of the month" process that incorporates a committee of peers and other staff. Make each selected employee of the month eligible for becoming an "employee of the year." Consider acknowledging this achievement with a plaque, dinner, recognition in newsletters, and monetary bonuses. This program must be well thought out and extensive. There should be internal guidelines on how it is run. Although performance should be measured without bias, it is incredibly important that you be thinking of every department on every shift, full time and part time. If a specific shift or department is consistently receiving the recognition, there is no question that mutiny will follow. Additionally, make parameters such as no one person can earn the employee of the month more than once in the same year. And, managers and department heads should be exempt from the program. Make some of the qualifiers difficult to achieve, such as no missed days during the month, successful completion of required training on time, no late arrivals, perfect punches on the time clock (meal breaks), proper attire, and subjective items like great attitude and always greeting guests, especially while on tours. Clearly, there is a lot to be considered here, it will require a significant amount of thought, as it should.

Display Special Postings

Consider having bulletin boards in the staff lounge area. Acknowledge births, engagements, weddings, or other special events. Welcome back employees from a vacation or another leave. Recognize the accomplishments of employees' children such as academic or athletic achievements and honors.

Scheduling Options
Flexible Scheduling

Make establishing a set schedule for full-time employees a priority. Allow employees to switch days with approval. Accept special requests prior to the completion of the schedule. Consider allowing job sharing positions and establishing an internal pool. Try to maintain set days off for senior staff.

Self-Scheduling

Ask employees their preferred workdays while keeping staffing requirements in mind. Guide employees in the scheduling process, but allow for them to work together to complete a schedule. Provide incentives for employee flexibility as a reward.

Increased Staffing

Know your community's busiest times. Try to have more staff available during the busiest times. Determine what duties may be delegated to other employees (however, ensure compliance with regulations).

Vacation Scheduling

Post a vacation schedule for employees to be able to see the possible times available to them. Have a policy that indicates that employees must sign up at least 30 days in advance for vacation. Consider seniority and sign-up dates when approving requests for vacation time off. Try to accommodate vacations based on seniority.

Opportunities for Growth

Professional Development

Provide on-sight educational in-services relative to professional development (see Chapter 7 for additional information). Consider topics that would be mutually beneficial for the employees and the community such as teamwork, conflict resolution, cultural awareness, organizational skills, and communication skills. Seek input from employees on topics of interest.

Skills for Personal Growth

Invite guest speakers to discuss topics important for life skills and coping. For example, educational in-services on stress management, parenting, finance, and motivation may be helpful. Create partnerships with local community organizations that may be willing to offer discounts for employees. Provide assistance for costs as a reward or benefit. Develop support groups that might meet before or after work.

Off-Site Education

Offer tuition support for off-site educational programs. Allow an employee to attend an off-site program as a reward for good performance.

Scholarships

Provide scholarships for continued education in any healthcare field. Seek contributions for the scholarship fund and support staff fund-raisers for the scholarship.

Written Materials

Publish a newsletter and include useful information for the staff. Subscribe to geriatric newsletters and journals for employees to share. Provide a staff library.

Tuition Assistance

Provide tuition assistance and link payback to longevity and continued service. Formalize tuition assistance as a benefit. Promote partnerships for discounted tuition for students.

Employee Assistance Programs

Provide referrals for counseling services. Partner with churches and community agencies for staff support services. Provide informational material in staff lounges on topics such as parenting, divorce, alcohol and drug abuse, wellness, and financial planning.

Career Ladders

Develop career ladders for all positions. Develop criteria for each level within each careered ladder. Offer training for specialized units. Promote from within the community when possible.

Post Open Jobs

Post all job openings and keep the posts updated. Search for qualified individuals from within your community.

Peer Review

Encourage employees to participate in the development of standards for in-services, attendance, scheduling, routines, and policies. Allow for peer input at job performance reviews.

Promote Health and Wellness

Have intermittent health screenings available. Have wellness programs available both on and off site. Provide health insurance. Negotiate discounts for employees at local gyms. Provide employees access to on-site exercise equipment. Identify employees who are willing to facilitate walking or exercise groups. It is more than likely that the healthcare provider you choose for your benefits program will not only partner with you to create a program but will incentivize it by lowering the rates. One such popular program that has been effective is biometrics, which promotes healthier living and monitors positive lifestyle change in staff.

Other Incentives

Treats

Provide free coffee or tea in the employee lounge. Provide a refrigerator and microwave for staff use. Sponsor an ice cream social or pizza party on occasions. Sponsor celebratory meals in honor of staff recognition awards. Always have food at all-staff meetings, and this food should never be provided by your internal culinary team; it should be from a third-party provider and voted upon by the team.

Transportation

Assist employees to create carpools. Arrange for pickup of staff at certain locations on a set schedule with a shuttle service. Arrange for discounted purchases of bus passes. Transportation is a critical issue for today's long-term care workforce.

Uniforms

If possible, pay an allowance for uniforms. Negotiate discounts for employees at local uniforms shops. Is volume ordering feasible? Can uniforms be provided? Ask your worker's compensation insurance provider what type of deals they may offer as incentive for safety apparel, such as nonskid shoes.

Child Care

Have a list of childcare providers for employees with children. Support employee efforts to assist each other with childcare issues. Is it feasible to create an in-house day care with reduced fees for employees?

Meals

Allow employees to purchase meals at community cost. Consider free meals, especially for staff working extra shifts. Provide inexpensive vending items.

Teams

Sponsor employee sports teams. Purchase shirts printed with the community logo.

Discounts

Seek discounts for employees with all vendors associated with the community. In addition, try to negotiate discounts at local grocery stores, department stores, and local services.

Staff Empowerment

Empowerment is the process of enabling individuals to think, behave, take action, and control work and decision-making in autonomous ways. It is empowering to take control of one's own destiny. The empowerment of employees can result in increased initiative, innovation, involvement, enthusiasm, and efficiency. Empowerment involves enabling employees to make decisions on their own, involving employees to take responsibility for improving things, and encouraging employees to take an active role in their work.

Bowen and Lawler (1992, p. 32) offer a common definition of *empowerment* as: *"the sharing with frontline employees four organizational ingredients: 1) information about the organization's performance; 2) rewards based on the organization's performance; 3) knowledge that enables employees to understand and contribute to organizational performance; and 4) power to make decisions that influence organizational direction and performance."*

Hahklotubbe (2005) suggests that long-term care communities often overlook the concept of employee empowerment and hence are missing a key component of both employee productivity and job satisfaction. His research linked empowerment to morale and productivity in long-term care environments, and identified employee empowerment as being frequently ignored as a way to potentially improve quality of care.

Because job satisfaction is linked with retention, understanding and promoting employee empowerment is crucial for the assisted living community. There are some considerations that the administrator may take into account in an effort to promote employee empowerment.

Overall Picture

Help your employees understand the overall picture of the community. Educate employees by sharing your mission, strategic plans, public relations, and financial status. Teach customer service. Explain how public image and reputation are linked to community success. Stress the importance of the employees' role in creating success for the organization.

Input on Care Decisions

All employees should be asked for and encouraged to provide input to supervisors and managers. The input of direct-care staff in the formation of care plans is critical. Seek the participation of direct-care staff in resident-specific concerns, such as behavioral or feeding problems.

Input on Policies and Procedures

Request and accept input from employees for changes to policies and procedures.

Input on Quality Assurance/Improvement

Include employees of all levels in your quality assurance/improvement teams. Include issues such as training and orientation, retention, staffing policies, documentation tools, and scheduling. Ask for employee assistance, and ask staff to share their problems and successes. Invite and encourage all staff levels to be involved in staff meetings. Safety should be a priority for staff and residents. All personnel should be invited to be a member of the internal safety committee and attend the monthly meeting.

Benefits

Request input from employees about benefit concerns. When possible, allow options and choices. Periodically review the benefits package and adjust accordingly. Invite the benefits provider to attend an all-staff meeting on a semi-annual basis to discuss new programs, announce open enrollment dates, and answer any questions staff may have.

Residents

Encourage suggestions regarding residents, such as room assignments and scheduling. Frontline staff will have valuable information on residents, such as resident conflicts and current problems. Seek ideas for improving care. Assist employees in the improvement of communication skills. Ask open-ended questions that promote the sharing of ideas. Communicate directly with employees about resident care, such as personal care and activities. Seriously consider the ideas of the staff with respect.

CONCLUSIONS

This chapter illustrates the importance of retaining and empowering quality employees in the assisted living community. The reader learned the definitions, risks, and factors associated with and adverse consequences of staff turnover in long-term care communities. Job satisfaction is the most important factor in retaining quality staff. Job satisfaction is influenced by many factors, including wages and benefits, working conditions, respect, and morale. Retention strategies are described and illustrated with examples that the reader may want consider when developing a successful retention plan.

REFERENCES

Bowen, D., & Lawler, E. (1992). The empowerment of service workers: What, why, how and when. *Sloan Management Review, 33,* 31–45.

Castle, N. (2006). Measuring staff turnover in nursing homes. *The Gerontologist, 46*, 210–219. https://doi.org/10.1093/geront/46.2.210

Castle, N., & Engberg, J. (2005). Turnover and quality in nursing homes. *Medical Care, 43*, 616–626. https://doi.org/10.1097/01.mlr.0000163661.67170.b9

Castle, N. G., & Anderson, R. A. (2011). Caregiver staffing in nursing homes and their influence on quality. *Medical Care, 49*, 545–552. https://doi.org/10.1097/MLR.0b013e31820fbca9

Decker, F. H., Harris-Kojetin, L., & Bercovitz, A. (2009). Intrinsic job satisfaction, overall satisfaction, and intention to leave job among nursing assistants in nursing homes. *The Gerontologist, 49*, 596–610. https://doi.org/10.1093/geront/gnp051

Hahklotubbe, D. (2005). Empowerment and long-term care: A contradiction in terms. In D. Yee-Melichar & A. Boyle (Eds.), *Aging in contemporary society: Translating research into practice* (pp. 165–185). XanEdu Publications.

Hospital and Healthcare Compensation Service. (2019). *Assisted living salary & benefits report.* https://www.hhcsinc.com/hcs-reports.html

Institute for the Future of Aging Services and the American Association of Homes and Services for the Aging. (2010). *Direct care worker retention: Strategies for success.* https://www.leadingage.org/sites/default/files/Direct%20Care%20Workers%20Report%20%20FINAL%20%282%29.pdf

Lescoe-Long, M. (2000). Why they leave. *Nursing Homes Long Term Care Management, 49*(10), 70–74.

Paraprofessional Healthcare Institute. (2019). *Growing a strong workforce: A recruitment and retention guide for employers.* https://phinational.org/resource/growing-strong-direct-care-workforce-recruitment-retention-guide-employers

Parsons, S., Simmons, W., Penn, K., & Furlough, M. (2003). Determinants of satisfactions and turnover among nursing assistants: The results of a statewide survey. *Journal of Gerontological Nursing, 29*, 51–58. https://doi.org/10.3928/0098-9134-20030301-11

Riggs, C. (2001). A model of staff support to improve retention on long-term care. *Nursing Administration Quarterly, 25*, 43–54. https://doi.org/10.1097/00006216-200101000-00009

Stone, R. I., & Dawson, S. L. (2008). The origins of better jobs better care. *The Gerontologist, 48*, 5–13. https://doi.org/10.1093/geront/48.Supplement_1.5

CONTINUING EDUCATION

WITH CONTRIBUTING AUTHOR DAVID HAHKLOTUBBE

LEARNING OBJECTIVES

Upon the completion of Chapter 7, the reader will be able to:

- Define *continuing education*.
- Identify the importance of continuing education as a key component of professional staff development.
- Understand the regulatory requirements surrounding continuing education in assisted living.
- Learn about types and models of continuing education.
- Identify best practices for continuing-education requirements.
- Consider the impact of professional development on millennials.
- Understand the importance of professional conferences and associations.

INTRODUCTION

This chapter focuses on continuing education, a key component of professional staff development for both assisted living administrators and direct-care staff. Continuing education is defined, and its importance is discussed. Regulations for continuing-education requirements by state are summarized. The chapter then continues with descriptions of types and models of continuing-education programs from professionals in the industry. The chapter goes on to discuss various factors associated with the effectiveness of continuing education in long-term care. Best practices and practical suggestions complete the chapter.

CONTINUING EDUCATION

Continuing education is an integral part of professional development (Puetz, 1981). Although it is often a requirement for certification or licensure renewal, it should not be viewed as just a necessity. As discussed in Chapter 6, professional development is the key to retaining valuable employees. For decades, most professional groups, such as physicians, nurses, teachers, and engineers, aim to improve the quality of their professional performance by continuing professional development, often in the form of continuing-education classes (Todd, 1987). Long-term care professionals, specifically assisted living administrators and staff, also benefit from continuing education.

Continuing education is an all-encompassing term within a broad spectrum of postsecondary learning activities and programs. Recognized forms of postsecondary learning activities within the domain include degree credit courses, nondegree career training, workforce training, formal personal enrichment courses, self-directed learning (such as through internet interest groups, clubs, or personal research activities), and experiential learning as applied to problem-solving.

Within the domain of continuing education, professional continuing education is a specific learning activity generally characterized by the issuance of a certificate or continuing-education units for the purpose of documenting attendance at a designated seminar or course of instruction. Licensing bodies in a number of fields impose continuing-education requirements on members who hold licenses to practice within a particular profession. These requirements are intended to encourage professionals to expand their knowledge and stay up-to-date on new developments. Depending on the field, these requirements may be satisfied through college or university coursework, extension courses, or conference and seminar attendance.

Methods for Delivering Continuing Education

The method of delivery of continuing education can include traditional types of classroom lectures and laboratories. However, continuing education makes heavy use of distance learning, which not only includes independent study, but can also include videotaped/CD-ROM material, broadcast programming, online/internet delivery, and online interactive courses. Menne, Ejaz, Noelker, and Jones (2008) acknowledge the benefits of emerging technologies in providing more options for delivering continuing education. Besides lectures, alternatives now exist, like web-based training, videos, group activities, and articles. Although there are many benefits to the latest technologies, such as the ability to stop and start a course, learn at a specific pace, take the class in a native tongue, or go back and reinforce a concept, the argument exists that secondary gains of attending a classroom-style format are lost. These gains are having real-time questions answered by the facilitator or by a peer, seeing real examples of what is happening currently in other communities, and having the ability to troubleshoot a challenge you may be having in your community with other professionals and peers. Furthermore, there is value to expanding your network of other providers who may be a valuable resource in the future.

Vital Need for Continuing Education

The U.S. Department of Health and Human Services (2018), in the publication *Healthy People 2030*, included objectives related to health education and professional development. Furthermore, *Recreating Health Professional Practice for a New Century*, a landmark report for the Pew Health Professions Commission (O'Neil & Pew Health Professions Commission, 1998), listed 21 specific competencies necessary for all professionals in the changing healthcare environment, with seven competencies directly related to education and professional development (Allegrante, Moon, Auld, & Gebbie, 2001). The demographics of the aging population highlight the need to anticipate an increase in need for both long-term care services and professionals (U.S. Department of Health and Human Services, 2000). Menne et al. (2008) emphasize the significance of providing continued education and training to direct care workers, and how these two areas are tied to job satisfaction of these workers, and alleviating employee turnover. Certainly, assisted living professionals will continue to be an integral part of meeting the needs of the aging population.

Continuing Education: What Administrators Say

Cristina Flores (2005), in a California study, surveyed certified assisted living administrators to identify their perceived need for additional knowledge in specific areas of practice. Areas in which *maximum need for knowledge* was identified by most participants included:

- Health and aging
- Mental health and aging
- Behavioral/dementia management
- Activity programs
- Marketing
- Regulatory updates
- Management and staffing
- Elder abuse

Areas in which *moderate need for knowledge* was identified by most participants included:

- Public policy for the aged
- Death and dying
- Hospice regulations
- Dementia regulations
- Meeting the cultural needs of residents
- Biology of aging
- Nutrition and aging
- Healthcare and service
- Pharmacology
- Exercise physiology
- Women's health and aging

There were no areas for which *minimal or no need for additional knowledge* was identified by most participants.

REGULATORY REQUIREMENTS

The requirements for continuing education are fueled by government and laws, professional organizations, and standards of care/practice. Societal pressures for improved quality of care and regulatory agencies, such as state agencies, are responsible for the oversight of assisted living communities. These types of demands give rise to the need for quality continuing-education courses.

As noted throughout this book, regulations vary state by state. Table 7.1 summarizes the annual direct-care staff training requirements (i.e., continuing education) by state. Information regarding the annual continuing-education requirements for assisted living administrators by state are described in Chapter 4.

TABLE 7.1 ANNUAL CONTINUING-EDUCATION HOURS FOR DIRECT-CARE STAFF

HOURS UNSTATED	1–5 HOURS	6–10 HOURS	11+ HOURS
Kansas	California	Arkansas	Alaska
Kentucky	Indiana	Hawaii	Connecticut
Louisiana	Iowa	Idaho	Delaware
Maine	Minnesota	Illinois	District of Columbia
Mississippi		Massachusetts	Georgia
New Hampshire		Nevada	Nebraska
North Dakota		Ohio	North Carolina
South Carolina		Oklahoma	Oregon
South Dakota		Rhode Island	Pennsylvania
West Virginia		Texas	Vermont
			Virginia
			Washington
			Wisconsin

Source: Carder, P., O'Keeffe, J., & O'Keeffe, C. (2015). *Compendium of residential care and assisted living regulations and policy: 2015 edition.* U.S. Department of Health and Human Services, Office of the Assistant Secretary for Planning and Evaluation, Office of Disability, Aging and Long-Term Care Policy and Research Triangle Institute. https://aspe.hhs.gov/basic-report/compendium-residential-care-and-assisted-living-regulations-and-policy-2015-edition

MODEL CONTINUING-EDUCATION PROGRAM

David Hahklotubbe, MA, has developed a model of seven continuing-education classes for assisted living administrators and staff. Descriptions of the courses he has developed and improved over time are noted in Exhibit 7.1.

EXHIBIT 7.1

SEVEN MODEL COURSES FOR ADMINISTRATORS AND DIRECT-CARE STAFF

1. You Have Openings, You Need This Marketing Class
An in-depth look into the principles of marketing, sales, and business development. Most operators of long-term care communities are equipped to provide quality care, but do not have the education, ability, or interest in managing the sales and marketing side to their businesses. The overall impact on neglecting the marketing of their services are far reaching; utilizing system's theory, we can see that a lack of marketing effects budgets for staffing, quality of care for residents, perception in the community, life span of the business, capital ppgrades, and the perception that the general public will form of long-term care living. Designed to help empower students with tools to recognize that marketing is a necessary component to running a quality care home; , assist students to recognize what services are marketable; help students understand how to create a successful marketing plan, accentuating their individual points of difference; help students understand the importance of execution, maintenance, and constant penetration into the market; and to, show tips and tricks for utilizing referral sources effectively and knowing who to steer clear from.

2. The Best Dementia Class You Will Ever Take
Designed as an overview of various dementias, Alzheimer's disease, and other memory impairments. It identifies the most difficult recurring behaviors to manage in persons suffering from these impairments. It introduces an intervention that treats the difficult behavior as a system rather than as a random occurrence. The behaviors focused on are anxiety, agitation, hallucinations, wandering, "wanting to go home," paranoia, dressing/ bathing, inappropriate sexual behaviors, sleeping problems, incontinence, and eating issues. It allows students to become comfortable applying techniques through studying fictitious case studies and then acting out the management techniques in a group role-playing format. This course has a segment dedicated to sundown syndrome. There is no reason why learning about dementia can't be fun!

(continued)

EXHIBIT 7.1

SEVEN MODEL COURSES FOR ADMINISTRATORS AND DIRECT-CARE STAFF (*CONTINUED*)

3. The Best Activities Class You Will Ever Take Designed as an in-depth overview of various approaches to activities for those suffering from dementia, Alzheimer's disease, and other related cognitive impairments. It identifies the most difficult recurring behaviors to manage, placing a special spotlight on the role of activities in managing sundown syndrome. It shows how activities can be utilized to redirect or even prevent behaviors from occurring. It introduces assessment techniques for both the care staff and the client. It applies the system approach toward managing behavior, introducing different levels of activities designed to stimulate and redirect certain behaviors. It addresses the physical/psychological and emotional components of each activity. It spotlights knowing when to abandon an activity and when to move on to the next. It introduces activities as a marketing tool. It discusses and maps out how to create an activity calendar. Last, and most fun, failure-free activities created by Hahk Training and Consulting are introduced, participated in, and led by students.
4. The Staffing Class You Hope Your Competitors Aren't Taking Designed to assist the management team in acquiring, empowering, and retaining quality personnel. Consists of group activities designed to tackle common staffing issues utilizing real-life mistakes as functional case studies. The concept of **empowerment** and how it fits in long-term care is discussed. The students learn techniques and strategies about how to employ the empowerment concept in their facilities. The systems approach is discussed in terms of cyclical rewards gained by employing the concept. In-depth discussions about how empowerment has a direct relationship with morale, productivity, and effectivity are explored. Techniques for building effective teams from the ground up by successful staffing are given. The fact that training and education are necessary ingredients in retention is covered. Finally, management paradigm change and the results of being a proactive/hands-on manager are shared.
5. Successfully Managing Your Biggest Challenge: Families of Your Clients Designed as an in-depth, hands-on tutorial on how to manage familial psychodynamics. Understanding the pressure, emotional stress, and a bevy of other influences on the behavior of the family members of clients in long-term care. The class begins with an empathic exercise and leads into discussion about common psychological issues that afflict families. Clinical definitions of common psychological issues are presented as a foundation. Discussion about how these psychological issues can influence behavior and the types of behavior that are commonly manifested is shared. Most important, a discussion about how to avoid the behaviors from occurring is presented. Finally, there is great emphasis on a cutting edge concept of "Viewing a Complaint as a Gift." Role plays and fictitious case studies are used to create an interactive environment.
6. Burnout: If You and Your Staff Are Immune to It, You Don't Need This Class The foundation is laid by providing the grim statistics of how burnout affects the physical, emotional, and financial well-being of the long-term care provider. Systems theory is applied to how burnout ultimately affects the quality of life of our clients and staff. The clinical definition of *burnout* is provided as are relaxing group activities designed to empower the student with the ability to identify burnout, identify its source, and implement a program to manage and prevent it. Specific, effective stress-management and prevention techniques are discussed and engaged in. Applied activities include purposeful breathing, smudging (spiritual Native American cleansing), releasing the demons through drumming, visualization, and aroma therapy. The discussion of creating ritual and forming "good habits" is discussed. The goal of this class is to educate while relaxing, recharging, and rejuvenating. The dress code is "relaxed" (sweats, pajamas, and slippers are recommended).
7. Maintaining Compliance Through Safe Food Handling Practices (ServSafe®) Designed as an in-depth look into safe food handling and satisfying dietary requirements. This course is nationally recognized and required certification training for compliance with the Department of Health. This course covers principles and detailed instruction on preparing, storing, and serving food to paying clientele. In addition, a segment has been added to cover the dietary needs of clients of long-term care. This course is accompanied by an optional exam, which provides the opportunity for those who wish to be in complete compliance by having a ServSafe® certified employee in their building. This course is approved for 8 hours of continuing-education units as well as satisfying the Department of Health curriculum. The class duration is 8 hours; exam time is an additional I hour. It is highly recommended that the student take the exam and receive the ServSafe® certificate; however, this is not required.

Source: From Hahk Training and Consulting. (n.d.). *Continuing education for license renewal.* Author.

FACTORS ASSOCIATED WITH THE EFFECTIVENESS OF CONTINUING EDUCATION IN LONG-TERM CARE

As mentioned earlier, continuing education is an integral part of professional development (Puetz, 1981), so it is crucial to understand the factors that may influence its success. The administrator plays a key role in ensuring that continuing education has a positive effect throughout the community. Stolee et al. (2005) designed a two-part study; thie first study included a sample of 17 management and 18 staff participants in long-term care facilities in Ontario study. The second study resulted in the development of a list of organizational and system factors in the effectiveness of continuing education in long-term care. Their sample consisted of 34 experts in long-term care. Results indicated that various factors like workforce issues, which include a changing resident population with more difficult care needs, require more knowledge, skills, and different models of care. In addition, staff resistance to change, like keeping their old ways and refusing change, was one of the factors hindering the effectiveness of continuing education in long-term care. Stolee et al. (2005) found management support to "be the most important factor impacting the effectiveness of continuing education." Administrators were acknowledged as the most instrumental people in long-term care, in terms of creating a better work environment that supports change. A participant in the study supported this finding by stating: "If you don't have an administrator that is going to support it, you're not going to get the funding. You're not going to get the time and energy that is going to promote that education." The importance of collaboration between administrators and staff was also emphasized. Stolee et al. (2005) emphasized the need for collaboration to meet goals at both an organizational and individual level to create a work environment that empowers staff to improve care. Supporting this statement, the study listed ways in which management could support continued education, like providing more funding for access to continuing education, and the required staff coverage. Overall, multifaceted organizational support was placed at the top of the list to the success of continuing education. Organizational support was quoted to play a central role when it came to "the development of a workplace environment that fosters innovation and change."

BEST PRACTICES IN CONTINUING EDUCATION: REFORM IN CALIFORNIA

In response to several investigative reports about the failure in oversight and enforcement regarding assisted living communities in California, the RCFE (Residential Care Facility for the Elderly) Reform Act of 2014 was introduced (California Advocates for Nursing Home Reform, n.d.). The reform bills focused on improving care, empowering residents, and providing the licensing agency with new tools to ensure compliance with regulatory standards. Specifically, legislative bill SB 911 (Block) expanded and specified continuing-education requirements for staff in assisted living communities.

Direct-Care Staff

In addition to the increased initial training direct-care staff receive, direct-care staff now must receive an additional 20 hours each year on specific topics. See the list of topics required annually for direct-care staff as determined by the California Assisted Living Association (http://caassistedliving.org/provider-resources/laws-regulations/staff-training/).

For those direct-care staff providing care to residents with dementia, in addition to initial training, they must receive an additional 8 hours of education annually. See the list of topics required annually for direct staff providing care to patients with dementia as described by the California Assisted Living Association (http://caassistedliving.org/provider-resources/laws-regulations/staff-training).

Administrators

Although the number of continuing-education hours remained the same (i.e., 40 hours every 2 years), for administrators, the Reform Act specified minimum required knowledge for administrators in California. See the list of minimum knowledge requirements for continuing education for administrators as described by the California Assisted Living Association (http://caassistedliving.org/provider-resources/laws-regulations/staff-training/). Furthermore, 8 hours of education must be specific to dementia.

THE IMPACT OF PROFESSIONAL DEVELOPMENT ON MILLENNIALS

It is no surprise that the workforce is currently going through generational change. It is important for administrators to acknowledge the shifting workforce when offering continuing-education and professional development opportunities to their employees. Tim Clark (2013), Brand Contributor at Forbes, explains the three-generation workplace: Baby boomers (a generation 76 million strong) are reaching the traditional retirement age, but many are continuing to work well into their 60s and 70s (and sometimes beyond). At the same time, Millennials (a generation 80 million strong) are advancing in their careers and beginning to take on leadership roles. Add in the Gen Xers (those in their mid-30s and 40s), and for the first time we are seeing a workplace full of three generations (Clark, 2013).

An article titled, "Forget Work Perks. Millennial Employees Value Engagement," written by Mackenzie Kassab (2018) at Harvard University, explains that millennials value engagement at work, which consists highly of training and personal development in their jobs. It is important for administrators to understand that a new work force is coming in, which values continued education and opportunities for purpose and fulfillment in the organization. With a workforce that values opportunity, administrators must be prepared to guide professional growth in their employees and provide resources for career planning.

IMPORTANT CONFERENCES FOR ADMINISTRATORS AND DIRECT-CARE STAFF

Attending conferences is an important aspect of continuing education for both administrators and direct-care staff. Many conferences provide continuing-education credits toward different certificates and licenses. In addition, conferences provide a networking opportunity for strong professional connections. There are dozens of conferences that providers can choose from. Below is a list of some popular conferences to attend:

1. Argentum Senior Living Executive Conference https://conference.argentum.org
2. California Assisted Living Association Conference and Trade Show—https://caassistedliving.org/education-events/trade-shows/exhibitor-information
3. International Council on Active Aging Conference, Summit, & Trade Show—https://www.icaa.cc/conferenceandevents/overview.htm
4. Leading Age Annual Meeting and Expo—https://www.leadingage.org/leadingage-annual-meeting-expo

5. Pioneer Network Conference—https://www.pioneernetwork.net/conference
6. Senior Living 100 Conference—https://www.seniorliving100.com
7. University of Southern California Senior Living Executive Course—http://gero.usc .edu/event/2018-senior-living-executive-course

THE IMPORTANCE OF JOINING AN ASSOCIATION

There are a number of benefits to joining a professional association. Like selecting a training vendor or attending a conference, the potential member must perform due diligence to find the right association for them. Associations range in membership size from a quorum of 10 to over 10,000. Depending on the needs, it is not unusual to belong to more than one association. Many providers belong to a local association with only local members while simultaneously belonging to a larger association that is statewide or even national.

Consider the smaller associations first; getting to know your local providers in the spirit of working collaboratively for a common goal is a great way to establish yourself and not only gain access to potential referral sources, but also to pipelines for staff recruitment. Local associations also are able to identify pertinent issues that will directly affect providers of that region, where statewide and national associations provide similar information on a macro-scale. While all associations are unique in their agenda and purpose, some common threads are education, alliances, community service, member support, and networking.

Bridging the gap between the smaller, community-based associations and the national ones are the large organizations that have local chapters. Larger statewide or national organizations have a bit more to offer on a grander scale. Although many small associations have some local influence and offer continuing education, the larger organizations have a strategically planned advocacy program, often visiting lawmakers in their state capitals in large numbers to lobby for senior living. The larger associations will also have access to information like bills that are in the pipeline to become law so that the providers can prepare, take action, and remain in compliance. Conferences are a large part of the statewide and nationwide associations where well-organized programs are offered ranging from the expected continuing-education courses to sessions with state licensing, practicing elder-law attorneys, and popular authors who keynote the events. Of course, a driving force of the conference is to generate revenue to keep the association functioning properly. They achieve this by high attendance fees, corporate sponsorship, and vendor expositions. Although there has been a bit more focus on attracting the smaller operator, these larger associations are mainly run by and focused on the larger providers and may not be the right choice for smaller operators.

As an administrator, it is important to choose the right association and consider not just being a member, but a functioning committee or chair. Overall, associations are beneficial and should be taken into consideration by assisted living administrators.

CONCLUSIONS

This chapter demonstrates the importance of continuing education for assisted living professionals, specifically, administrators and direct-care staff. Continuing education is discussed so as to assist the reader in understanding the benefits of excellent continuing-education programs, as well as the legal requirements that vary by state. Leaders in the continuing-education field share their model programs, both with traditional classroom and online curriculum descriptions.

Researchers and professionals continue to identify ways to improve the quality of care and quality of life of residents living in assisted living communities. Continuing education is an important way to maintain and update the knowledge and skills necessary to run a successful assisted living community. It is the attendee's responsibility to share all information with their teams and to perform due diligence by vetting the best vendors and conferences for their educational needs. Becoming a member of a professional association may have many benefits, but it is critical to choose wisely to maximize the return on the investment.

REFERENCES

Allegrante, J., Moon, R., Auld, E., & Gebbie, M. (2001). Continuing education needs of currently employed public health education workforce. *American Journal of Public Health, 91*(8), 1230–1234. https://doi.org/10.2105/AJPH.91.8.1230

California Advocates for Nursing Home Reform. (n.d.). *Introducing the RCFE Reform Act of 2014.* http://canhr.org/publications/newsletters/Advocate/FrontArticle/adv_2014Q1.htm

California Assisted Living Association. (n.d.). *Staff training.* http://caassistedliving.org/provider-resources/laws-regulations/staff-training

Carder, P., O'Keeffe, J., & O'Keeffe, C. (2015). *Compendium of residential care and assisted living regulations and policy: 2015 Edition.* U.S. Department of Health and Human Services, Office of the Assistant Secretary for Planning and Evaluation, Office of Disability, Aging and Long-Term Care Policy and Research Triangle Institute. https://aspe.hhs.gov/basic-report/compendium-residential-care-and-assisted-living-regulations-and-policy-2015-edition

Clark, T. (2013). *The 3-Generational Workplace: It's (Really!) A Good Thing.* https://www.forbes.com/sites/dailymuse/2013/12/02/the-3-generational-workplace-its-really-a-good-thing/#53c9259b965c

Flores, C. (2005). Assessing the needs of RCFE administrators. In D. Yee-Melichar & A. Boyle (Eds.), *Aging in contemporary society: Translating research into practice* (pp. 17–25). XanEdu Publications.

Hahk Training and Consulting. (n.d.). *Continuing education for license renewal.* Author.

Kassab, M. (2018). *Forget work perks. Millennial employees value engagement.* https://www.extension.harvard.edu/professional-development/blog/forget-work-perks-millennial-employees-value-engagement

Menne, H., Ejaz, F., Noelker, L., & Jones, J. (2007). Workers' recommendations for training and continuing education. *Gerontology & Geriatrics Education, 2,* 91–108. https://doi.org/10.1300/J021v28n02_07

O'Neil, E. H., & Pew Health Professions Commission. (1998). *Recreating health professional practice for a new century.* Pew Health Professions Commission.

Puetz, B. (1981). *Continuing education for nurses: A complete guide to effective programs.* Aspen Publications.

Stolee, P., Esbaugh, J., Aylward, S., Cathers, T., Harvey, D., Hillier, L., Keat, N., & Feightner, J. (2005). Factors associated with the effectiveness of continuing education in long-term care. *Gerontologist, 45,* 399–405. https://doi.org/10.1093/geront/45.3.399

Todd, F. (Ed.). (1987). *Planning continuing professional development.* Croom Helm.

U.S. Department of Health and Human Services. (2018). *Healthy people 2030.* Author. https://www.healthypeople.gov/2020/About-Healthy-People/Development-Healthy-People-2030/Framework

INTERPROFESSIONAL PRACTICE: ISSUES FOR ASSISTED LIVING ADMINISTRATION

LEARNING OBJECTIVES

Upon the completion of Chapter 8, the reader will be able to:

- Identify the need for interprofessional care in assisted living communities.
- Define *interprofessional care* and *interprofessional teams*.
- Identify the benefits of interprofessional practice for assisted living administrators.
- Describe the roles of selected interprofessional team members.
- Describe issues faced by assisted living administrators working with interprofessional teams.

INTRODUCTION

Interprofessional practice teams are important in the provision of high-quality, person-centered, and team-based care. These methods of care delivery are relevant for elders with the complex and interconnected problems frequently found in residents of assisted living facilities. Interprofessional workers include physicians, nurses, physical therapists, occupational therapists, dentists, pharmacists, social workers, dieticians, chaplains, and others. This chapter provides an introduction to interprofessional practice within assisted living communities. Definitions of *interprofessional practice* and benefits and challenges of this practice model are further explored as is the role of the assisted living administrator in the promotion of this team-based care model.

Need for Interprofessional Care

A series of reports from the Institute of Medicine (IOM) in early 2000 revealed concerns about the quality of the U.S. healthcare system. Quality healthcare delivery was determined to be compromised in part by rising costs, care-provider shortages, and rising medical error rates resulting in significant morbidity and mortality for patients across the healthcare system (Kohn et al., 2000). Many of these concerns followed changes in healthcare delivery as a result of federal Medicare and Medicaid legislation in 1965. This legislative change resulted in increases in healthcare access and insurance coverage for impoverished U.S. citizens and those individuals aged 65 and older (Centers for Medicare & Medicaid Services, n.d.).

At the present time, healthcare in the United States is not only one of the most costly systems in the world, but also has poorer outcomes than many other developed and developing countries (Josiah Macy Jr. Foundation, 2013). Concerns about health professionals unable to provide essential care in teams rather than in individual silos were also identified (Institute of Medicine, 1972). A lack of teamwork, inadequate communication, and limited collaboration were identified as responsible for many adverse health system and patient outcomes (Brandt, 2015). Poor communication was also often identified as a major source of medical errors and was connected to quality and safety problems (Vega & Bernard, 2016).

External forces facilitating change in U.S. healthcare delivery have been associated with an increase in quality-improvement measures, additional patient-safety initiatives, an increased need for improved care transitions, escalating healthcare costs, healthcare practice redesign, and initiation of federal and state healthcare policies (Brandt, 2015). Recent passage of the Patient Protection and Affordable Care Act (ACA) has created government-based incentives for healthcare providers to improve quality and safety outcomes, placing the patient at the center of value-based care rather than volume-based care (Nester, 2016). These changing conditions underscore the need for team-based, interprofessional practice in all settings, including assisted living facilities. The proposed team-based approach to patient care promotes coordinated care, patient education to improve overall health, early interventions in the treatment of health problems, and assistance with effective management of chronic health conditions such as congestive heart failure, diabetes, asthma, and chronic obstructive pulmonary disease (COPD; Nester, 2016).

The need for healthcare system change has also resulted in an emphasis by accrediting agencies, quality care experts, corporate and insurance stakeholders, and policy experts at both the national and state levels on healthcare system redesign (Brandt, 2015). Strategies to improve and redesign healthcare systems have focused on system improvements and an emphasis on teamwork and collaboration across members of health professions (Brandt, 2015). In addition, there is an emphasis on holistic strategies to keep individuals healthy through recognition of the social determinants of health and inclusion of services to deal with wellness as well as illness in multiple settings, including transition, home-care, long-term care, and community-based settings (Brandt, 2015).

DEFINITIONS OF *INTERPROFESSIONAL PRACTICE*

The term *interprofessional* was first used in the United States in 1975 to communicate shared decision-making across a number of professions (Kane, 1975) and this definition supplanted terms such as *interdisciplinary care*. The World Health Organization stated that interprofessional practice takes place when health workers from different professional backgrounds deliver comprehensive care services through collaborative work with patients, families, caregivers, and community settings. The goal is the highest quality of care delivery across settings (World Health Organization, 2010).

Interprofessional practice is collaborative by design. Collaborative practice in varied healthcare settings occurs when multiple professionals engage in work with patients and families; includes clinical and nonclinical work such as disease diagnosis and treatment, health surveillance, management, and communication; and focuses on improvement of health outcomes (World Health Organization, 2010).

The terms *multidisciplinary* and *interdisciplinary care* are now being replaced by *interprofessional care*. Mutual respect is a critical element of this approach with individuals managing patients and complex problems through connections, relationship building, and interdependencies (Nester, 2016). This approach is also based on an understanding that professionals who consider other perspectives are able to deliver better healthcare services (Vega & Bernard, 2016). Bridges et al. (2011) further note that an interprofessional approach may improve healthcare outcomes through combined professional resources.

In response to quality and safety healthcare concerns and in an attempt to refine understanding of interprofessional practice, the national associations of six health professions developed a series of interprofessional practice competencies. These core competencies were built around a central goal of intentionally building a safe, improved, person-centered, and population- and community-based healthcare system (Schmitt et al., 2011). Four identified core competencies include: (a) values/ethics for interprofessional practice to maintain a climate of mutual respect and shared values; (b) roles/responsibilities to support a team approach to maintain health and treat disease; (c) interprofessional communication with patients, families, communities, and other health professionals to support a team approach to maintain health and treat disease; and (d) teams and teamwork through the application of relationship-building values to perform effectively in different team roles and deliver care that is safe, timely, effective, equitable, and efficient (Schmitt et al., 2011).

Defining interprofessional practice as related to care of elders is of critical significance to assisted living administrators. In a 2008 report, the Institute of Medicine envisioned care that is responsive to an aging U.S. society. This care model, delivered in assisted living facilities, ensures an adequate supply of healthcare workers working together in healthcare teams on improved healthcare delivery systems (Institute of Medicine, 2008). Team care delivery occurs in systems that are intentionally designed around the importance of a core and central relationship between elders and their caregivers (Young & Siegel, 2016).

Defining interprofessional practice also requires that care providers from continually expanding professional teams be required to address disease processes as well as functional status and quality-of-life issues (Young & Siegel, 2016). The use of interprofessional collaborative practice also has the potential to improve the health of all Americans, especially in the areas of aging, mental health, and dementia. This can be accomplished through team-based educational models focused on reduction of healthcare costs per capita through improvement of patient care experiences, improving provider experiences, and improving population health outcomes (Farrell et al., 2018).

BENEFITS OF INTERPROFESSIONAL PRACTICE

Assisted living administrators need to consider the benefits of this practice approach for care delivery in their facilities. Research evidence presented by the World Health Organization Framework for Action on Interprofessional Education & Collaborative Practice (World Health Organization, 2010) revealed a number of benefits, including: (a) improvement in access to and coordination of many health services; (b) appropriate utilization of clinical specialist resources; (c) improved health outcomes for individuals with chronic illnesses; and (d) improvements in patient safety and overall patient care. The use of collaborative practice was additionally shown to decrease (a) patient illness outcomes, (b) staff turnover, (c) conflict and tension among caregivers, (d) clinical error rates, (e) hospital readmission rates, and (f) mortality rates (World Health Organization, 2010). The National Center for Interprofessional Practice and Education noted benefits associated with high functioning collaborative teams as improving the costs, outcomes, and experiences of healthcare (Vega & Bernard, 2016).

Distinct benefits from the use of interprofessional care models in health systems include reduced costs for elders with chronic illnesses such as heart failure. Benefits also include the reduction of redundancy and costs of medical testing (World Health Organization, 2010). Healthcare system benefits have also been shown for professionals and for workers in nonregulated areas such as nursing assistants, community health workers, and managers (World Health Organization, 2010).

Research findings on the benefits of interprofessional practice in a number of countries, including Australia, Belgium, Sweden, the United Kingdom and the United States, reveal that interprofessional practice may slightly improve patient functional status, healthcare resource utilization, as well as care provider adherence to recommended practices (Reeves et al., 2017). A number of studies also suggest that interprofessional practice may improve overall healthcare processes as well as overall patient outcomes (Zwarenstein et al., 2009).

Additional research reveals improved quality outcomes with the use of interprofessional healthcare teams throughout many healthcare systems (Lutfiyya et al., 2016). One problem noted in current systematic reviews is that much of prior research has been focused on individual-level short-term changes, and changes to practice-based processes rather than practice outcomes or overall population health (Lutfiyya et al., 2016). Additional research is needed to support large-scale benefits of an interprofessional approach to clinical practice.

INTERPROFESSIONAL PRACTICE TEAMS

Assisted living administrators employing interprofessional teams for elder care require an understanding of the healthcare workers participating in this important collaborative practice. Interprofessional teams are composed of individuals, including physicians, nurses, physical therapists, occupational therapists, social workers, dentists, pharmacists, and dieticians—all of whom are qualified to work with elders. Brief descriptions of selected interprofessional team members working in many assisted living settings are presented as follows.

Physician

The physician is a professional with a doctorate in allopathic or osteopathic medicine. Training for the degree follows medical training, clinical residency, and board certification in a specialty area. Physicians are licensed by the state where they practice (Mauk, 2018). Many physicians working in assisted living settings are specialized or subspecialized in geriatrics.

The physician is responsible for oversight of medical care for residents, including diagnosis and management of illnesses, prescription management for all chronic and acute illnesses, and prescriptions for medical treatments as needed. Physicians work in collaboration with nurses, physical therapists, occupational therapists, pharmacists, dieticians, social workers, and psychologists. Physicians may supervise physician assistants (PAs) who are educated at the postbaccalaureate or master's level, licensed at the state level, and board certified at the national level (Mauk, 2018). The PA joins the interprofessional team member working collaboratively with the physician.

Nurse

Assisted living facilities employ nurses at different levels of educational preparation. Advanced practice nurses with either master's or doctoral-level preparation as gerontology primary care or acute care nurse practitioners or clinical specialists frequently work as members of interprofessional teams. Advanced practice nurses hold state licensure and national certification.

The roles of advanced practice nurses in assisted living communities include the provision of primary care and acute care services, the diagnosis and management of illnesses, treatment (including prescription management) of acute and chronic illnesses, and patient and family education (Mauk, 2018). In selected assisted living communities, the advanced practice nurse works independently to directly provide patient care. Other settings may employ both advanced practice nurses and physicians for patient care management.

The RN is educated at the associate degree, baccalaureate, master's, or doctoral level and licensed by the state of practice following completion of a state board examination (NCLEX-RN®). The roles of RNs are varied and include assessment, planning, coordination, and evaluation of care to elders with a focus on health, optimal wellness, disease prevention, education, and patient advocacy (Mauk, 2018). Assisted living RNs may act as direct-care providers depending on state regulations for assisted living facilities. Direct-care provision also includes assistance with mobility, activities of daily living, and management of patient's social and emotional needs (Nursing Licensure.org, 2019).

Assisted living nursing practice requires that the RN employ a holistic practice approach to improve or maintain an elder's independence, function, well-being, and quality of life through activities, including counseling, health education, direct clinical care, access and advocacy within healthcare systems for appropriate policies promoting respect and values for elders, and guiding end-of-life care for elders and family members as needed (Scope and Standards of Assisted Living Nursing Practice, 2006).

The assisted living RN provides direct supervision to licensed vocational nurses and nursing assistants in the form of oversight and evaluation of direct patient care delivery, including patient assessments, hygiene, mobility, and personal care, and in some settings, this includes medication administration. State regulations determine RN supervisory activities, staffing ratios, and role responsibilities within each state's assisted living facilities. The RN may also work as an administrator of the assisted living facility and in this capacity develops, monitors, supports, and evaluates systems necessary for patient care implementation (Scope and Standards of Assisted Living Nursing Practice, 2006).

The RN works in collaboration with all members of interprofessional teams, delegating decisions and treatment recommendations to licensed practical nurses and nursing assistants as needed to provide comprehensive care to residents. The RN is responsible for safe delegation of care to licensed vocational nurses as well as unlicensed personnel such as nursing assistants (Mauk, 2018). Delegation of specific care activities is governed by individual state boards of nursing with RNs adhering to state regulations and policies on assistive personnel delegation. Understanding of RN delegation and supervision issues is relevant for administrators in many states because the nursing workforce in assisted living facilities is composed mainly of licensed vocational nurses and unlicensed workers.

Physical Therapist

The physical therapist is educated at either the master's level or the doctoral level (DPT). The physical therapist completes a state licensure examination and many clinicians also complete specialty certification such as gerontology certification. The role of the physical therapist includes assessment for mobility and functional capacity and treatment, including strengthening, mobility, use of assistive devices, and rehabilitation (Mauk, 2018). Activities connected with this role also include review of each patient's medical history, development of individual care plans outlining patient goals, and use of exercises and hands-on therapy to relieve and prevent pain (U.S. Bureau of Labor Statistics, 2019).

The physical therapist is viewed as a leader in rehabilitation allowing patients with disease or chronic health conditions, impaired body functions, injuries, or activity limitations to improve their functional status (American Physical Therapy Association, n.d.). Restorative therapy programs may provide elders with exercises to improve range of motion and muscle strength.

Physical therapists work as members of interprofessional care teams, collaborating in assisted living settings to provide elders with comprehensive treatments and preventive therapy programs. Supervision of physical therapist assistants and aides is also an important component of this role (U.S. Bureau of Labor Statistics, 2019). The assisted living administrator benefits from an understanding of the many roles of the physical therapist.

Occupational Therapist

The occupational therapist (OT) is educated for practice at either the master's degree or doctoral-degree level. State licensure and national certification are also requirements for OT practice. Many OTs also complete specialty certification in a number of content areas, including gerontology for clinicians working with elders. The OT assesses and treats sensory, perceptual, cognitive, and functional deficits impacting an individual's abilities to complete activities of daily living. The OT also assesses the need for assistive devices and rehabilitative services (Mauk, 2018).

The OT who works with elders provides a blend of mental, psychological, and physical exercises to enhance performance of activities of daily living. Additional benefits of occupational therapy include assistance for elders with arthritis to promote use of joint function; increased range of motion in joints through exercises; use of exercises in vision therapy to improve specific visual impairments; coping strategies for chronic pain through improved body mechanics, ergonomics, neuromuscular re-education, muscle tension reduction, proactive pain control, and communication skills trainings (PT Solutions, 2019). The OT can also assist elders with improvement of memory and cognitive skills. Sensory stimulation, reading books, solving puzzles, and a focus on simplified activities are examples of activities that the OT can introduce into care management for these individuals (PT Solutions, 2019).

The OT works in collaboration with members of interprofessional teams providing care for elders in assisted living facilities. Assisted living administrators understand that many state regulations vary in the provision of specific OT treatments such as assistive devices for elders. It is important for administrators to note the significance of the OT as an important member of an interprofessional approach to care management in assisted living facilities.

Social Worker

Social workers are educated at both the baccalaureate level for an LSW (licensed social worker) degree and at the master's level for an MSW (master of social work) degree. State licensure is required for the social worker to engage in healthcare delivery. The increasing and expanding roles of the social worker involve the provision of counseling and psychotherapy as well as the provision of coping strategies for individuals and families dealing with many of the changes associated with aging and chronic illness (Mauk, 2018). The social worker is trained in systems perspectives with a focus on care delivery for society's most underserved, marginalized, and vulnerable individuals (de Saxe Zerden et al., 2019).

The role of the social worker on the interprofessional care team is underscored by an expanding body of evidence showing the impact of social factors, including employment, income, education, and discrimination on mental, physical, and behavioral health outcomes for individuals.

The perspective of the social worker allows the social worker to address health equity, the social determinants of health, and the adoption of behavioral healthcare methods in healthcare settings (de Saxe Zerden et al., 2019). Elders in assisted living communities have been shown to benefit from services provided by social workers operating in an interprofessional approach to care delivery.

Dietician

The dietician is educated at the baccalaureate level, completing a national examination prior to practice in healthcare settings. The registered dietician (RD) is an individual who meets specific academic and clinical requirements determined by the American Dietetic Association (ADA). The focus of this education is food science, nutrition science, alternate feeding modalities, and counseling for behavioral changes (Institute of Medicine, 2000). The RD serves as a nutrition specialist with in-depth knowledge of the role of food and nutrition in the prevention, treatment, and progression of both acute and chronic illnesses. Dieticians also provide additional understanding of the psychological, educational, and socioeconomic factors impacting food and nutritional behaviors of individuals across the lifespan (Institute of Medicine, 2000). Requirements for licensure of the RD vary among states and in some states licensure is not required for dieticians.

The RD serves as an important member of interprofessional teams. Physicians prescribe nutrition therapy as a Medicare Part B service (Institute of Medicine, 2000) and work in collaboration with the RD. The RD also serves in a supervisory capacity for oversight of the certified dietary manager (CDM). The CDM who frequently works in long-term care or assisted living settings may screen for nutrition risks, provide preventive nutrition services, and manage interventions for individuals with less complex nutritional needs (Institute of Medicine, 2000). The assisted living administrator needs to understand how the RD can best work as a member of interdisciplinary teams.

Dentist

The dentist is a professional educated at the doctoral level and licensed at the state level. The dentist provides dental care and supervises dental hygienists in all aspects of oral care provision.

State policy and regulatory requirements for dental care have evolved under federal mandates (Oral Health Workforce Research Center, 2016). The Older Americans Act of 1965 was reauthorized in 2016 to include oral health in approved screenings (Romaszewski, 2017). The U.S. Surgeon General's Report on Oral Health identified the unmet oral health needs of elders, many living in long-term care or assisted living facilities.

Health disparities for vulnerable elders in the area of oral health are now widely recognized and the need for enhanced dental services, especially in these facilities for the elderly, is now identified (Romaszewski, 2017). Although disparities have been noted, there are currently no uniform standards for dentistry provision in long-term care or assisted living settings. The provision of dental services to elders in these settings is more difficult than is care delivery to elders in other types of settings (Oral Health Workforce Research Center, 2016).

The assisted living administrator needs to have an awareness of best practices associated with delivery of dental care to elders in assisted living settings. Best practices in dental care require complex and collaborative interprofessional efforts by all team members (Oral Health Workforce Research Center, 2016). The administrator working with interprofessional teams will need to recognize the significance of including dentists with other professionals in interprofessional teams.

Pharmacist

Educational preparation for pharmacists includes 2 years of specific undergraduate study. Four years of additional study are required for the Pharm D degree. National examination is required for pharmacy practice and all pharmacists are required to hold state licensure. Many individuals working with elders obtain additional certification in the field of geriatric pharmacotherapy (Mauk, 2018).

The role of the pharmacist includes the preparation and dispensing of medications. Medication education and clinical consultations for patients, families, and healthcare team members are also important elements of the pharmacist role (Mauk, 2018). Pharmacists serve as pharmacotherapy experts in the rapidly expanding and complex field of medication development, administration, and evaluation and are a critical resource for both patients and providers.

Although administrators do not provide direct healthcare services to elders in assisted living settings, they should be aware of the importance of the role of the pharmacist in elder care. This is underscored by an increase in medication errors, now documented in increasing frequency at multiple practice locations. The presence of the pharmacist on the care team can reduce or prevent the morbidity and mortality associated with costly medication errors.

Chaplain

A chaplain is an individual who is grounded in initiating, developing, and fostering mutual and empathic relationships with patients, family members, and staff (Standards of Practice for Professional Chaplains in Long-term Care, 2012). The board-certified chaplain has a baccalaureate degree or master's degree in theological studies, is ordained or commissioned by one of a number of religious authorities, has completed four units of clinical pastoral education, has a minimum of 1 year of experience in the chaplain role, and maintains membership in a certifying body (Standards of Practice for Professional Chaplains in Long-term Care, 2012).

Although the roles of the chaplain vary institutionally, there are common elements to the services provided to patients and families, including: (a) assessment of individualized care plans for elders, (b) provision of spiritual and religious resources, (c) relationship building with local faith communities, (d) facilitation of religious rituals and prayers, (e) provision of education and consultation for patients and staff, (f) provision of leadership within the healthcare setting, (g) contributing to ethical decisions as needed, and (h) participation in interdisciplinary collaboration and teamwork (Standards of Practice for Professional Chaplains in Long-term Care, 2012).

Administrators need to understand the importance of including a board-certified chaplain as a member of the assisted living healthcare team. The role of the chaplain adds value to an interprofesional approach to elder care.

ISSUES FOR ASSISTED LIVING ADMINISTRATORS

The assisted living administrator interested in facilitating interprofessional teams into service delivery will face a number of issues with this care approach. Issues related to the benefits of interprofessional teams, costs associated with care delivery, and challenges associated with interprofessional team care are briefly addressed.

Benefits of Interprofessional Team Care

Administrators planning to integrate an interprofessional approach to elder care in assisted living communities will need to identify the benefits associated with this practice approach. A major benefit of an interprofessional approach is the provision of patient-centered care designed to address the entire person, the environment and context in which the care is delivered, and the problems of each patient (Mauk, 2018). The professionals who provide care to elders are experts in their fields and are able to address the many complex, interconnected problems of elders residing in assisted living facilities. The administrator will note the benefits of team members who have shared values, shared responsibilities, and shared goals for the elders they treat in the care setting. Care delivery associated with this approach is more comprehensive, less fragmented, more likely to reduce errors while increasing success in overall elder care and management. Quality and continuity of care as well as better overall health outcomes are results that the administrator can directly observe from this approach (Mauk, 2018). An interprofessional approach also allows professionals to engage in opportunities for personal growth and learning through collaboration with colleagues. The administrator can benefit from the creation of a workplace environment that facilitates these positive outcomes for professional employees.

Interprofessional Practice Costs

Both direct and indirect costs associated with interprofessional practice vary institutionally. In general, the use of an interprofesional team approach can reduce overall costs of care delivery as a result of less service duplication and less redundancy of elder services. An interprofessional approach to patient care also has the potential to reduce medical errors, especially in the area of medication errors. This results not only in administrative cost savings but also in cost savings associated with improved healthcare and improved elder health outcomes.

Administrators should also note cost savings and improved care delivery from a team approach to care. Although overall costs of adding professionals to an interprofessional team may be increased, potential increased productivity and time saving in overall care delivery can counter team member personnel costs. Reductions in waiting times for consultations, understanding about the availability and effective use of resources, and reduction in service duplication are all cost-saving benefits of inteprofessional team care (Mauk, 2018). Administrators can also maximize cost savings through the use of a team approach rather than through individual patient encounters.

Interprofessional Team Challenges

Assisted living administrators should be aware of potential challenges associated with the use of interprofessional teams. Because staffing in the majority of assisted living settings involves the use of unlicensed personnel, professionals may not be hired as full-time employees. This requires professionals to focus on the supervision of unlicensed employees. For example, the assisted living RN would be required to spend time in the supervision of licensed vocational nurses and nursing assistants and would then add teamwork to an existing workload.

Many assisted living settings have employee staffing appropriate for their facility size. Although there are benefits of interprofessional teams composed of professionals from a number of disciplines, hiring these individuals into a small setting may not be feasible. Team building with professionals from different institutions or hiring professionals on a part-time rather than a full-time basis also presents challenges to the overall team functioning and cohesiveness as well as overall team communication and problem-solving capabilities. Professionals from some disciplines may not be readily available or interested in working in assisted living communities and this can also present challenges to assisted living administrators. Issues of quality and safety with use of part-time or volunteer professionals may also be problematic for administrators.

CASE STUDY

MC is a frail 86-year-old female retired school teacher who entered a small assisted living community several years ago primarily because she had no close family and felt very isolated in her prior home. Her health had been stable and she had been able to enjoy many of the facility's social activities, including working with local school children in the facility flower garden, nature walks with a local group of elders, and regular travel for lunch and movies with facility friends. MC was very happy living in the assisted living facility.

During the past 6 months, MC has been experiencing a number of falls, both in the facility and out in the garden and on her walking tours. Falls are a new problem for MC who has not had any prior difficulties with walking or balance. Although the recent falling episodes have not resulted in serious injuries, MC is at risk for significant problems if the falls continue. MC is now worried that if she continues she will be unable to continue her social activities. She also fears that she will have to leave the assisted living community for placement in a long-term care facility.

MC had completed an annual physical about 10 months prior to her falling episodes. The results of the exam were essentially normal. MC's physician conducted another exam which revealed that MC was mildly anemic and that she had experienced a 5-pound weight loss. Because MC was frail, the physician treated her mild anemia and ordered a wheelchair for use when out on her nature walks and traveling with her friends. The assisted living nurses initiated a protocol for falls precautions in MC's room. These strategies helped reduce the number of MC's falls but left her feeling anxious and depressed. The use of the wheelchair meant that MC was no longer able to work in the flower garden. While MC could continue her nature walks, she noted that the walks were not the same.

The RN providing comprehensive care for MC remained concerned about her risk for falls, her weight loss and increasing frailty, and her new and worsening depression connected to the falls and recommended use of a wheelchair. The RN discussed MC's status with the assisted living administrator. Both the RN and the administrator supported an interprofessional approach to care for elders in assisted living facilities.

An interprofessional team consisting of MC's physician and RN, a physical therapist, occupational therapist, social worker, chaplain, dietician, and dentist was convened, and each of the team professionals collaborated on a comprehensive treatment plan for MC. The physical therapist noted that MC would benefit from gait training and muscle strengthening exercises. The occupational therapist felt that MC would not have to only use a wheelchair but could also use a walker or cane to provide stability and could also use a kneeling chair in the flower garden. The social worker identified the importance of MC's social interactions and discussed other possible social activities including a weekly card group and a choir for elders. The chaplain offered to initiate regular visits to informally chat with MC. The dietician identified the need for a comprehensive nutrition analysis for MC to further investigate her weight loss. The dentist noted MC had not been examined by a dentist in many years and recommended a routine exam.

Although the recommendations from each professional on the team provided a comprehensive team-based approach to MC's problems with falls, the assessment data from

(continued)

CASE STUDY

both the dietician and dentist proved to be instrumental in addressing underlying reasons for her falls. MC told the dietician that hard foods hurt her mouth so she drank mostly tea and coffee for each of her meals. MC was not eating enough calories to maintain her weight and was eating foods that resulted in her mild anemia. The dental examination revealed that MC had several severe dental caries that were creating her oral pain and decreased nutritional status. MC was then placed on a high-calorie, high-protein diet and a treatment plan to treat her dental caries was implemented by the dentist. These interventions resulted in a reduction in MC's oral pain, and an ability to increase her intake of nutritionally adequate foods. MC's anemia resolved, she regained several pounds, and stated that she felt stronger. Since implementing the collaborative recommendations from the interprofessional team, MC has not experienced any falls, is less frail, less depressed, and has been able to resume her social activities with her friends.

CONCLUSIONS

Interprofessional care is a team-based and patient-centered comprehensive approach to patient care. For the aging patient, this approach is especially beneficial in addressing the multiple and often complex problems faced by this age group. The benefits of this approach include improved care delivery and reduced costs. Members of interprofessional teams include physicians, nurses, physical therapists, occupational therapists, dieticians, dentists, pharmacists, social workers, and chaplains.

The assisted living administrator can provide an environment for improving care delivery for patients in assisted living settings. Although many smaller facilities will not be staffed with many professionals, administrators can develop strategies to provide a comprehensive team-based approach for elders in assisted living communities.

REFERENCES

American Physical Therapy Association. (n.d). *The role of the physical therapist in national health care reform.* https://www.apta.org

Brandt, B. F (2015). Interprofessional education and collaborative practice: welcome to the "new" forty-year old field. *Advisor,* 9–17. https://doi.org/10.3402/meo.v16i0.6035

Bridges, D. R., Davidson, R. A., Odegard, P. S., Maki, I. V., & Tomkowiak, J. (2011). Interprofessional collaboration: Three best practice models of interprofessional education. *Medical Education Online, 16*(1).

Centers for Medicare & Medicaid Services. (n.d). *History.* http://www.cms.gov/About-CMS/Agency -Information/History/index/html

de Saxe Zerden, L., Lombardi, B. M., & Richman, E. L. (2019). Social workers on the interprofessional integrated team: Elements of team integration and barriers to practice. *Journal of Interprofessional Education & Practice, 17,* 100286. https://doi.org/10.1016/j.xjep.2019.100286

Farrell, T. W., Luptak, M. K., Supiano, K. P., Pacala, J. T., & De Lisser, R. (2018). State of the science: Interprofessional approaches to aging, dementia, and mental health. *Journal of the American Geriatrics Society, 66,* 40–47. https://doi.org/10.1111/jgs.15309

Institute of Medicine. (1972). *Educating for the health team.* National Academy of Sciences.

Institute of Medicine U.S. Committee on Nutrition Services for Medicare Beneficiaries (2000). *The role of nutrition in maintaining health in the Nation's elderly: Evaluating coverage of nutrition services for the Medicare population.* National Academies Press.

Institute of Medicine. (2008). *Retooling for an aging America: Building the health care workforce.* The National Academies Press.

Josiah Macy Jr. Foundation. (2013). Conference Recommendations from: *Transforming patient care: Aligning interprofessional education with clinical practice redesign.* Josiah Macy Jr. Foundation. http://macyfoundation.org/docs/macy.pubs/Transforming Patient Care_ConferenceREc.pdf

Kane, R. (1975). *Interprofessional Teamwork.* University of Syracuse School of Social Work.

Kohn, L. T., Corrigan, J., & Donaldson, M. S. (2000). *To err is human: Building a safer health system.* National Academy Press.

Lutfiyya, M. N., Brandt, B. F., Cerra, F. (2016). Reflections from the intersection of health professions education and clinical practice: The state of the science of interprofessional education and collaborative practice. *Academic Medicine, 91*(6), 766–771. https://doi.org/10.1097/ACM.0000000000001139

Mauk, K. (2018). *Gerontoligical nursing: Competencies for care* (4th ed.). Jones & Bartlett Learning.

Nester, J. (2016). The importance of interprofessional practice and education in the era of accountable care. *N.C Medical Journal, 77*(2), 128–132. https://doi.org/10.18043/ncm.77.2.128

Nursing Licensure.Org. (2019). *Nursing licensure requirements.* http://www.nursinglicensure.org

Oral Health Workforce Research Center. (2016). *Evolving delivery models for dental care services in long-term care settings: 4 state case studies.* School of Public Health University at Albany, State University of New York. www.Oralhealthworkforce.org

PT Solutions. (2019). *Key benefits of occupational therapy for older adults.* https://ptsolutions.com/key-benefits-of-older-adults

Reeves, S., Pelone, F., Harrison, R., Goldman, J. & Zwarenstien, M. (2017). Interprofessional collaboration to improve professional practice and healthcare outcomes. *Cochrane Database of Systematic Reviews.* https://doi.org/10.1002/14651858.CD000072.pub3

Romaszewski, J. K. (2017). The journey to improving access to dental services for individuals in assisted living facilities across North Carolina. *North Carolina Medical Journal, 78*(6), 398–401. https://doi.org/10.18043/ncm.78.6.398

Schmitt, M., Blue, A., Aschenbrener, C.A., & Viggiano, T. R. (2011). Core competencies for interprofessional practice: Reforming health care by transforming health professionals' education. *Association of American Medical Colleges, 86*(11), 1351.

Scope and Standards of Assisted Living Nursing Practice for Registered Nurses. (2006). www.alnursing.org

Standards of Practice for Professional Chaplains in Long-term Care. (2012). https://professionalchaplains.org/file/professional_standards_of_practice/sop_longtermcare.pdf

U.S. Bureau of Labor Statistics. (2019). *Occupational outlook handbook, physical therapists.* https://www.bis.gov/ooh/healthcare/home.htm

Vega, C. P., & Bernarnd, A. (2016). Interprofessional collaboration to improve health care: An introduction. *Medscape.* www.medscape.com

World Health Organization. (2010). *Framework for action on interprofessional education and collaborative practice.* Author. http://www.who.int/hrh/resources/framework_action/en

Young, H. M., & Siegel, E. O. (2016). The right person at the right time: Ensuring person-centered care. *Generations: Journal of the American Society on Aging, 40*(1), 47–55.

Zwarenstein, M., Goldman, J., & Reeves, S. (2009). Interprofessional collaboration: Effects of practice-based interventions on professional practice and healthcare outcomes. *Cochrane Database of Systematic Reviews, 2009*(3). https://doi.org/10.1002/14651858.CD000072.pub2

BUSINESS AND FINANCIAL MANAGEMENT

BUSINESS, MANAGEMENT, AND MARKETING

WITH CONTRIBUTING AUTHOR JOSEPH F. MELICHAR

LEARNING OBJECTIVES

Upon the completion of Chapter 9, the reader will be able to:

- Describe management theories and how they can be implemented in assisted living community (ALC) administration.

- Discuss how creating a management method and style is important to ALC operations.

- Implement a planning framework in order to provide a basis for efficient and effective ALC management and organizational structure.

- Understand business and operational plans, and how they can be used in the management and operation of an ALC.

- Understand the need for and integration of information and technology support systems.

- Understand the importance of marketing, and how it fits into the management and operation of an ALC.

INTRODUCTION

An organization's managers seek the efficient use of resources to meet the end goals and objectives of the organization. For ALCs, the end objectives are related to the provision of residential services tied to the well-being of residents. Knowing the desired outcomes, the issue(s) faced by ALC managers are how to undertake management tasks and then plan for success. Management has been defined as "both science and art" (Buttaro, 1994). There are numerous textbooks and articles addressing the topic of management for an ALC (J. Allen, 1999; Singh, 2010).

This chapter presents an overview on specific management methods that might be used in managing ALCs. The effective use of any management approach is dependent on the description of the organization and its business, operational, and marketing plans. These plans describe the selection and application of an effective management methodology and style. Irrespective of management style, there are constraints that must be met (e.g., budget, schedule, services, etc.); however, the planning system approach is a way of describing operations, expectations, and limitations to enable the execution of an effective ALC management.

This chapter contains fundamental information on (a) management theories; (b) management method and style; (c) general constraints on management and operations; (d) organizing principles; (e) "system" as the basis for organization, management, and evaluation; (f) a framework to create a business and operation plan enabling evaluation of outcomes; (g) evaluation and quality control; (h) business plans; (i) operational plans, (j) information and technology support services, and (k) marketing plans and approaches.

MANAGEMENT THEORIES

Managers control resource transformations into services and the implementation of those transformations. There are a large number of management methodologies with some common threads that include participatory versus nonparticipatory styles, quality control, and constant evolution of product quality. Recurrent themes are also seen in the different methodologies, and in some cases, some of the "latest methodologies" almost appear like fads. It is best to remember the song lyric about everything old being new again (P. Allen & Sanger, 1979), and to develop a management strategy from a mix of approaches, both old and new. The following text outlines some of these management strategies.

Scientific Management

"Scientific management" stems from the work of Taylor (1911), and was developed in a period that reflected "reductionism" as a principle. Taylor described a management approach that reduced management to controlling tasks with a high degree of division of labor. The focus is on producing well-defined tasks within the work profile making it is easier to train and assign workers to the task. The approach initially was focused on activities within a production process of physical objects, but has grown to be used more generally, and is embedded in many subsequent methodologies. Its value to an ALC is the concept of looking at tasks and the division of labor and how these definitions affect the services provided within a broader and more facilitative management process.

Bureaucratic Method

The bureaucratic organizational form (March & Simon, 1958) was first described by the sociologist Max Weber (1947). It features clearly delimited functions that include component elements with rigid boundaries, and well-defined tasks and lines of authority and reporting. A top-down chain of command is created with separation of an organization into functions and outputs. The categorization of function creates rigidity and limits decision-making within each organizational unit.

There is less room for individuality, adaptation, and ability to innovate than in most other forms of management, which spawned the concept of the bureaucratic personality (Merton, 1940). People working in bureaucracies can become authoritative within their small portion of the organization and typically stay within the boundaries created for them. This form tends to be hierarchical, and the amount of authority and control grows as you move up the hierarchy.

There have been a series of analyses that suggest that bureaucratic method can be used without the rigidity and strong control (Alder & Borys, 1996). This view suggests that some of the strong points of this method can be used without accruing its negative aspects. Organizational units can have delimited functions, a clear statement of boundaries, and enunciation of job descriptions. The use of team concepts and internal communications can avoid the rigidity of pure bureaucratic forms. An ALC can use this concept to help frame its organizational structure, and define processes, lines of communication, and the expected lines of authority in different components.

Theory X and Theory Y

During the 20th century, the role of the interpersonal and behavioral aspects of organizational operation and management grew. It could be seen in Merton's (1940) description of bureaucracy and escalated during he 1960s (e.g., Hodge & Johnson, 1970). One major step in this growth was Theory X and Theory Y (McGregor, 1960), which stemmed from Maslow's (1943, 1954) "hierarchy of needs" (i.e., physiological need, safety needs, social needs, esteem needs, and self-actualization). The lowest level indicated a need for control that decreased across the hierarchy to self-actualization at the highest level. Theory X represents an approach that requires external direction and is reflective of a strong top-down authoritarian approach. Theory Y reflects an approach that seeks to develop each person's higher motivations and results in a participatory management style in which people are seen as assets.

Theory X seems to reflect most aspects of a rigid pure bureaucratic form. It assumes employees avoid work when possible, will not take responsibility, need reward systems to perform, and require a high degree of control. Theory Y presents the employee in an opposite manner. The employee becomes a source of support to the organization and is more participatory and can provide a degree of self-management and creative support. The role of the manager changes from controlling and highly directive (X) to facilitative, sharing decision-making, accepting input, and inviting interaction with employees (Y) who are viewed as assets.

Theory Z

Theory Z (Ouchi, 1982) has often been thought of as a blend of Theory X and Y, having more in common with Theory Y. Theory Z was published over 20 years after McGregor's (1960) work and after much of Deming's (1989) work proved successful in Japan. The theory underscores a "management style that focuses on strong company philosophy, a distinct corporate culture, long range staff development, and consensus decision making" (Ouchi, 1982). Theory Z provides many benefits, specifically including an increase in commitment, job satisfaction, and morale.

There is a strong emphasis on participatory management, shared decision-making, a strong organizational commitment, hiring the correct people, and giving them a focal role in their jobs. Ongoing training is important including cross-training of jobs. The managers and employees need to have a shared vision. As changes occur, all members of the organization adapt.

Deming's Management Method

Deming's (1989, 1990, and 1993) management methodology grew from Deming's work in the mid-20th century and focuses on quality of management as well as production outcomes. The framework for producing quality is the Deming cycle (Deming & Walton, 1989): *plan, do, study, and act (PDSA).* A set of 14 points was defined by Deming and became the hallmark of the worldwide application of the Deming concepts. Deming's ideas were initially best received in Japan and many writings on the subject credit this approach as playing a large role in the revival of Japan's post-war economy.

Rienzo (1993) discusses the Deming method, and cites four interacting and interdependent bases for the approach: appreciation for systems, understanding of variation, appreciation and use of knowledge, and insights into human behavior and relationships. Deming's 14 points (2010) are:

(a) create constancy of purpose for improvement of product and service; (b) adopt the new philoso-phy; (c) cease inspection, focus on evidence, and share information; (d) improve the quality of supply and resource and do not focus solely on price; (e) improve constantly improve the system of produc-tion and service; (f) institute education and training (including concept of variation and statistics); (g) adopt and institute leadership and a culture of helping; (h) drive out fear and instill confidence; (i) break down barriers between staff areas; (j) eliminate slogans and targets for the workforce; (k) eliminate numerical standards for the workforce and management; (l) remove barriers and bound-aries that rob people of pride of workmanship; (m) encourage education and self-improvement for everyone; and (n) take action to accomplish the transformation and ever-improving quality.

Deming's work has spawned a number of adaptations of his framework. For example, Anderson et al. (1994) synthesize the steps into seven constructs: visionary leadership, internal and external cooperation, learning, process management, continuous improvement, employee fulfillment, and customer satisfaction. Rienzo (1993) presented a method for applying the Deming management method using a planning framework for service organizations and processes, and is representa-tive of a broad number of application approaches. Deming was well known as a statistician and wrote about the use of statistical methods (1981/1982), and, as pointed out by Grant et al. (1994), the methods developed by Deming evolved from statistical process control with connections to the scientific method. Deming's overall approach is not limited to statistical approaches and has focuses on long-term planning and cooperation between all members of an enterprise (owners, managers, employees, and customers).

Total Quality Management

Total quality management (TQM) places quality and customer satisfaction as an organization's primary focus and is also attributed to Deming (2010). The TQM process was defined by the International Organization for Standardization (ISO) as: "a management approach for an organi-zation, centered on quality, based on the participation of all its members, and aiming at long-term success through customer satisfaction, and benefits to all members of the organization and to society" (ISO 8402, 1994).

TQM was first widely used in Japan and then spread internationally. TQM follows four distinct process steps: (a) continuous improvement, (b) a belief in the process working, (c) understanding how the product is used, and (d) having an aesthetic property.

The TQM step of "continuous improvement" termed *Kazien* (Imai, 1986; Japanese Human Relations Association, 1995; Kotelnikov, 2010) has evolved into a focus of management styles. It is specifically focused on a team-based approach. In Japan, the concept is often imbedded in TQM and is attributed to Deming (1989) and the Deming cycle (namely, *plan, do, study, and act* done in a continuous cycle). The focus is on maintaining continuous improvement in management and the production process (or for an ALC, service processes and outcomes).

Six Sigma

Six Sigma, developed by Motorola in the mid-1980s, is based on improving output quality through reducing defects in output products (DeFeo & Barnard, 2004) and is an outgrowth of TQM. This management procedure evolved from many of the methods described herein and uses the Deming PDSA cycle in the form of: define, measure, analyze, improve, and control. The meth-odology is based on a continuous monitoring of processes and products for control and quality improvement (Juran, 1992).

Six Sigma relies on statistical methodologies based on standard deviations (sigma) from the mean of a normal distribution to achieve its goals. The methodology looks for deviations using a statistical analysis procedure aimed at process control and quality outcomes, and seeks to remediate the problems discovered. This method is usually applied by external consultants, tends to be costly, and is dependent on the ability to define end outcomes in forms adaptable to statistical analysis. The concepts of this approach are useful for an ALC, even if the statistical methodology is less of a fit. A review of its functioning at GE and other large companies is discussed by Morris (1996), and would be useful for ALC managers to review.

Reengineering or Business Process Reengineering

Reengineering or business process reengineering (BPR) involves a review and redesign of an organization and its processes. According to Hammer and Champy (1993, p. 109), reengineering is "the fundamental rethinking and radical redesign of the business processes to achieve dramatic improvements in critical, contemporary measures of performance." BPR is considered a means of significant change in perspective or direction of the organization. Improvements can be sought in the output, production process, product quality, rapidity of production, and management of an enterprise. The focus is on the production or business processes that produce the organization's outcomes, and seem to bear some similarity to the reductionism approach suggested by Taylor (1911). The enthusiasm for the methodology seems to be waning (Davenport, 1995; Weicher et al., 1995), but the concept of periodically looking at the organization and its business and management strategies with a process focus has value for an ALC.

Planning–Programming–Budgeting System

The Planning–Programming–Budgeting System (PPBS) is a methodology (Fisher, 1966; Gorham, 1967) aimed at defining a project or organization, as well as its plan, and looks to see whether the resources are adequate to the task. It also looks to see whether there are scheduling conflicts that would reduce the chances for timely success. If there is an inadequacy, the PPBS process is repeated until a balance is achieved. PPBS was developed in the Department of Defense in the early 1960s to better manage resources relative to desired outputs. Typically, its use was aimed at hardware development in large programs and most often used to develop a budgeting process.

One limitation for a service program is that the PPBS starting point does not sufficiently address context or the desired service direction that is often the basis of human service programs (Melichar, 1972a). One approach to remedying this deficiency is to begin with a description of environment, context, goals, and objectives. Another is to link these elements to each part of the organization, service, and people receiving the service. The methodology suggested for this approach was NOBS (Melichar, 1972a), which was a blend of PPBS and "the systems approach." Not only is it important to reach a balance between input resources and output products in an optimal manner, but it also must identify how the processes are used meet the organization's goals.

Management by Objective

Management by objective (MBO) is a process (Odine, 1965; Drucker, 1981b) of relating outcomes to objectives. Managers hone processes until they produce outcomes defined by initiating objectives. This approach works best when imbedded with a PPBS type of system. One of the problems found by the author is that it is possible to achieve objectives without getting the outcomes desired. At least three potential sources of error occur: (a) the objectives can be badly written and not match the function or operation to which they are related, (b) the objectives may not add up to the goals and expected outcomes (please refer to the goal/objective hierarchy described later in this section), and (c) the measurement to determine the objective specified is in error. The concept is useful if these errors are avoided and is helpful in evaluation and quality control.

Zero Defects

Zero Defects is a methodology for developing quality control in the process of manufacturing products (Crosby, 1982). The goal is to reduce the number of defective products and thereby decrease the cost of production, improve the quality of the end product, increase customer satisfaction, and reduce time spent on inspection and evaluation of the products. This approach has value within an ALC when used within a larger management framework and when the service outcomes are clearly defined.

Likert's Management Approach

Likert (1961, 1967) defined four types of management systems: the *exploitive authoritative system managers decide direction and make decisions based on an organizational hierarchy*; the *benevolent–authoritative system*, which is *similar to the exploitive authoritative system except a reward system is provided within the hierarchy*; the *consultive system*, in which *there is up and down communication within the hierarchy, but decisions are still hierarchical*; and the *participative (group) system*, in which *directions and decisions are made across the organization hierarchy, and there is a shared responsibility for the specific direction and actions taken.*

MANAGEMENT METHOD AND STYLE

A management method can be a mix of multiple methods (see, for example, Hall's [1963] discussion of bureaucracy as a continuum). The method selected should fit the organization as it is defined in the organization's business plan, and should have the support of upper managers. A basis for conflict would exist if a participatory management style was selected and upper managers were focused on authoritative rigidity and control.

In contemporary management, there is a strong focus on team-centered approaches, high degrees of communication, information flow, information support systems, and continuous improvement (plans, outcomes, management, and organization). An ALC needs to frame a management method that fits its goals, approach, and services.

Management Styles

Management often has been defined in terms of participatory versus nonparticipatory styles. In a participatory style, all levels of management can provide input to operations, and thereby produce a horizontal organization structure. A nonparticipatory style has a clearly defined supervisory-subordinate structure (e.g., the bureaucratic form) and follows a vertical framework.

Management styles can also be defined in terms of leadership. Lewin et al. (1939) defined three types of leadership: authoritative, participative, and delegative. The styles also define how an organization will be formulated and managed. The amount of control and delegation of responsibility are implicit. The definition of *management* is similar to that of Likert (1967), who identified four types of leadership: exploitive authoritative, benevolent authoritative, consultative, and participative.

The management methodology selected places limits on the management styles available The style selected will have a large impact on roles, reporting lines, organizational communication, operating tenor of the organization, task definition, and assigned responsibilities. The style defines who makes the decisions and and how decisions will be made in the ALC, and, in turn, shapes the character of the service process of delivery. The nonparticipatory and participatory styles of management are discussed in the following subsection. Lewin's delegative style is not included as it reduces the amount of control available, which seems appropriate for a service organization, except with regard to highly specific services (e.g., medical).

Top-Down or Nonparticipatory Management

The top-down or nonparticipatory management style is typically defined as following Theory X (McGregor, 1960, 2002) and the bureaucratic form of management. Lines of authority are clearly delineated starting from the upper levels of management to the lower levels. There are clearly defined roles, delineated boundaries, and very strict lines of authority, control, and reporting. Any ideas and all control and decisions flow from the top down. There are times where rigidity is important, for example in life-threatening situations when consensus management may be inappropriate.

Likert (1967) also described a "benevolent authoritative" leadership style that had a reward system as its basis. This style still has top-down control, and limits control and participation in decision-making by subordinates. This style does not provide very good communication to others about problems noted, as it lacks feedback and isolates innovation from subordinates.

There are useful concepts in the bureaucratic form that can be used without absorbing their weaknesses. By loosening the rigidity of the form, the delineation of roles, lines of communication, definition of tasks and processes, creation of organizational units and structure, and lines of authority can be useful in considering how the ALC creates its management. For example, the definition of tasks does not mean there cannot be shared responsibility and decision-making.

Participatory Management

A participatory management style is part of McGregor's (1960, 2002) Theory Y and also is described in TQM and Kaizen methods (Wilson, 2013). This management styles uses a horizontal structure with weaker lines of authority and supervisory control. The management of the enterprise is more team focused with shared input and decision-making

Team building has become part of the participatory management landscape. The use of a team includes a broader range of inputs and talents for management, planning, operations, decision-making, and quality control. There is shared responsibility across the team and within the organization. One example of this approach is the use of Kaizen (Wilson, 2013).

The team approach places a high value on knowledge and stresses the need to educate team members. The team approach still maintains lines of control, definition of roles, lines of authority, and information as well as flow. Constraints do exist on the team and its activities in the form of budgetary limitations, for example. Team participation is aimed at consensus, but there are times when a decision must be made and requires a determination of who will make it. As a service organization, an ALC cannot become dysfunctional, nor can a lack of a team decision negatively influence the residents.

Mixed Management Styles and Style Selection

A pure form of any management style is unlikely to exist. A better approach is to define a mixed management approach, based on all of the different management methods. In the planning framework suggested later in this chapter, there are references to almost all of the management methods defined earlier. For example, the overall structure of the planning system is a variation of the PPBS approach, and includes elements of the bureaucratic form, has a goal-tree structure, is amenable to the use of MBO, and is consistent with TQM. The goal tree is a simple exercise that can help take a customer from a specific stated requirement to a more general and valuable goal, then back to the correct specific requirement. This is done to establish that the stated requirement, and the real underlying goal (business goal), are in fact linked.

Rather than first selecting a specific management method, it would be more fruitful to decide how management will be used in the ALC. An ALC might consider what type of control structures it will use, and how decisions will be made within and across the organization. The approach also might include some areas of management in which the residents have input. An ALC has different focuses at different parts of the organization, and the mix of styles can vary by amount, focus, organizational level, or other organizational parameters. The selected management framework, a mix of styles, and how they will be used should be made known across the ALC.

MANAGEMENT AND ORGANIZATIONAL STRUCTURE

The management method and style selected need to be integrated into the overall organization and its operation. The development of management and organizational structures needs to include the following: (a) line staff relationships—who reports to whom and for what functions, (b) staffing of the organization, (c) organization chart, (d) a delineation of decision-making and authority as well as control, (e) internal and external feedback systems, (f) functions of the components of the organization with a clear delineation of responsibilities, and (g) definition of the information flow lines and how they are to be used.

It has been argued (J. Allen, 1999) that an ALC can be separated into an upper, middle, and lower-level management structure with staff to carry out the directions of the managers. In a more horizontal organizational structure with a participatory style, these conceptual distinctions are less clear.

Constraints on Management and Operations

An ALC is managed under some fixed constraints, methodological limitations, and a large number of truisms:

1. The management approach must fit within the budgetary limitations of the ALC. Management should remain the means to achieve success and not be the end purpose.

2. The implementation of the management functions must fit the size of the organization. The discussions of the leadership roles often are by identification of key managers (e.g., executive, operating, financial, and compliance officers each with staff support). An ALC may not afford this executive staffing level, yet management must still fulfill the functions through existing staff sharing responsibility for the functions.

3. There is no universally accepted "best management approach." The best fit could vary with the ALC, its staff, and the management team's personalities. In some cases a highly structured top-down organization is appropriate; in most situations it is the antithesis of a good approach.

4. The management approach and methodology should fit the needs and services of the ALC as opposed to selecting a management methodology, and then fitting the needs and services to the management methodology.

5. When examining both the overarching ALC organization and its specific components and activities, it is good to remember the often-stated truism "everything is connected to everything else" (generally paraphrasing John Muir [1911]). It is important not only to define the ALC's goals, activities, components, and functions, but also to describe how they are connected and reliant upon each other, and on the information requirements, flows, and exchanges needed to efficiently operate the ALC and its services. For a general review of management operations, see Lewis and Black (2003).

Organizing Principles

As many of the management methods share common elements, it seems best to facilitate this chapter's intended discussion by creating an appropriate management style, methodology, and approach for an ALC using the following organizing principles: (a) management is an ongoing and dynamic process; (b) adaptation and evolution are integral to developing the management process, the ALC organization, and the services it provides; (c) management and staff must focus on the quality of service outcomes and the well-being of residents; (d) feedback from across the organization into the management process is central to the improvement of outcome quality, management, operational service processes, and organizational development; (e) in order for feedback to occur there must be a set of organizational directions and an overarching plan, a set of operational plans, clarity of goals and objectives, a monitoring and measurement system, and clearly defined feedback and information flow lines; (f) communication within and across the organization is critical to successful management; and (g) information collection, flow, availability, control, and reporting are important to the communication process, oversight, and management. In simple terms, you cannot fix a problem of which you are unaware.

There is a broad collection of literature that defines the concept and creation of an organization that stems from the seminal work of March and Simon (1958, 1993). An organization must be structured and have a stated purpose and direction. A review of the literature finds the term *system* used repeatedly. The "systems" concept (Churchman, 1968; Von Bertalanfy, 1968) refers to the principles selected to plan and review an ALC's organization and its business and operational plans. Supportive and broadening views of the "systems concept" can be found in descriptions of "purposeful systems" (Ackoff & Emory, 1972), "observing systems" (Von Forester, 1981), and "inquiring systems" (Churchman, 1971).

System as the Basis for Organization, Management, and Evaluation

In the heuristic chosen, *system* is joined by *structure* and *process* (Melichar, 1972a, 1972b) in a method for framing the organization, its services, operation, and projects. A systems representation of a management framework, business, and operational plans are models of the ALC and its operation. An evaluation framework is included and should ascertain how closely operations match the organization's plans and models.

A systems model of the organization includes all the organizational components as contributing subsystems, which, in turn, can have subsystems. A hierarchy is created that includes relationships and connections within the system model that is representative of the organization's structure within its environment and context. Each component and its activities, tasks, and processes can be identified along with timelines and outcomes attached that form the service processes. The framework creates a basis for planning, evaluation, information flow, service provision, and management. The system diagrams make it possible to trace the flow of events, resources, and directives, as well as organizational connections, lines of authority, resource flows, and information flows. In using this single approach it is possible to outline: (a) a business model; (b) an operational plan and planning system; (c) an evaluation system; (d) a resource management framework; (e) an organizational chart clearly defining jobs, responsibilities, staff, and so on; (f) service process models, including definition of desired outcomes; (g) information systems; and (h) what the residents should expect in addition to definitions of their well-being.

The approach used in framing the organization, its components, and activities acts as a foundation for the business plan and then the operational plan. The framework helps to address the full range of an ALC's organization and operation, and provides a way to tie the pieces together and form the basis for its management. This includes evaluation, a focus on quality, cost containment, and efficient use of resources. In the next section, a common planning framework for all aspects of an ALC is therefore presented.

Planning Framework

The following is a framework for planning, operation, and management of an ALC under the system-type model (for an alternative, see Siegal et al., 1993). The framework (Melichar, 1972a) includes a direct link to the evaluation process and feedback loops that facilitate a constant improvement process, leading to improved quality. Each part of the framework enables better use of management practices by indicating "what is to be managed" and the ALC's structure with integration of all its parts and activities. The planning process is a means for improving management, operations, and service outcomes and is not an "end" outcome. The components of the planning framework are presented in Figure 9.1 and are briefly discussed in the text that follows.

The *environment* sets the *context* and boundaries of the unit being described or planned. The business plan would differ from either the view of the overall operations or a unit of the organization. The ALC as an organization is responding to a *need* within the environment that also helps define its purpose. The lack of clear need limits the potential for the success of the ALC. The clearer the statement of need within the ALC environment, the more focused the business and marketing plans, and their operations.

The transition from need and purpose to set ALC directions occurs by defining *goals and objectives*. The format for developing the goals and objectives can best be done by developing them in a hierarchy in the form of a goal tree (for a description of the use of goal trees, see Kavakli & Loucopoulos, 2004). An example of a hierarchical goal tree is presented in Figure 9.2. The topmost level is an overarching, or supragoal, which is then broken into contributing goals, followed by subgoals, objectives, and subobjectives (if needed).

The creation of a goal/objective hierarchy should be consistent with the structure of the organizational components and their functions and activities (or organizational units such as departments). The individual components will share common goals and objectives, or in terms of the hierarchy, a branch of the goal tree. A good check on organizational direction is to define a separate set of *expected outcomes* to assure that the goals and objectives defined lead to produced services and outcomes.

The next step is to define *strategies* by which to transform the statement of intent, purpose, goals, and objectives into the activities required, in addition to the functions and tasks to be performed, and the organizational components needed to carry them out (this also creates an organization chart). The organizational components and their activities are the processes that form the services created. The description should include: reporting, lines of control, authority, support services, and information requirements and control. Once the activities, components, and services are identified, then the needed *staffing* can be identified. The type and amount of staff needed to carry the service outcomes can be described.

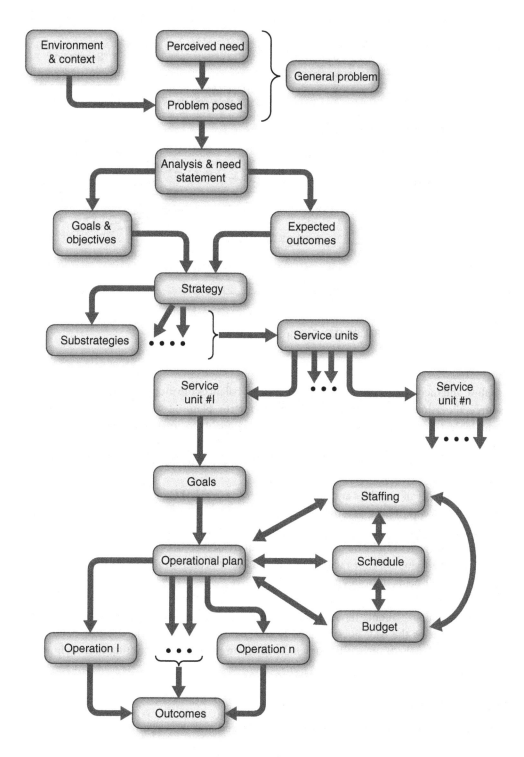

FIGURE 9.1 Planning format.

A *schedule* should be defined for the various service and nonservice activities, reports, operational milestones, decisions, and all other milestones. Based on the activities schedule, the *general resources* needed to operate them can be defined and may include: staff, facility, maintenance,

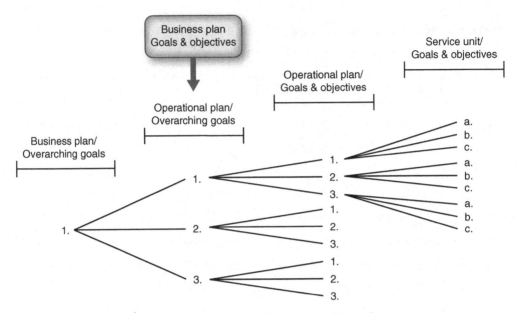

FIGURE 9.2 Example of a goal-tree hierarchy.

cash flow, and income sources. The *budgeting* process balances the income needs, income sources, resource allocations, and resource requirements for the planning unit being considered. The overall budget must ensure that income and expense are at the least equal. The preceding definitions create the basis for an *evaluation system* (Figure 9.3) that provides the measures of performance, outcomes, and client satisfaction, and establish the basis for quality control and effective management.

The multiplicity of variables and competing interests in an ALC require an *iterative* use of the planning framework. Using iterative planning will balance a budget, reduce conflicts between organizational elements, and produce better resource allocations to organizational components and services. Changes can be made in the ALC if future occurrences differ from those forecasted in planning the framework, or the evaluation and quality control program concerning services and resident well-being indicates problems.

The planning framework provides a means of looking at the ALC or any component and its operation and management. The manner in which that framework is used and implemented is a decision made by the ALC governing body and management team. The decision could range from simply using the framework, informally reviewing the ALC, or drafting thorough written plans.

Evaluation Systems and Quality Control

Once business and organization plans are implemented and the organization is operational, a tendency can occur to let the operation simply continue and to only deal with problems that arise. The system model presents an alternate strategy using a continuous system of evaluating performance of both the total operation and its components. The purpose of this system is to ensure that goals and objectives are being met, the overall facility and its components and services are effective, residents are receiving appropriate care, residents' well-being and outlook are positive, resources are adequate and effectively controlled, and all laws and regulations are met.

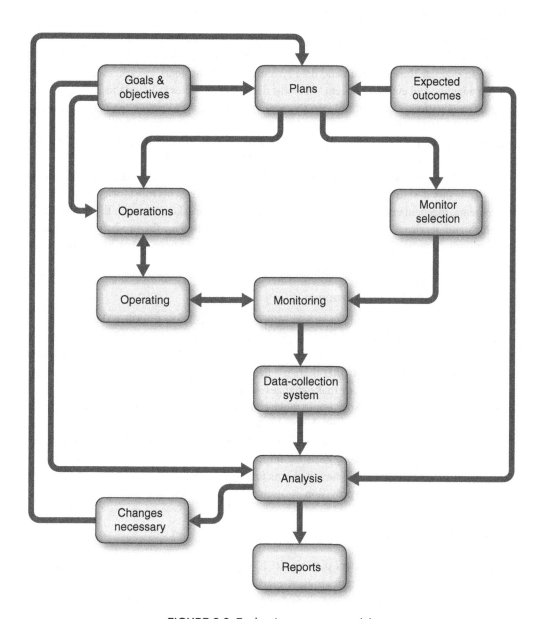

FIGURE 9.3 Evaluation process model.

Evaluation Strategies, Feedback Loops, and Quality Management

An evaluation process provides a clear picture of how the facility operates and should provide feedback to aid in managing service and support processes and identify problems. The development and maintenance of an evaluation system and quality management plan is dependent on monitoring defined parameters and their reporting to management. The feedback loops need to be developed in the operational plan along with the needed measures and procedures for transmitting evaluation results to management and the ALC operational units.

An effective information system will enable both capture and control of data and can become the repository for feedback. One caveat of this system is that simply providing data and feedback does not assure action on that information. The overall evaluation design must include: the methodology, techniques, reports, and schedules needed to ensure the data accrued are effectively used.

The evaluation system is integral to the information system. A profile of who needs what information, and when they need it, is an important part of the design. The design must also include methods to evaluate the evaluation and data systems. One of the goals, as earlier defined, was to create an adaptive and evolving system—it is this design that enables meeting this end.

For any evaluation or measure of effectiveness, it is important to define the target measures (e.g., goals, objectives, intents, and types of information). Evaluation and management support information are based on having a meter to measure against. In simplistic terms, one cannot determine what "end" was accomplished if that "end" was never defined. Ad hoc afterthoughts do not offer overly effective information; the information requirements need to be designed as part of the facility design and management system. These requirements must include compliance requirements, mechanisms to protect residents, and support an ALC's focus on the quality of its operations and services. A TQM-type methodology that focuses on the production of quality in a continuous manner, by looking at process outcomes and customer satisfaction, requires an appropriate evaluation and information support system.

Evaluation and the Change Process

Once an evaluation is completed, an organization must decide how to utilize the information gathered to better its operation and ensure quality. An ALC has been presented as a multi-tiered organization that has multiple component activities, supports, and services. The evaluation data must be weighed to determine whether there is a need to change the overall structure of the organization, alter the system model, or make changes in components, processes, or services. A decision is also required as to whether or not to make small corrections on a continuous basis (typical of TQM approaches), or more abrupt changes as in the BPR methodology. Whatever decision is made, any change must focus on service processes and their outcomes; include an adaptive process for the organization; offer a basis for improvement; provide ways to adapt to changing conditions or new knowledge; and have a means to correct failure to meet goals and objectives, correct less than optimal service provision, or improve its cost basis.

THE BUSINESS PLAN

An ALC operates under a business plan model (Osterwalder et al., 2004; Ing, 2009) that also serves as an ongoing overarching or strategic plan for the organization. The operational plan is a separate entity but uses the business plans direction to guide the operation of the facility and functions as a mechanism to transform input resources into resident-centered outcomes. The two plans serve the organization differently, and although they share a common interface, they must be kept separate.

The business plan should address exactly what is expected from the business and its creation as described in Figure 9.4. The expectations should address: (a) fiscal resources such as expected income and cash-flow requirements; (b) the expectation of added resources from external agencies and community sources; (c) the services expected from the board of directors; (d) the expected mix of residential types and expected occupancy rates; (e) reporting of progress of the organization toward expectations by management; (f) the services to residents, their well-being, and the quality expected to be provided; (g) management performance; and (h) potential staff availability and the community's demographic profile.

The business plan focuses on the viability of the organization, the oversight of the ALC's operation, and is used to review the effectiveness of its operation. Typically, the business plan is focused

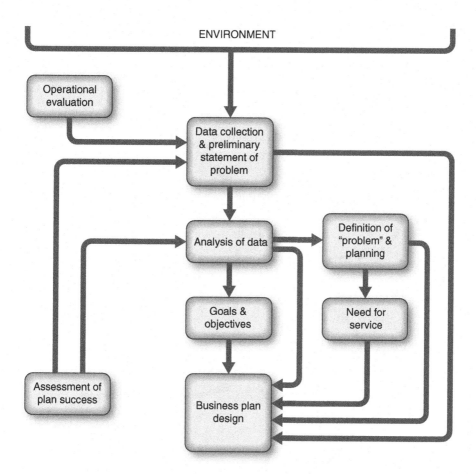

FIGURE 9.4 Business plan development.

on issues addressed by investors, owners, and/or the board of directors. This section reviews some of the main aspects of the business plan, but due to space limitations, it is not put into the planning system framework as earlier described.

Business Plan Perspectives

An organization is a system of interacting parts (as described earlier and summarized in Figure 9.5). This system (ALC) can be viewed from many different aspects, and may appear different to various viewers (operators, providers, residents, families of residents, staff, managers, and external agencies), each with a unique perspective and desired set of outcomes from the ALC. In total, they create an overall sense of the organization and its operation, and yet they all are a part of it. The organization's management must take these perspectives into account while maintaining or producing a steady organizational framework, ongoing operations, the input resources needed to underwrite the operations, marketing and acquiring residents, and the desired outcomes from the business model.

The identification of organizational and management approaches, along with organizational components, begins with the business model. The business model addresses how the overall organization is formulated, the desired operational strategy, and the financial model needed to

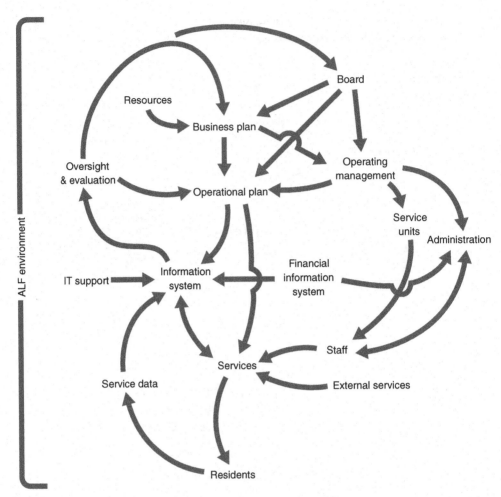

FIGURE 9.5 Business plan overview schematic.
ALF, assisted living facility.

maintain operations. The business plan presents what the facility intends to produce, its resource utilization approach, and a timeline for major outcomes. From that framework, the business plan can develop, monitor, and maintain a plan of operation to actualize its goals.

The business plan should show organizational components and the interrelation of those components that is needed to make each part of the organization a performing entity within the overall ALC system. Each operation is integrated with the other operations to provide the residential care services. Management is the control element of these processes and occurs relative to the entire organization or to any of its components. Each component must fit into the overall system that is the facility, and thereby the management of each component must synergistically fit within the overall ALC management.

Business Plan Issues

The first step in creating a business plan is to develop and/or maintain a viable business model. A business model evolves from the following questions: What is the organization to be? What are its goals? How will it maintain itself economically? How will it operate? A business plan should at a minimum answer these questions in a clearly written statement that becomes the organization's framework for its existence and operation. The business plan should also be viewed as a strategic plan that at a minimum includes: (a) the context and environment for the organization, including competing services; (b) the purpose and goals of the organization and the services it will provide; (c) the resources required and how they will be used, including cash-flow requirements, estimated income and expenses, and sources of income; (d) who is/will be served, including a target popu-lation profile; (e) the time frame of the business plan and its components; (f) business strategies; (g) facility operation; and (h) an understanding of consumers and their expectations.

Furthermore, the real estate market in the area should be surveyed. One reason for this is that the ALC either owns a real property or is leasing a real property. The business plan needs to address how the real property is treated as an asset and cost item, which includes its cost basis, assets, and liabilities. Competing services that may affect income streams should also be identified, and as well as the number of clients served, cost profile, type of clients served, the res-idential-unit mix, and a general organizational structure. This information along with knowledge about the target population should also help identify an advantageous residential-unit mix and becomes an internal resource for the facility's planning, financing, and marketing.

The data should determine whether it is advantageous to target populations that are differ-ent from those sought by competing services, to focus on private clients versus public support, low- versus high-income groups, or consider focusing on underserved populations. Marketing of the facility should be addressed. Even if an effective facility is created, there is little social or eco-nomic value if the facility is not populated with residents. The issue is described in the Marketing Approaches section found at the end of this chapter.

The community in which the facility exists helps to define some of the parameters in planning. It enables planning to take advantage of community resources or lack thereof. Will the residents be drawn only from the community? Does the community accept and encourage this type of facility? What is the pool of workers available for staffing needs? Is there adequate housing in the community for the staff? What is the cost of living in the service area? Links to other organiza-tions in the community (including a parent company if a chain or franchise) should be identified as well as potential partners and services available to the ALC and its residents.

The preceding framework is useful as both a start-up guide and prospectus, but should be updated as the facility evolves. It should provide a basis for assessing how a facility is doing for both management and its oversight board. The framework also provides a set of parameters in planning the operation and services of the facility and is an important element in maintaining the ALC's focus over time.

Once operational, a facility must look at how it is performing from the multiplicity of per-spectives described in the business plan. Is it meeting the goals and objectives as outlined in the business plan, in addition to the processes of the operational activities? Are resources being used effectively and are costs being controlled? Can the facility and its services be improved? Are the needs of residents, resident's families, and staff being met? Is the operation meeting all regulatory requirements? The business plan should provide methods for continuously looking at these ques-tions systematically, and how to best make changes based on the assessment of performance as was earlier addressed.

Business Plan Directions

The ALC exists for a specific reason and should be defined as part of the business plan (or overall strategy) in a clear statement of purpose, goals, and expectations to substantiate the "why" of the organization. The ALC's core ideology should be clear and part of the basis for determining the direction set by the board. The business plan should include residents' perspectives and the ALC's expectations for maintaining the well-being and satisfaction of residents.

The definition of expectations should include how the organization will adapt to change (economic, cultural, informational, capital, and technological). If the organization is not in a static environment, it should have an adaptive potential built into its strategic plan. Lack of adaptive potential means that at some point the organization will become uncompetitive and unresponsive to the needs that it addresses.

A clear set of financial goals and objectives (including time frames) used to rate accomplishments should be identified. This identification should form the basis for the overall financial operation of the ALC and represent the requirements and outcomes expected by owners, investors, and the board. The financial plan's goals and objectives should be identified, and include the organization's operational, financial, and management strategies.

A set of goals and objectives needs to be defined for the board of directors. This is a statement of intent, and should frame the expectations of the board, criteria for board membership, and expected performance guidelines. The role of the board with respect to the business plan, how the board will evaluate the achievement of the business plan, and how the board itself will be evaluated should be included in the set of goals and objectives.

The business plan should address exactly what is expected from the business. The expectations should address: (a) financial issues such as income and cash-flow requirements; (b) the expectation of added resources from external sources; (c) the services expected from the board of directors; (d) the expected mix of residential types and the expected occupancy rates; (e) reporting oft progress of the organization toward expectations by management; (f) the services to residents, their well-being, and the quality of care to be provided; and (g) the internal management performance.

Implementation Strategy

The business plan should address the framework and methods needed to implement the plan. This strategy is focused on the creation and maintenance of the ALC, and not the operational level strategies. The basis for the marketing of the ALC should be identified. The method for transitioning the business plan into the operational and marketing plans should be addressed.

The strategy should address the physical building as well as how the insurance requirements of the business plan will be addressed. The mix of housing types within the ALC operation and the business model used need to be addressed as well. The framework for any financial arrangements should be addressed. The way the ALC will relate to other services in the area needs to be taken into consideration. A strategy for developing a management framework for the operation of the ALC should be defined.

Activities and Services to Be Provided

The result of the preceding suggestions should enable description of the organizational framework, including its main components and the activities needed to maintain viable operation of the ALC and any constraints or limitations it faces. The structure of the board should be identified along with its operational guidelines and the roles to be ascribed to the board. A similar description should be provided for the operational units and any activities needed to meet the ALC goals, objectives, expectations, and strategies. The differentiation of positions and roles, flow of resources, information, services, and authority should be identified, which in turn will create the basis for identifying activities within the operational plan and their execution. A framework for the ALC's information system should be addressed along with the technological framework required for the physical building, services offered, management and administrative needs, and technologies to be offered to residents.

Resources: Available Income and Input–Output Expectations

The operation of the facility has been described as the transformation of input resources into outputs. The business plan should outline the expectations of the output creation to the input resources. The determination of input–output transformation is based on the sources of the input flow of resources and monies, and the determination of output is defined by the operational plans across the organization. The budget process involves matching these inputs and outputs.

The business plan should define the expected and existing resources of the facility. Resources include the facility, equipment, staff, community resources, and income. The resources also should include the cash flow and monies needed to supplement income flow and lags in payment. Specific definitions of access to cash, via loans or other sources, need to be explicitly defined. The definition of resources should be extended to include existing and expected sources of income.

Organizations acting as resources to the ALC include those related to services in the community or those that might exist within the ALC. Additionally, these resources may be external if the facility is a franchise or chain. Some of the most basic external services are the healthcare and social services systems. Links to educational facilities and other training sources should be identified as these programs are needed to maintain licensure in many different disciplines, as well as providing the ALC with interns and graduates.

The business plan should also identify general categories of expenses: facility costs, administrative costs, management costs, overhead ratio, operational cost profiles, and the ability to carry out the operation(s) during periods when expenses exceed income. The adjustment of income and expenditure on a scheduled basis should be a part of the business plan. The budget also should review the value of the real property of the ALC and provide a periodic financial report.

The budgeting process has to be iterative. Part of the input resource flow is the income stream from the residents. The sources of income per resident must be defined, as well as the expected total population. The definition of the output or services provided is the basis of the cost estimates and the monies that must be accrued. The timelines for all financial parameters, fiscal reports, and general performance reports should be included.

Evaluation and Quality Control

The business plan should define how the organization as a whole deals with the concept of quality and evaluation of quality, customer satisfaction, operational performance, cost-effectiveness, and management performance. The board and those in top management positions need to identify how they want to be informed of quality and performance matters.

The business plan evaluation process will lead to necessary revisions of the plan to maintain effective operation of the facility. Performance assessments and analysis of operations must be provided in a feedback loop to the board and upper management. If target goals are not being met (financial, operational, service, etc.), then the business plan needs to be reviewed and appropriate changes made. In turn, the operational plan and the actual operation must be adjusted. These revisions could alter the business model or any of the various operations undertaken within that model. Cost-benefit and cost-effectiveness can be included in the evaluation.

Implementation Design

The business plan should also address the implementation to form operational units and processes. There need to be links between the strategic business and operation plan, and activity. Defining how the broad targets and directions are transformed into the specificities of an operational plan and process is important. The goal of the implementation design is to provide a basis for the operational plan and service operation.

OPERATIONAL PLAN AND PLANNING SYSTEM

The business plan focuses on overall strategies, whereas the operational plan and planning system focus on the organization and operations that make the facility function (Figure 9.6). The operational plan takes direction from the business plan, but transforms the broad strategy into an organizational structure with an organization chart, goals and objectives, management, administration, financial and bookkeeping activities, functioning service units, output processes and services, and operational control mechanisms. The control mechanisms also aid in determining effectiveness measures for any component, component activity, and service, as well as their use of resources.

Managers must maintain control, effectiveness, and focus within the organization. Some control points are resource utilization and the budget, service program control, monitoring process, quality controls, and resident inputs. Inherent to management is providing leadership for the ALC and supporting leadership within the components of the organization.

The Environment and Context

The external environment, context, and general constraints can be drawn from the business plan. On the operational level, it is the physical building; support services; board directives; internal support; and community inputs, services, and resources that form the operational environment. These elements are the resources management can draw upon to inform the constraints on operations, ancillary service availability, and the ALC's overall environment. The environment will vary between ALCs, communities, and even the neighborhoods in the same community.

The strengths and weaknesses of the ALC should be identified along with its neighborhood and the safety of that area. Local community resources available to residents (e.g., banks, library, markets, post office, restaurants, stores, etc.) should be identified along with the availability of transportation, healthcare, and recreational services. The impact of local weather on residents should be reviewed, along with methods for adjusting services offered for either good or bad weather according to season.

Goals, Objectives, and Expectations

Goals and objectives should be set for overall management and for individual services and they should remain consistent with the business plan. A goal tree should be used to enable increasing specificity of goals for service operations. Each branch of the goal tree should reflect one component of the ALC (e.g., maintenance or food services). The upper portions of the goal structure should provide common links across the organization and to the business plan.

After defining subgoals in each branch, an objective hierarchy should be crafted with the final objectives being specific to each service. The definition of objectives includes: "who will do, by what, by when, as measured by" helping to define a specific direction and basis for evaluation. The lower level objectives should combine to form the ones above them. Providing a separate

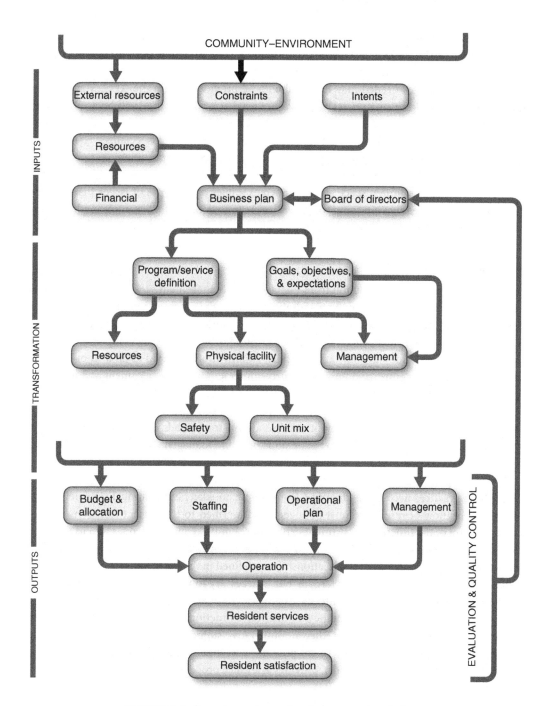

FIGURE 9.6 Overview schematic of an operational plan.

statement of expected outcomes for the ALC and each service offered will enable an assessment of the effectiveness of the operational plan's goals and objectives.

Strategies, Component Units, and Activities

A strategy is needed to implement the various goals and objectives for specific organizational units (e.g., reception or food services) and their services. The strategy should comprise all parts of the organization and the services offered to residents. The management of the ALC and each component should be defined, in addition to the planning, coordination, and integration of components into one service and operating system.

The support services needed may not be able to be provided within the ALC. Management must identify the lacking support services that *are* needed, and how they will be acquired and then integrated into the organization. Some possible examples of contracted services are accounting, bookkeeping, payroll, billing, maintenance, food services, reception, specialized resident services, information services, technology support, nursing service, transportation, and safety.

Each of the organization services needs to be addressed independently. As addressing each cannot be done in the limited space available, two examples of the types of issues that must be addressed for each organization component/service are provided. The first example is administration, and information and technology services are discussed in the following subsection.

Administration Example

Administration is a separate function from management. Management seeks to provide the best use of resources in a facilitative manner. Administration is the combination of support services needed to maintain the organization and its operation. Administrative services generally do not include direct client services, with the possible exception of support in the completion of forms needed to maintain residents' status at the facility. Administration serves as an arm of management to maintain the control and flow of resources, interaction with government and insurance agencies, banking services, and internal control of personnel and budgeting issues.

Like management, there is a multiplicity of definitions of administration and its functions. What is important to the ALC is how it defines administration, administrative functions, the support it provides, its integration into the organization, and management's expectation for input from the administrative unit.

Maintaining control of the flow of monies into and through the organization is needed. Accounting practices need to be identified from simple bookkeeping to annual statements. The inflow and outflow of resources must be logged and ascribed to the correct functions/departments; control of the function/department expenditures must be maintained, as well as methods to develop and maintain payroll, billing, and control of receivables. There also must be a strategy for defining banking and borrowing relationships as defined in the business plan. The accounting function can be met internally or externally but is necessary to use resources expeditiously and produce good cost-benefit and cost-effectiveness.

Personnel services also are part of the administrative function. The services must be provided as part of the management design. Other administrative support services also must be identified. For example, a personnel department provides personnel support services (e.g., taxes and insurance), provides employee support, provides grievance procedures, and remains current with human resources requirements.

Schedule, Staffing, Resources, and Budget

The schedule for each activity identified should be defined to ensure that processes/activities are completed in a timely manner. The schedules for different functions may have a large variation (e.g., schedules for daily, weekly, monthly, and annual time horizons).

A staffing profile needs to be created for all the components and activities within the ALC. The staffing profile needs to identify the education, skills, and experience required for each staff position. Job descriptions should be produced from the staffing profile, as well as the resources for finding appropriate staff, and the methods needed to locate them. Interviewing methods should also be identified, and a salary profile for the staff types must be set.

The budget and resources needed to operate the ALC, by component and activity, should be defined and matched to the activities defined, including staffing and the schedule. The balancing of activity and resources should be an ongoing process. The ALC needs to provide guidelines to the components and activities of the resources allocated to them, and create a feedback loop for those expenditures that need to be identified.

It is important to define how the information from the units will flow back to management and administration. Control systems need to be identified, and support systems for the ALC's activities need to be provided. The link to management, administration, record and reporting systems is important to define and maintain.

Evaluation and Quality Control

An evaluation system for the entire ALC and each of its components and activities should be designed from the goals and objectives. The operational plan needs to define how to measure the progress toward the objectives and performance quality established. Measures of some performance, such as maintenance, can be made using hard measures, but measures of resident well-being and satisfaction will be harder to define. In both instances, quality of the organization's output is dependent upon these monitors, and how the data retrieved is reported and used. These feedback loops are the basis for ongoing planning and quality control.

INFORMATION AND TECHNOLOGY SUPPORT SERVICES

The technical nature of our society is such that any ALC will house multiple technological systems. These systems provide support to the ALC's administrative, management, financial, and direct care services. The physical facility also includes a range of technologies that include heating and air-conditioning, safety, and security. Patient services include both support systems for the provision of care, but also for the use of residents' recreation and communication. The facilities are likely to have a wireless network, patient data online, medication control systems, and many other support services.

The management team needs to be aware of technological advances and new methodologies. The goal is to increase and improve service levels, and to utilize technologies that help to control costs. The internet has also become a resource for management, staff, and residents.

As with every benefit, there are associated costs. The facility is responsible for locating, evaluating, securing, and maintaining the system, in addition to training users. The ALC must have an IT department or equivalent services. The technical support staff becomes an increasing cost, while the technologies themselves become less expensive per unit function.

Information Systems

Organizations run on information. Systems are needed to accrue, manage, and make this information available in appropriate reports and queries. The sustainment of various organization functions is dependent on the information system chosen. Equally important is that the information system be integrated into the operational and management system. Cost savings come from synergy and meeting the needs of the entire staff. The system design must look at how the various organization processes use the information, and how the information gathered is put back into the system.

The information management system should be created as part of the overall facility design. The information system must be an integral part of the management and operational plans. The information system design process includes identifying (a) the supported processes within the organization; (b) how the information will be used by various staff, departments, and management; (c) the monetary costs and staff time costs of information (designing a system that increases staff demands over gains is not desirable); (d) the information needs of the evaluation, compliance, and quality- control system implemented by the facility; (e) the security needed at different levels of the organization; (f) who will share what information (e.g., administration may only need a portion of patient information, and direct services will not access personal and payroll records); and (g) who has overall responsibility for the information and information system.

Records Systems

One function of an information system is to maintain an organization's records. Part of an ALC's design is to determine what records are required to be maintained, and what additional information will be required by the organization to operate effectively. Information collection, control, management, and storage all have costs. The concept of "necessary and sufficient" should be a controlling concept but must be applied to all parts of an organization. What is necessary for the service process may be soporiferous for administration and vice versa.

Once a data system has been designed, built, and implemented, perhaps the most costly aspect of its operation is the collection of data. A careful review is needed to determine how the data will be gathered on a continuing basis, and what technologies can be used to reduce the costs in both monies and staff time. The definition of when and how data is collected may also determine its utility and uses.

The selection of information gathered has to be developed by department, section, function, or task. It must also fit within the processes undertaken by each component/service both in terms of their operational and functional needs, and how the recording of the information will fit into their day-to-day operations. These definitions also determine the parameters of the information system: input processes, data availability, reporting, interactive data, and patient support services. Some elements may have common uses; for example, provision of medications and their control provide support to service staff, protection of patients from wrong medications, inventory control, and fiscal reporting.

Resident Records System

The management system must identify which records about each resident are needed, and how the data will be recorded and accessed. There should be implemented a reliable set of standards concerning the amount and type of personal information, medical information, medication history, services provided, location, schedules, and support services assigned to each resident. Any compliance data (HIPAA) required must also be integrated. This records system is typically integrated into the overall information system of the facility with privacy and security safeguards.

The more technology is used, the more the facility is responsible for providing adequate support staff that is knowledgeable about "computing." As the ALC's resident records, medication lists, and schedules become computerized, the amount of time that the computer system can be down decreases without it influencing ALC operations. The need for available and knowledgeable staff increases in order to gain the rapid response in maintaining the information technology. The availability of computer support staff makes responses to problems timelier and better, but at the cost of providing the support.

Technical and Technology Support

The main support requirement will be in the information technology and computing areas. The various technologies utilized will be to improve systems and will require upgrades and staff support of these systems. The facility itself will have a series of technological systems in addition to the information systems. These systems also are increasingly computer based, more reliable, and often easier to repair, but still require maintenance, error recovery, and updates. The management plan must include the manner in which these systems will be maintained and what support is needed. For example, is the facility large enough to have technical staff or should it find support through an independent consulting agency?

Critical systems need to be identified, including a definition of acceptable downtimes for each. Data backup and recovery should be defined for each system, including the individuals responsible for addressing any problems. The facility should expect that its residents will want and need computer and internet access. The residents should have access to each to facilitate communication with family, information gathering, and entertainment. The amount and range of services needs to be defined by the facility as part of its management plan, in addition to how much technological support will be provided to residents.

MARKETING APPROACHES

Successful operation of an ALC is dependent upon maintaining an inflow of resources, which is related to the admission of new residents. The flow of income is resident based unless the facility is a nonprofit, in which case the ALC might also receive donations and/or grants. A base level of income is needed to meet necessary expenses and overhead, which equates to a base level of occupancy. A marketing program must focus on attaining and then exceeding this base occupancy level to ensure the facility can remain in existence.

Marketing Strategies

A first step in developing a market strategy is to define the marketing targets. A strategy then needs to be formed to undertake the actual marketing. An implementation plan is needed, which will be enacted by the staff. The last step is to define an evaluation strategy to determine the effectiveness of the marketing strategy. For overviews of ALC marketing, see Dixon et al. (2001) and J. Allen (1999).

The business plan should provide a community profile, types of services to be offered, competitors and their characteristics, the market segment targeted, and a clear delineation of the ALC from a nursing home (Dixon et al., 2001). The potential means for reaching the target population is part of the marketing strategy along with the community links for the ALC (especially if co-marketing is desired).

The marketing plan needs to identify the types of living arrangements available in the facility, including the cost of each option. Based on the cost structure and housing types available, the marketing plan and marketing strategy can be focused toward an appropriate segment of the population. The mix of living arrangements and the physical structure of the facility will have been identified in the business plan.

Marketing Message

The marketing plan should have a clearly identified message: This is who we are, these are the services we provide, these should be your expectations of our facility. The potential client can better evaluate the ALC if all the parameters of living at the facility are known. Potential assistance in presenting the facility should be identified; working with community organizations may help to create these links.

The marketing effort needs to provide advertising through media or mailings, links to community and healthcare organizations, tours of the facility, brochures, an online presence (e.g., a website), e-marketing (Strauss & Frost, 2008), e-marketing effectiveness (Ranchhod et al., 2001), and virtual tours and/or DVDs/CDs about the ALC and its services. Developing a specific marketing team is essential because team members know about the preceding efforts in relation to current goals and future focus of the overall marketing plan. In addition, staff responsibilities for each part of the marketing plan should be identified.

Ultimately, marketing should locate potential residents, provide a message about the ALC's existence, provide information to people interested in the ALC, send follow-up information to interested parties, and then offer an onsite tour. A specific team of people should be identified in order to ensure the implementation of all aspects of the marketing strategy. Roles should be defined and appropriate training provided.

Marketing Team and Activities

The onsite and interactive aspects regarding inquiries about the facility, requests for more information, or visitation need to be identified. Reception is the initial face of the ALC for either telephone inquiries or people arriving. The role needs to be clearly identified, and appropriate training given. The responsibility for responses to the inquiries needs to be identified. A similar responsibility needs to be offered to postal mail or email inquiries.

The marketing team should include assignments for provisions of onsite tours. The ability to answer both potential resident and family concerns needs to be considered. The team should have a clear understanding (and training if necessary) regarding the process of conducting tours and explaining the resources available within the ALC as part of the overall presentation of the facility to a potential resident. Each member of the team should understand the types of units offered, the size of each unit, and what is physically included (the services provided by the ALC) and all associated costs. The team should also be able to answer any questions about services available within the community: such as healthcare, recreation, cultural resources, transportation, and any unique aspects of the community. This discussion should also include the way in which residents can access these external services.

All presentations should address safety issues either within the facility, within the residential units, or in the community. The safety features of the facility should be presented, and the team must be able to answer questions. Safety should address both resident-based issues such as falls or health emergencies, as well as external threats to the facility. The team should also be prepared to address concerns about the safety of resident belongings.

The team should also present the services available within the facility. The food services (if offered) should have a clear description along with sample menus. Shopping facilities for food and other necessities need to be identified for potential residents, along with how they might access those services. Other services offered should be detailed (e.g., broadband, resident nursing, exercise facilities and programs, and visitor areas).

Assessment of Marketing Effectiveness

The ALC should have a method to evaluate marketing activity (Churchill, 1978). Is it meeting the goals of the business plan? Are the methods used cost-effective? How do the methods compare with those of competitors? How will the information from the evaluation be used to improve marketing, and what parts of the evaluation should be provided to other parts of the organization?

CONCLUSIONS

This chapter provides the reader with information on the ongoing process of management, including built-in quality control and resident satisfaction measures. An ALC should have business, operational, and marketing plans. A systems perspective is useful in developing these plans and should include the systematic aspects of the ALC as well as evaluation and quality-controls method. Management methods and styles need to be selected from the broad range of existing methods. Information systems and technology are important components of an ALC. Marketing must be matched to the business and operational plans, as well as to the specific target populations they define.

REFERENCES

Ackoff, R., & Emery, F. (1972). *On purposeful systems*. Intersystem Publications.

Adler, P. S., & Borys, B. (1996). Two types of bureaucracy: Enabling and coercive. *Administrative Science Quarterly, 41*(1), 61. https://www.questia.com/library/journal/1G1-18441679/two-types-of-bureaucracy-enabling-and-coercive

Allen, J. (1999). *Assisted living administration: The knowledge base*. Springer Publishing Company.

Allen, P., & Sanger, C. (1979). Everything old is new again [Song]. *On All that jazz* [Album]. A&M Records. www.oldisnew.org/playlists/160626_playlist.html#:~:text=LABEL%20%22Everything%20Old%20Is%20New%20Again%22%20PETER%20ALLEN%3A,the%20gumm%20sisters%3A%20SWAN%20SONGS%2C%20FIRST%20FLIGHTS%3A%20Hallow

Anderson, J., Rungtusanatham, M., & Schroeder, R. (1994). A theory of quality management underlying the Deming management method. *Academy of Management Review, 19*(3), 472–509. https://doi.org/10.5465/amr.1994.9412271808

Buttaro, P. (1994). *Basic management for assisted living and residential care centers*. HCF Educational Service Publishers.

Churchill, Jr., G. A. (1979). A paradigm for developing better measures of marketing constructs. *Journal of Marketing Research, 16*(1), 39–53. https://doi.org/10.1177/002224377901600110

Churchman, C. W. (1968). *The systems approach*. Delacorte Press.

Churchman, C. W. (1971). *The design of inquiring systems: Basic concepts of systems and organization*. Basic Books.

Crosby, P. (1982). *Zero defects subjective vs. objective, step 7 of Philip Crosby's 14-step quality improvement process*. https://www.brighthubpm.com/methods-strategies/94048-fourteen-steps-of-crosby

Davenport, T. (1995). Will participative makeovers of business process succeed where reengineering failed? *Planning Review, 23*(1), 24–29. https://doi.org/10.1108/eb054496

DeFeo, J., & Barnard, W. (2004). *Juran's six sigma breakthrough and beyond*. McGraw-Hill.

Deming, W. E. (1981–1982). Improvement of quality and productivity through action by management. *National Productivity Review, 1*(1), 12–22. https://doi.org/10.1002/npr.4040010105

Deming, W. E. (1990). A system of profound knowledge. *Actionline*, 20–24.

Deming, W. E. (1993). *The new economics for industry, government, education*. MIT Center for Advanced Engineering Study.

Deming, W. E. (2010). *Deming's 14-point plan for TQM*. http://www.1000advices.com/guru/quality_tqm_14points_deming.html

Deming, W. E., & Walton, M. (1989). *The Deming management method*. Dodd, Mead & Co.

Dixon, G., Parshall, P., Pratt, D., Salinger, J., & Young, D. (2001). The foundations of marketing referral development and successful strategies. In K. H. Namazi and P. K. Chafetz (Eds.), *Assisted living: Current issues in facility management and resident care* (pp. 65–76). Greenwood Publishing.

Drucker, P. (1981). Management by objectives: As developed by Peter Drucker assisted by Harold Smedly. *Academy of Management Review, 6*(3), 225. https://doi.org/10.2307/257878

Fisher, G.H. (1966). *The world of program budgeting. P-3361.* Rand Corporation

Gorham, W. (1967). PPBS: Its scope and limits—Notes of a practitioner. *National Affairs: The Public Interest.* https://nationalaffairs.com/public_interest/detail/ppbs-its-scope-and-limits-notes-of-a-practitioner

Grant, R., Shani, R., & Krisman, R. (1994). TQMS challenge to management theory and practice. *Sloan Management Review, 35*(2).

Hall, R. (1963). The concept of bureaucracy: An empirical assessment. *American Journal of Sociology, 69*(1), 32–40. https://doi.org/10.1086/223508

Hammer, M., & Champy, J. (1993). *Reengineering the corporation: A manifesto for business revolution.* Harper Business.

Hodge, B., & Johnson, H. (1970). *Management and organization behavior: Multidimensional approach.* John Wiley.

Imai, K. (1986). *Kaizen, the Kaizen: The key to Japan's competitive success.* McGraw Hill/Irwin.

Ing, D. (2009). Value creating business models. Message posted to coevolving.com ISO 8402:1994. International Organization for Standardization. *International Organization for Standardization (2000) Quality Systems Model for Quality Assurance in Design, Development, Production, Installation and Servicing.*

ISO 8402. (1994). Quality management and quality assurance—Vocabulary. *ISO 9000* (2015), 108. https://www.iso.org/standard/20115.html

Japanese Human Relations Association. (1995). *The improvement engine: The Kaizen Teian approach.* Productivity Press.

Juran, J. M. (1992). *Juran on quality.* Free Press.

Kavakli, E., & Loucopoulos, P. (2004). Goal modeling in requirements engineering: Analysis and critique of current methods. In J. Krogstie, T. Halpin, & K. Siau (Eds.), *Information modeling methods and methodologies* (pp. 102–124). Idea Group. https://www.igi-global.com/chapter/goal-modeling-requirements-engineering/23011

Kotelnikov, V. (2010). *Kaizen and total quality management.* http://www.1000ventures.com/business_guide/mgmt_kaizen_tqc_main.html

Lewin, K., Lippit, R., & White, R. (1939). Patterns of aggressive behavior in experimentally created social climates. *Journal of Social Psychology, 10,* 271–301. https://doi.org/10.1080/00224545.1939.9713366

Lewis, M., & Black. N. (Eds.). (2003). *Operational management: Critical perspectives on business and management.* Routledge.

Likert, R. (1961). *New patterns of management.* McGraw-Hill.

Likert, R. (1967). *The human organization: Its management and value.* McGraw-Hill.

March, J., & Simon, H. (1958). *Organizations.* John Wiley.

March, J., & Simon, H. (1993). *Organizations* (2nd ed.). Blackwell Pub.

Maslow, A. (1943). A theory of human motivation. *Psychological Review, 50*(4), 370–396. https://www.academia.edu/9415670/A_Theory_of_Human_Motivation_Abraham_H_Maslow_Psychological_Review_Vol_50_No_4_July_1943

Maslow, A. (1954). *Motivation and personality.* Harper & Row.

McGregor, D. (1960). *The human side of the enterprise.* McGraw-Hill, Inc.

McGregor, D. (2002). Theory X and Theory Y. *Workforce, 81*(1).

Melichar, J. F. (1972a). *NOBS: New or better systems.* URS Corp.

Melichar, J. F. (1972b). *An evaluation system structure.* URS Corp.

Merton, R. (1940). Bureaucratic structure and personality. *Social Forces, 8*(4), 560–568. https://doi.org/10.2307/2570634

Morris, B. (1996). *New rule: Look in not out.* http://money.cnn.com/2006/07/10/magazines/fortune/rule4.fortune/index.htm

Muir, J. (1911). *My first summer in the Sierra.* Houghton Mifflin.

Odine, G. S. (1965). *Management by objective.* Pilman Publishing.

Osterwalder, A., Parent, C., & Pigneur, V. (2004). *Setting up ontology of business models.* Faculty of Computer Science and Information Technology, Riga Technical University, Riga, Latvia. https://dblp.uni-trier.de/rec/conf/caise/OsterwalderPP04.html?view=bibtex

Ouchi, W. G. (1982). *Theory Z.* Avon Books.

Ranchhod, A., Zou, F., & Tinson, J. (2001). Factors influencing marketing effectiveness on the web. *Information Resources Management Journal, 14*(1), 4–12. https://doi.org/10.4018/irmj.2001010101

Rienzo, T. (1993). Planning Deming management for service organizations. *Business Horizons, 36*(3), 19–29. https://doi.org/10.1016/S0007-6813(05)80145-4

Siegal, E., Ford, B., & Bernstein, J. (1993). *The Ernst & Young business plan guide.* John Wiley.

Singh, D. A. (2010). *Effective management of long-term care facilities* (2nd ed.). Jones & Bartlett.

Strauss, J., & Frost, R. (2008). *E-Marketing.* Prentice Hall. http://www.ibiblio.org/eldritch/fwt/ti.html

Taylor, F. (1911). *The principles of scientific management.* http://strategy.sjsu.edu/www.stable/pdf/Taylor,%20F.%20W.%20(1911).%20New%20York,%20Harper%20&%20Brothers.pdf

Von Bertalanfy, L. (1968). *General system theory: Foundations, development, applications* (rev. ed.). George Brazllier.

Von Forester, H. (1981). *Observing systems.* Intersystem Publishers.

Weber, M. (1947). *The theory of social and economic organizations.* Oxford University Press.

Weicher, M., Chu, W. W., Lin, W. C., Le, V., & Yu, D. (1995). *Business process reengineering: Analysis and recommendations.* http://citeseerx.ist.psu.edu/viewdoc/summary?doi=10.1.1.94.8207

Wilson, M. (2013). *Total quality management and Kaizen principles in Lean management.* https://www.kaizen-news.com/total-quality-management-and-kaizen-principles-in-lean-management/#:~:text=TQM%20%28total%20quality%20management%29%20is%20among%20the%20key,kaizen%20process%20that%20engages%20everybody%20in%20the%20workplace

FURTHER READING

Champys, J. (1995). *Reengineering management.* http://en.wikipedia.org/wiki/HarperCollins

Davenport, T. (1995). *The fad that forgot people.* Fast Company.

De la Vera Gonzalez, J., & Sanchez Diaz, J. (2004). *Business process-driven requirements engineering: A goal based approach.* http://citeseerx.ist.psu.edu/viewdoc/download?doi=10.1.1.92.4477&rep=rep1&type=pdf

Deming, W. E. (1975). On some statistical aids toward economic production. *Interfaces, 5*(4), 1–15. https://doi.org/10.1287/inte.5.4.1

Deming, W. E. (1986). *Out of the crisis.* MIT Center for Advanced Engineering Study.

Drucker, P. (1981). What results should you expect? A user guide to MBO. *Public Administration Review, 36*(1), 12. https://doi.org/10.2307/974736

Drury, H. (1915). *Scientific management: A history and criticism.* Columbia University.

English, J., & Morely, H. (1968). *Cost-effectiveness: The economics of engineered systems.* John Wiley.

Erez, M. (1977). Feedback: A necessary condition for the goal setting relationship. *Journal of Applied Psychology, 62*, 624–627. https://doi.org/10.1037/0021-9010.62.5.624

Hammer, M. (1990). Reengineering work: Don't animate, obliterate. *Harvard Business Review*, 104–112.

Ignizio, J. (1994). *Goal programming and extension.* Lexington Books.

International Standard ISO 9001:2000(E). http://en.wikpedia.org/wiki/International_Organiztion_for_Standardization

Locke, E., Shaw, K., & Brawley, L. (1981). Goal setting and task performance 1969–1980. *Psychological Bulletin, 90*, 125–152. https://doi.org/10.1037/0033-2909.90.1.125

Maslow, A. (1965). *Eupsychian management: A journal.* Irwin-Dorsey.

Maslow, A. (1970). *Motivation and personality.* Harper & Row.

Namazi, K., & Chafetz, P. (Eds.). (2001). *Assisted living: Current issues in facility management and resident care.* Greenwood Publishing.

Reengineering Reviewed. (1994). *The Economist Wiki.* https://en.wikipedia.org/wiki/Business_process_re-engineering

Taylor, F. W. (n.d.). *The Principles of Scientific Management 1910.* http://americainclass.org/wp-content/uploads/2013/03/Taylor-Scientific-Management-1910-excerpt.pdf

Walton, M. (1986). *The Deming management method.* Putnam Publishing.

FINANCIAL MANAGEMENT IN ASSISTED LIVING COMMUNITIES

WITH CONTRIBUTING AUTHORS RAYMOND YEE AND MARK J. CIMINO

LEARNING OBJECTIVES

Upon the completion of Chapter 10, the reader will be able to:

- Describe accounting systems (cash basis and accrual basis) and accounting records (accrued expenses, accrued income, revenue, deductions from revenue, expense accounting).

- Discuss the organization of an accounting system (chart of accounts, documentary evidence of financial transactions, a journal, and general ledger).

- Define common accounting job titles and positions that exist in assisted living communities (ALCs).

- Describe financial reports (balance sheet, cash flow statement, and profit and loss statement).

- Discuss financial standard operating procedures for cash, accounts payable, resident accounts receivables, and credit and collections.

- Understand the need for account records such as payroll records, time and earnings records, federal payroll taxes, payroll journal, and employee personnel files.

- Describe budget preparation in relation to operating, the physical facility and equipment (capital), and cash.

- Discuss ratio analysis (current ratio and quick ratio) as an indication of future solvency problems.

- Understand risk management, including commercial insurance, liability insurance, property insurance, consequential loss insurance, and theft insurance.

- Understand the nature of different types of legal entities.

- Understand the value of collecting industry financial data.

- Understand the relationship dynamics of real estate, operations, and management companies.

INTRODUCTION

This chapter presents a summary of information on financial management in ALCs accounting systems, organization, financial reporting, department titles and staff, the use of accounting and financial software, standard accounting procedures, accounts records, budget preparation, financial ratio analysis, risk management, and common accounting terms and definitions. The information contained in this chapter will help administrators and operators of ALCs to learn about basic financial concepts and accounting terminology.

This chapter also relates the functions of accounting and accounting systems to ALC management. Planning and controlling are two management functions previously considered. One of the purposes of the planning function is to make very basic decisions concerning the types of services to be provided by the ALC. In addition to management objectives, ALCs must also be concerned with fiscal objectives in order to have adequate funds to carry out the purposes and goals of the communities. Fiscal objectives should take into consideration both income and expenditures within the various organizational units or departments, and should be expressed in monetary or statistical terms to allow coordination of operations in the various departments.

ACCOUNTING SYSTEMS

To have effective management functions relative to the planning and controlling of an ALC, a strong organizational structure must be established for fiscal operations. There must be some sort of information and statistical data relating to each department or aspect of the business. Accounting is the system which accumulates data of quantitative nature relating to the activities taking place in the communities. Senior management and the financial administrator must be able to utilize this information to make key and sound managerial decisions. Accounting is also the interpretation of the results of the data, involving not only accumulation, but the correct interpretation and then effective communication within the organization. Accumulation means the mechanical process of actually recording financial transactions. Interpretation responds to the analysis of the information (key financial ratios and trends) in order to assist senior management in making correct financial decisions of the ALC. Lastly, communication corresponds with the reporting of this information, and presenting the data in a manner to help senior management understand and then make decisive financial decisions.

The accounting system should accurately reflect detailed aspects of the assisted living industry. Sophisticated methods of accounting are not required. The system, however, should be able to allow for basic cost accounting so that senior management will be aware of all expenses and revenues relating to each department. The accounting system should also be able to collect data, such as the number of admissions, readmissions, resident transfers (upgrades/downgrades), and discharges, in order to help senior management perform their strategic planning.

Accounting is a discipline that is based on basic that should be understood by the financial manager. Some of these basic concepts are:

1. The ALC is considered a legal entity that can buy, sell, and carry out additional business activities.

2. The ALC is capable of continuity of activity; it has both a life of its own and a business life divided into parts. These parts are timed measurements to determine the amount of dollars earned and the expenditures in each piece.

3. The facts ascertained by the accounting process must be capable of being objectively documented. That is, an accounts payable invoice should be supported by the proper documentation that includes a purchase order (PO), vendor invoice, receiving report, and a paper check issued in payment of the bill.

4. The accounting system must be consistent year to year. Consistency means that standardization and uniformity of accounting policies and procedures are used in the accounting process every year.

5. Full disclosure relating to accounting procedures is essential. That is, all pertinent and important financial information used to generate each accounting report must be reported by the ALC.

6. *Historical cost* is the accounting term for the evaluation of assets and the recording of most expenses. The term *cost* signifies that the amount of cash or cash equivalent given in exchange for property or services.

7. Any acquisition of donated property does not involve cost; this property should be recorded at fair market value (FMV) when it is obtained. Failure to do so will result in the underreporting of assets, revenues and expenses.

When establishing an ALC entity, there are two basic systems of accounting that can be used: Cash basis or accrual basis. Figure 10.1 depicts one way to select the right accounting method:

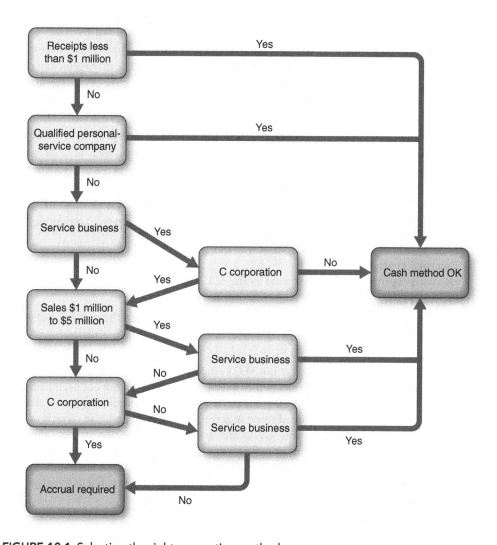

FIGURE 10.1 Selecting the right accounting method.

Source: From Jennings, R. (2001, May 1). *Cash or accrual?* https://www.journalofaccountancy.com/issues/2001/may/cashoraccrual.html

Cash Basis

In a cash-basis accounting system, revenues are recognized when the cash is received by the ALC, whereas expenses are recognized when the payment is actually made by the ALC. All expense and asset items are *not* recorded until the cash is actually disbursed. The operating statement, or the profit and loss statement, that results from cash basis accounting methodology is the summary of cash receipts and disbursements or a recording of cash flow. Items, such as accrued income, accrued expenses, depreciation, expense accounting, revenues, and deductions, are *not* included. A cash-basis system is more popular because it is much simpler than accrual basis. For example, it does not demand as many bookkeeping records. One advantage to cash basis is that it is suggested for companies that primarily deal with cash. A simpler accounting method is better and/or appropriate for the ALC, so when choosing the "optimal" method of accounting, one must weigh numerous factors as described in Figure 10.1.

Accrual Basis

In an accrual-basis accounting system, the primary accounting method used by ALCs (especially large ALCs and those communities that are part of a nationwide chain), the information that is provided can be developed into more meaningful data, giving senior management a more detailed and expanded picture of the overall obligations and prospects of the ALC. The accrual system of accounting provides recognition to all revenues in the time period they are earned, and to all expenses when they are actually incurred. The cash flow has very little to do with recording these types of transactions as they are reflected when they take place irrespective to the flow of cash between the ALC, its residents, and vendors. One example of an advantage to accrual basis is that because it requires a more detailed description of the revenues and expenses, it increases the chances of an exact measurement of net income and loss.

Furthermore, the typical ALC accounting records should include the following six items: accrued income, accrued expenses, revenue, deductions from revenue, expense accounting, and depreciation.

1. **Accrued expenses**
   Accrued expenses are those incurred by the ALC, but not yet paid in cash.

2. **Accrued income**
   Accrued income is income that has been earned by the ALC, but the cash has not yet been received in-house.

3. **Revenue**
   Revenue is the income received at the ALC's established rates, or charges for all services rendered to the resident whether or not these amounts have not been paid to the ALC by the resident or third-party payee (e.g., state Medicaid, long-term care insurance carrier). The purpose of revenue accounting is to keep precise records of gross revenue earned. The revenue is allocated to the appropriate departments within the ALC, which establishes a meaningful comparison as to earning potential of the various departments in the communities. Those departments with earnings potential (e.g., physical therapy, home aide, cafeteria, etc.) may also be compared in terms of expense in order to determine which ones are making a profit.

4. **Deductions from revenue**
   At times, the ALC may receive less than its full charge for goods and/or services rendered to its residents. It is essential to note that the comparisons between potential

revenue and revenue losses due to partial resident payments at less than full charges be recorded in the accounting system. These revenue losses or deductions are of three basic types as follows:

- **Contractual allowances**
A *contractual allowance refers to*the uncollectable difference between the full established charges and what is actually paid by state Medicaid or the negotiated contractual rate by a long-term care insurer and the ALC. For example, the ALC posted charges for per-diem resident rate are $400, and the long-term care insurer negotiated payment rate is $300 per day. The $100 per day difference is considered to be the contractual allowance and thus deducted from resident revenue. The same methodology also exists for state Medicaid payment rates.

- **Deductions for charity care**
All charity care provided to a resident by the ALC is deducted from resident revenue. The charitable care should be first recognized by the ALC at the established rates. It should be noted that a charitable care deduction cannot be taken after a service has been billed to a resident.

- **Bad debt provision**
These are estimated accounts receivable amounts that cannot be collected by the ALC from the resident, and therefore are considered credit losses. The bad debt provision is *not* the same as deductions for charitable care. If there has been any collection effort by the ALC to obtain the monies owed by a resident and/or long-term care insurer and that effort is not successful, there would then be a reduction of resident revenues by utilizing the bad debt provision to offset the difference.

5. **Expense accounting**
Expense accounting is used to collect on an accrual basis. It is a meaningful record of the operating expenses that relates to the ALC and/or individual communities department.

6. **Depreciation**
All ALC assets, whether they are purchased or donated, must be included in the community's balance sheet. All assets (except land) depreciate, or lose value over time through use, wear and tear, or technological obsolescence. The assets would eventually need to be replaced and their replacement is considered an operating expense that reflects the actual cost to replace them. If an asset were recognized and its depreciation expense not taken into consideration, the assisted living community's real cost of operations would be significantly understated. Therefore, depreciation must be recorded as an operating expense. There are five depreciation methodologies that are recognized and allowed by the U.S. Internal Revenue Service (IRS) as follows:

a. **Line depreciation**
The straight-line depreciation method is the easiest to use and record, in addition to being the easiest to understand. It basically provides for equal periodic charges to expenses over the estimated life of the asset. For example, an ALC purchases physical therapy equipment for $5,000 to service its residents. This exercise apparatus has an estimated life span of 10 years. Therefore, for 10 continuous years, $500 would be the depreciation value each year.

b. **Units of production method**
   This depreciation method is based on asset usage. That is, the more an asset is utilized, the faster it depreciates. The asset life is expressed in terms of hours, miles, or number of operations. For example, in order to conserve energy and save monies, an ALC purchases compact fluorescent light (CFL) bulbs for its residents' quarters and common use areas. Each CFL light bulb costs $5, and has a life span of 5,000 hours. Therefore, each CFL light bulb would depreciate at a rate of .001 cents per hour.

c. **Declining balance method**
   The declining balance method is illustrated by a declining periodic depreciation charge over the estimated life of the asset. A common method is to double the straight-line depreciation rate and then apply the resulting rate to the cost of the asset. For example, the ALC bought a sonogram machine to use in the community's health clinic. The state-of-the-art diagnostic equipment cost $20,000, and you would double the straight 10% line depreciation rate, therefore depreciating 20% of the $20,000 which provides a $4,000 first year depreciation expense. At the end of the second year, the depreciation formula would be $20,000 subtracted by $4,000, or $16,000 times 20%, or $3,200, which is the second-year depreciation amount. Furthermore, the original formula is applied each year thereafter until $20,000 (the original amount) is exhausted.

d. **Sum-of-the-years digit method**
   This depreciation method can be best portrayed as a steaildy decreasing periodic depreciation charge over the life of the asset so that a progressively smaller fraction is used each year versus the original first year of the asset. For example, an ALC licenses an advanced drugtracking software for $15,000 in order to track resident medication dosages for its pharmacy department. The software developer guarantees that the application will have an estimated useful life span of five years. Therefore, the drug software is depreciated where the denominator is 5 + 4 + 3 + 2 + 1 or 15. For the first year, the numerator is five, for the second year it is four and so on, as illustrated in Table 10.1.

e. **Accelerated depreciation**
   Accelerated depreciation, like the declining balance method and the sum-of-the-years digit method allows for a higher depreciation charge in the early part of an asset's useful life, especially during the first year, as it then gradually declines thereafter. The accelerated depreciation method is preferred by the ALC along with most other institutions and companies in other industries because of the increased depreciation expense in the early years that help to reduce taxable earnings. Furthermore, under IRC Section 179 deductions (or first-year

TABLE 10.1 DEPRECIATION: SUM-OF-THE-YEARS DIGIT METHOD

YEAR	ASSET COST	DEPRECIATION RATE	DEPRECIATION AMT.
1	$15,000	5/15	$5,000
2	$15,000	4/15	$4,000
3	$15,000	3/15	$3,000
4	$15,000	2/15	$2,000
5	$15,000	1/15	$1,000
Total:			$15,000

expensing), the IRS would allow an ALC a full deduction for investments in depreciable business equipment during the year the property is placed in service. The **Section 179 deduction** is now $1,000,000 for **2019**. This means businesses can **deduct** the full cost of equipment from their **2019** taxes, up to $1,000,000, with a "total equipment purchased for the year" threshold of $2,500,000.

Furthermore, additional tax-law changes enacted at the end of 2018 by Congress on how to treat accelerated depreciation (Tax Cuts and Jobs Act), increased first-year accelerated depreciation to 100%. It went into effect for any long-term assets placed in service after Sept. 27, 2017. The 100% accelerated depreciation amount remains in effect from Sept. 27, 2017 until Jan. 1, 2023. After that, first-year accelerated depreciation decreases as follows:

- 80% for property placed in service after Dec. 31, 2022 and before Jan. 1, 2024,
- 60% for property placed in service after Dec. 31, 2023 and before Jan. 1, 2025,
- 40% for property placed in service after Dec. 31, 2024 and before Jan. 1, 2026,
- 20% for property placed in service after Dec. 31, 2025 and before Jan. 1, 2027.

The Tax Cuts and Jobs Act also has other related provisions, such as Section 168(k), which allows for bonus depreciation (100% expensing) on eligible equipment and property, thus allowing accelerated depreciation for a reduced tax burden, similar to Section 179. A company can take both Section 179 and Bonus Depreciation allowances, but Section 179 must be applied first, and any amount over the $1,000,000 limit to Section 179 may then be taken in bonus depreciation.

Before you take Section 179 and/or bonus depreciation deductions, always consult with your tax accountant or tax attorney. Although it is true the deductions effectively reduce your ALC's tax burden for the year in which the equipment was purchased, you may also give up future years' depreciation, thereby impacting subsequent years' tax burdens as well.

In addition, accelerated depreciation of an asset results in a lower book value for that asset, which will affect the debt-to-worth ratio of your balance sheet. While this may not have a major impact on your ALC, it could affect your ability to seek additional funding for the ALC.

Evaluating the short and long-term effects of your capital purchase decisions and tax strategies is important to running your ALC. Your tax professional can help you determine the effects of these tax strategies, so you can make the most informed decisions.

Accounting Standards: Generally Accepted Accounting Principles

As one might imagine, there are various accounting standards used throughout the world for reporting financial activity. Often, however, there is a need to be able to adequately rely on, and compare with, the way entities present their accounting. To that end, companies that are required to report to outside stakeholders, particularly publicly traded companies on the stock market in the United States, should follow generally accepted accounting principles (GAAP). GAAP is a combination of authoritative standards (set by industry expert boards) and the commonly accepted ways of recording and reporting accounting information. GAAP aims to improve the clarity, consistency, and comparability of the communication of financial information to the outside world (stockholders, banks, government regulators, etc.). The ultimate goal of GAAP is to ensure a company's financial reports are complete, consistent, and comparable.

ACCOUNTING SYSTEM ORGANIZATION

The accounting system itself contains the following items: chart of accounts, documentary evidence of financial transactions, a journal, and general ledger.

TABLE 10.2 SAMPLE CHART OF ACCOUNTS

Assets (items of value owned by the ALC)
101—Cash (money in banks and investments such as U.S. Treasuries that are very liquid) 102—Accounts receivable (monies owed to communities by residents for past services provided such as rent and physical therapy) 103—Inventory (stock such as the cost of unused supplies like food stuff, cleaning materials, and CFL light bulbs) 104—Investments (money market funds, certificates of deposit, and depreciation fund) 105—Land (the cost of land)
Liabilities (items of debts owed by the ALC)
201—Accounts payable (the amount of monies owed to creditors for supplies and services) 202—Salaries (the amount of monies and wages owed to full and part-time employees that have not been paid) 203—Interest payable (the amount of monies owed to financial institution on the loan principal) 204—Employee benefits payable 205—Taxes payable (can be separated into federal, state, and municipal)
Capital (items that are the equity of the owners of the ALC. It is the amount of the owners' investments. For a publicly traded company, it would be the corporate ownership rather than a proprietary ownership in private investor hands)
301—Owner's capital 302—Owner's withdrawals 303—Revenue and expense summaries
Revenues (items that are income for ALC)
401—Resident daily room charges 402—Resident cafeteria charges 403—Resident physical therapy 404—Resident nursing care charges 405—Gift shop revenues
Expenses (items that are expenditures for ALC)
501—Salaries 502—Consultation fees (e.g., outside auditor) 503—Employee health insurance 504—Communities telephone/internet 505—Employee travel

The ALC's finance department must establish a chart of accounts before any financial transactions can be recorded. The Chart of Accounts is basically the manner in which the financial information is recorded and classified. It helps to systematize data of a financial nature, as well as assist in meeting the reporting requirements of the U.S. Internal Revenue Service, state Medicaid, and other government regulatory agencies. A sample chart of accounts is shown in Table 10.2.

Furthermore, to illustrate a more detailed chart of accounts, a chart of accounts for the Kingsbridge Heights Assisted Living Community Corporation is depicted in Table 10.3. Note how detailed cash, accounts receivables, salaries, etc. are expanded and recorded compared to prior sample chart of accounts.

Documentary Evidence for Internal and Independent Auditors

Whenever the ALC dispenses monies for various transactions, it is an important requirement in the accounting cycle that these disbursements be recorded by various kinds of documentation.

TABLE 10.3 KINGSBRIDGE HEIGHTS ASSISTED LIVING COMMUNITY CORPORATION CHART OF ACCOUNTS

ASSETS		LIABILITIES	
Current Assets		*Current Liabilities*	
1101	Cash—petty	2102	Accounts payable—supplies
1103	Cash—payroll account	2104	Notes payable—short-term
1106	Cash—operating Fund	2107	Mortgage payable—short-term
1112	Investments—money market fund	2109	Debts payable—current
1114	Investments—certificates of deposit (less than 1 year)	2111	Employee benefits payable
1117	Investments—depreciation fund	2113	Employee health insurance payable
1122	Accounts receivable—medicare Part B	2115	Salaries payable
1123	Accounts receivable—medicaid/DSS	2201	Taxes
1124	Accounts receivable—resident self-pay	2204	Taxes payable—New York state
1126	Accounts receivable—other payers (e.g., commercial, VA, workers' compensation)	2205	Taxes payable—New York city
1163	Unexpired liability Iinsurance	2207	Taxes payable—federal
		2221	Interest payable
Noncurrent Assets			
1302	Land	*Noncurrent Liabilities*	
1305	Land improvements	2303	Notes payable—long term
1402	Building—primary	2313	Mortgage payable—long term
1414	Building—secondary	2323	Bonds payable
1426	Building—garage/storage	2401	Pensions payable
1430	Building improvements	*Capital*	
1502	Furniture—primary	3001	Shareholders' equity
1504	Furniture—secondary	3101	Net income (loss)
1512	Equipment—primary		
1514	Equipment—secondary	*Revenue (Healthcare)*	
1516	Equipment—office	4001	Medicare Part B
1518	Equipment—kitchen	4003	Medical department of social services
1519	Equipment—laundry	4005	Other payers (e.g., commercial, VA, workers' compensation)
1521	Transportation		
1524x	Equipment—land maintenance		

(continued)

TABLE 10.3 KINGSBRIDGE HEIGHTS ASSISTED LIVING COMMUNITY CORPORATION CHART OF ACCOUNTS (*CONTINUED*)

		Ancillary	
Contra Assets, Accumulated Depreciation		4212	Physical therapy
1602	Accum. depr.—primary building	4214	Occupational therapy
1604	Accum. depr.—secondary building	4216	Social services/activities
1606	Accum. depr.—garage/storage	4218	Speech therapy (contract)
1630	Accum. depr.—building improvements		
1642	Accum. depr—furniture maintenance	*Uncompensated care*	
1644	Accum. depr.—furniture (secondary building)	4311	Contractual alowance—Medicare Part B
1651	Accum. depr.—equipment (primary building)	4313	Contractual allowance—Medicaid 1651
1654	Accum. depr.—equipment (secondarybuilding)	4315	Contractual alowance—other payers (e.g., commercial, VA, workers' compensation)
1666	Accum. depr—office equipment	4332	Donated charitable care
1668	Accum. depr.—kitchen equipment	4341	Bad debts
		4315	Resident refunds
1669	Accum. depr—laundry		
1671	Accum depr—transportation		
1674	Accum. depr.—land improvements		
1680	Accum. depr.—building improvements		

Expenses

Administration

5001	Salaries—management
5002	Salaries—clerical
5003	Consultation fees
5006	Health insurance
5011	Payroll tax
5013	Taxes—income
5015	Taxes—property
5022	Insurance—liability
5026	Retirement fund
5032	Supplies
5034	Telephone/cellular/internet

(continued)

TABLE 10.3 KINGSBRIDGE HEIGHTS ASSISTED LIVING COMMUNITY CORPORATION CHART OF ACCOUNTS (*CONTINUED*)

5035	Travel
5037	Postage/mailings
5039	Licenses and professional dues
5042	Repairs
Plant Operation	
5101	Salaries
5106	Health insurance
5111	Payroll tax
5122	Utility—electricity
5124	Utility—gas
5126	Utility—water
5128	Utility—sewage
5132	Supplies
Healthcare Workers	
5201	Salaries—nurses
5202	Salaries—health aides
5206	Health insurance
5211	Pharmacy
5224	Laboratory
5237	Uniforms
5242	Repairs
Dietary	
5301	Salary—management, food services
5302	Salary—kitchen staff
5306	Health insurance
Assets Liabilities	
5311	Payroll tax
5332	Supplies
5342	Repairs
Laundry	
5401	Salaries
5406	Health insurance

(continued)

TABLE 10.3 KINGSBRIDGE HEIGHTS ASSISTED LIVING COMMUNITY CORPORATION CHART OF ACCOUNTS (*CONTINUED*)

5411	Payroll tax
5432	Supplies
5442	Repairs
5461	Contract services
Housekeeping	
5501	Salaries
5506	Health insurance
5511	Payroll tax
5532	Supplies
5542	Repairs
Rehabilitation (Physical Therapy)	
5601	Salaries (or contract)
5606	Health insurance
5611	Payroll tax
5632	Supplies
5642	Repairs
Occupational Therapy	
5661	Salaries (or contract)
5666	Health insurance
5671	Payroll tax
5682	Supplies
5692	Repairs
Social Service/Admissions	
5701	Salaries (or contract)
5706	Health insurance
5711	Payroll tax
5732	Supplies
5742	Repairs
Activities	
5801	Salaries—beautician
5802	Salaries—arts and crafts
5806	Health insurance
5811	Payroll tax

(continued)

TABLE 10.3 KINGSBRIDGE HEIGHTS ASSISTED LIVING COMMUNITY CORPORATION CHART OF ACCOUNTS (*CONTINUED*)

5832	Supplies—beauty
5833	Supplies—arts and crafts
5835	Transportation
5837	Special events
5842	Repairs
Capital Expenses	
5904	Interest—mortgage
5907	Interest—long-term debt
5914	Debt service—mortgage
5917	Debt service—long-term debt
5934	Depreciation—plant
5936	Depreciation—equipment

DSS, Department of Social Services; VA, Veterans Affairs.

For example, the items that would record the issuance of a bank check for an item bought by the ALC would be the store register receipt of the item, purchase order, vendor invoice, credit card statement, or other evidence that this transaction had occurred. The reliability and accuracy of the ALC's accounting systems is based upon the extent of the necessary documented evidence for the various transactions that occurred. The typical accounting cycle is described as follows:

1. First, the transaction is recorded in the billings journal on a daily or chronological basis.
2. Second, from the billings journal, there is a posting to the general ledger.
3. Next, from the general ledger, an electronic accounting spreadsheet (e.g., Microsoft Excel and/or Great Plains software, etc.) is produced.
4. Last, from the spreadsheet, various financial reports (e.g., profit and loss statement, balance sheet, and income statement) are generated.

Billings Journal

The billings journal is a chronological record of increases and decreases affecting transactions. Adjusted and closing entries are made at the end of each month. These entries do not reflect the account balances which are required to be documented as part of the various financial statements for the communities at the close of each month. The financial data in the billings journal must be transferred to a book called the *general ledger* Establishing journal entries in the general ledger helps to recognize revenue (Oracle, 2016).

General Ledger

A general ledger is kept for each community's account in the chart of accounts. At the close of each month (i.e., "closing the books"), the financial data recorded in the billings journal is transferred to their respective account in the general ledger. This accounting procedure is called *posting*.

Electronic Accounting Spreadsheet

After all financial transactions for the month have been journalized and posted, and after the balances have been determined for each general ledger account, an electronic accounting spreadsheet is prepared. The accounting spreadsheet is the worksheet from which the community's accountants compile important financial statements such as the profit and loss statement, the income statement, and the balance sheet.

DEPARTMENT TITLES AND STAFF

The following are a list of common accounting job titles and positions that one would encounter within the accounting department of an ALC. The larger the size of the ALC, the more departmental titles and accounting personnel are required.

Accountant

By analyzing revenues, costs, financial liabilities, and assets, accountants are able to calculate future cash flows fairly accurately. Financial reports such as balance sheets or profit-and-loss statements must be maintained and reported to administrators. The majority of an accountant's day is spent completing or analyzing paperwork, but communication among departments is also necessary.

Accounting Manager/Supervisor

Accounting professionals must often calculate, input, and verify data on a regular basis. Managers and supervisors oversee all of these basic functions in addition to maintaining all financial records. These positions may require a great deal of time spent researching or reviewing the work of others.

Assistant Controller

Controllers assist in leading the daily activities of an accounting organization. They are responsible for preparing, evaluating, and presenting budgets and reports directly to management. Their duties range from establishing to implementing company practices and procedures. Extensive knowledge of accounting principles is mandatory.

Auditor

Auditors are responsible for carefully analyzing reports, statements, and accounting software of an internal or external community to ensure accurate calculations. They must have a thorough knowledge of all laws and regulations relating to accounting practices, because their job is to detect and report any discrepancies within a company's financial records. If an error has occurred, it is their duty to trace it back to the source and make recommendations to ensure more accurate accounting in the future.

Bookkeeper

Familiarity with standard accounting procedures is required for a bookkeeper position, due to the fact that they are responsible for recording a company's business transactions. Bookkeepers are responsible for maintaining records within given ledgers or computer programs. They must keep accurate records and balance all reports and ledgers on a monthly basis.

Clerk

Associates planning on working towards higher level positions often start as accounting clerks. Duties are often redundant but allow candidates to learn the processes of an accounting office or department. Daily activities generally include ledger maintenance and the preparation of basic financial reports.

Controller

Developing and implementing efficient policies, procedures, and practices is the main priority of a controller. They must oversee all aspects of the accounting department, such as budget or report maintenance and preparation. Once they are positive data has been compiled properly, they are responsible for presenting the data to management.

Chief Financial Officer

Immense creativity and independence are necessary for chief financial officers (CFOs) because they are held accountable for organizing and directing the ALC's overall financial policies. Insurance, tax, treasury, accounting, budgeting, and many other aspects are included in this grouping. An in-depth education of accounting practices and higher education is needed for these professionals. A certified public accountant and/or MBA degree in accounting or managerial finance is helpful.

Director

Accounting, payroll, and cost accounting functions are direct responsibilities of the accounting director. They are responsible for a number of tasks and applications; therefore, extensive education and experience is generally mandatory. They must have the capability to lead others within the department as well as work within deadlines.

Financial Analyst

Reconciling and forecasting the internal accounts are a large part of an analyst's career. They spend an immense amount of time compiling data, ensuring accuracy, analyzing information, and creating reports. They monitor all documents and report any trends to management.

Office Administrator

The development of policies and procedures of all office activities is the primary responsibility of the office administrator. They supervise all associates and proceedings on a daily basis. Duties, including filing, typing, faxing, mailing, and dictating, are often delegated to clerks or administrative assistants. They must maintain order among all records.

Office Manager

These careers often require extensive experience and good judgment. Office managers are expected to direct the general duties of multiple business office operations. They must be capable of directing and coordinating others within their department.

Payroll Administrator

Although this position focuses mainly on payroll functions, a keen understanding of all accounting practices is necessary to adequately fulfill this role. Typical duties include compiling accurate records of timesheets within a software system, computing earnings, and withholding mandatory amounts such as taxes or benefits. Accuracy and attention to detail are traits a payroll administrator must possess.

Payroll Specialist

Payroll specialists are often in charge of compiling timecards within a computer system, or inputting data from hard copies of timesheets or production records. They have the ability to balance payroll when completed and ensure proper the state, federal, and local tax payments are made. Since pay is generally issued at a specific time, these professionals must be able to complete all work within a given deadline.

Principal

As the highest authority in the accounting department, principals assume numerous duties. They oversee all accounting functions from preparing reports and entering data, to collaborating with other departments and organizing special projects. Principals are commonly responsible for performing audits of departments, monitoring department workloads, and creating and monitoring databases. They handle any communication necessary among fellow administrators and management.

Specialist

Common duties for accounting specialists revolve around the direction and planning of financial statements, cost control systems, and ledger accounts. Basic accounting skills are mandatory for these positions, and immense organization is integral. They watch over all aspects of basic accounting tasks.

Staff Assistant

Duties are often varied for these occupations. Staff assistants may handle duties from basic administrative tasks, such as filing or organizing data to running reports. They take on more responsibility as experience is gained, but these are generally entry-level positions. An understanding of accounting principles is generally required.

Tax Specialist

It is often easier to maintain detailed tax information year round rather than attempting to organize wide-ranging information within a short period of time. As a result, many organizations employ tax specialists year round. Their duties are not only limited to preparing tax returns.

USE OF ACCOUNTING AND FINANCIAL SOFTWARE

Today, ALCs require state-of-the-art technologies and innovative processes to operate efficiently and cost-effectively. ALCs must have systems and processes in place that help them financially operate the communities with timely and accurate tracking of revenues and expenses information. The processing of invoices must be paid on time, collecting monies owed to them by residents should be done on a regular basis, and paying their employees accurately, as well as reporting critical financial and utilization data to federal and state government agencies, is important. Thus, in order to successfully operate an ALC the fiscal administrator must automate the financial function with computer technologies and accounting software.

Accounting software is application software that records and processes accounting transactions within functional modules such as accounts payable, accounts receivable, payroll, and trial general ledger balance. It functions as an accounting information system. It may be developed "in-house" by the ALCs, or it may be purchased from an outside software developer. It may also be a combination of a third-party application software package with homegrown modifications. Overall, accounting software varies greatly in its complexity and cost. For example, the Yardi Senior Living Suite is software designed specifically for ALCs. This program includes online health records and portals for residents as well as online management assistance (www.yardi.com/markets-we-serve/assisted-living).

The accounting software market has been undergoing considerable consolidation since the mid-1990s with many vendors ceasing to exist or being bought out by larger companies. Most software vendors today offer cloud-based accounting application software suites as well as data backup and storage capabilities to protect their clients' information.

Typical accounting software that is used in ALCs is composed of various modules with different sections. The most common modules are as follows:

Core Modules

- Accounts receivable—Where the communities enter money received from residents/patients
- Accounts payable—Where the communities enter their bills and pay money they owe vendors
- General ledger—The communities' "books" used to generate their monthly, quarterly, and annual financial statements
- Billing—Where the communities produce bills/invoices to residents and outside vendors
- Stock/inventory—Where the communities keep control of their inventory/supplies/parts
- Purchase order—Where the communities order their inventory/supplies/parts
- Sales order—Where the communities record resident sales for the patient census

Noncore Modules

- Debt collection—Where the communities track attempts to collect overdue resident bills (sometimes part of accounts receivable)
- Electronic payment processing
- Expense—Where communities' employee business-related expenses are entered
- Inquiries—Where the communities look up information on screen without any edits or additions to resident and/or vendor records
- Payroll—Where the communities track employee salaries, wages, and related taxes
- Reports—Where the communities print out management, financial, and utilization census data
- Purchase requisition—Where requests for purchase orders are made, approved, and tracked by the communities

In many cases, implementation (i.e., the installation and configuration of the accounting system at the ALC) is a bigger consideration than the actual software chosen when considering the total cost of ownership for the ALCs. Most midmarket and larger accounting software applications are sold exclusively through resellers, developers, and consultants. Those vendors generally pass on a licensing fee to the software vendor and then charge the communities for installation, customization, and support services. Communities' clients can normally count on paying roughly 50% to 200% of the price of the software in implementation and consulting fees.

Small-sized ALCs typically use inexpensive accounting software that is limited in function, but allows most general business accounting functions to be performed. The modules used are accounts payable type accounting transactions, managing budgets, and simple account reconciliation. Many of the low-end accounting software products are characterized by being "single-entry" products, as opposed to double-entry systems seen in many businesses. Some products have considerable functionality, but are not considered GAAP or International Financial Reporting Standards (IFRS)/Federal Accounting Standards Board (FASB) compliant. Some low-end systems do not have adequate security or audit trails.

The most complex and expensive business accounting software used by a larger ALC chain is frequently part of an extensive suite of software often known as *enterprise resource planning (ERP)* software. These applications typically have a very long implementation period, often greater than 6 months. In many cases, these applications are simply a set of functions that require significant integration, configuration, and customization to even begin to resemble an accounting system. The advantage of a high-end solution is that these systems are designed to support individual communities' specific processes as they are highly customizable and can be tailored to exact business requirements. This usually comes at a significant cost in terms of money and implementation time.

Crane (2007) describes the importance of accounting software in ALCs and states that:

> Yardi Senior Housing Management software, from Yardi Systems in Santa Barbara, CA, is a Web-based program that does it all —from running financial reports to managing residents' care schedules. For those services, there are substantial start-up costs and annual license fees. Initial costs, including implementation and training, might start at $30,000 for smaller operators; annual fees are in the neighborhood of $4,000 per community and include hosting through Yardi servers, plus product updates and some telephone support.

FINANCIAL REPORTING

There are three major financial reports that all businesses produce: the balance sheet, the cash-flow statement, and the profit-and- oss statement. Descriptions of these reports and other tables an ALC generates follow.

The Balance Sheet

The balance sheet is used to depict the entire financial operation of the ALC in terms of its assets, liabilities, and capital (stockholder's equity) at a given period in time. It is usually prepared and reported monthly, quarterly, and annually. The items in the balance sheet are : (a) assets, including current assets, long-term investments (such as stocks, bonds, etc.), and fixed assets (property, equipment, and assets having a value to the communities over a long period of time), as well as liabilities, including both current liabilities and long-term liabilities (debts that are due in 1 year or more), such as mortgages, capital equipment loans, and corporate debt (long-term bonds).

Capital or stockholder's equity is the amount of money provided by the owner(s) of the business. This can come from the sale of company stock, retained funds (earned for the owner[s] but left in the business) and equity funds (considered a long-term and/or permanent investment by the owner[s]). The net worth of the ALCs can be calculated as the total assets minus total liabilities equal the owners' equity. Therefore, the total liabilities plus the owner's equity must represent the total assets of the ALC.

The balance sheet is the essential financial statement that reports the main types of assets owned by the ALC. Assets are only half of the picture; the ALC also borrows money. At the date of preparing the balance sheet, the community owes money to its financial lenders who will be paid sometime in the future. Also, most ALCs purchase many things on credit and owe money to their vendors, which will be paid in the future. Amounts owed to lenders and suppliers are called *liabilities*. A balance sheet reports the main types of liabilities of the communities and separates those due in the short-term and those due in the longer term.

At times, an ALC might have its total liabilities greater than its total assets. This would occur if the ALC has been losing money. In the vast majority of cases, a community has more total assets than total liabilities. That is true because (a) its owners have invested money in the business, which is not a liability of the business; and (b) the business has earned profit over the years and some of the profit has been retained in the business (profit increases assets). The sum of invested capital from owners and retained profit is called *owners' equity*. The excess of total assets over total liabilities is traceable to owners' equity. A balance sheet reports the make-up of the owners' equity of a business.

The balance sheet usually has the following format:

Assets

Assets are the economic resources of the business. Examples are cash on deposit, long-term investments, equipment, and buildings.

Liabilities

Liabilities arise from borrowing money and buying things on credit from banks and investment firms.

Owners' Equity

Owners' equity arises from two sources: money invested by the owners, and profit earned and retained by the ALC.

One reason the balance sheet is called by this name is that the two sides balance, or are equal in total amounts:

$$\textit{Total recorded amount of assets} = \text{Total recorded amount of liabilities} + \\ \text{total recorded amount of owners' equity}$$

Owner's equity is sometimes referred to as *net worth*. You compute net worth as follows:

$$\text{Assets} - \text{liabilities} = \text{net worth}$$

Net worth is not a particularly good term because it implies that the ALCs are worth the amount recorded in their owners' equity accounts. Though the term may suggest that the business could be sold for this amount, nothing is further from the truth. An example of a typical balance sheet is shown in Table 10.4.

TABLE 10.4 KINGSBRIDGE HEIGHTS ASSISTED LIVING COMMUNITY CORPORATION BALANCE SHEET

	JULY 31, 20XX	JULY 31, 20XX
Assets		
Current assets		
Cash	$182,100	$8,502
Accounts receivable (less bad debts of $27,096)	160,551	184,191
Securities	675,825	31,500
Inventory	186,018	164,640
Prepaid insurance	7,200	10,800
Total current assets	1,211,694	399,211
Noncurrent assets		
Equipment	5,949,000	5,943,600
Plant	17,301,012	17,301,012
Less accumulated depreciation	8,316,576	7,086,900
Building and equipment property	14,933,436 7,950,000	16,157,712 7,950,000
Total fxed assets	22,883,436	24,107,712
Total assets	**24,095,130**	**24,507,345**
Liabilities		
Current liabilities		
Accounts payable	8,556	73,818
Notes payable	100,875	1,065,813
Benefits [ayable	74,529	2,114,751
Current portion of long-term debt		
Mortgage	692,040	576,699
Long-term debt	225,000	225,000
Total current liabilities	1,101,000	3,832,494
Noncurrent liabilities		
Mortgage payable	10,380,606	11,072,649
Debts payable	2,025,000	2,250,000
Total noncurrent liabilities	12,405,606	13,322,649
Total liabilities	**13,506,606**	**17,155,143**

(continued)

TABLE 10.4 KINGSBRIDGE HEIGHTS ASSISTED LIVING COMMUNITY CORPORATION BALANCE SHEET (*CONTINUED*)

	JULY 31, 20XX	JULY 31, 20XX
Net worth		
Retained earnings		
Year to date	106,875	82,521
Total	1,112,868	1,005,993
Shareholder's equity	9,368,781	6,263691
Total net worth	10,588,524	7,352,205
Total liabilities and capital	**24,095,130**	**24,507,345**

The Cash-Flow Statement

The cash-flow statement for an ALC presents a summary of the sources and uses of cash during a financial period. *Essentially, it is a record of payments.* Successful financial administrators have to manage both profit and cash flow. ALCs are like a two-headed dragon in this respect. Even with a successful profit-making approach, ignoring cash flow can bring ruin upon an ALC. Still, some financial managers become preoccupied with making profit and overlook cash flow, thus causing vendor bills, and then employee payroll, to be paid late. For financial reporting, cash flows are divided into three basic categories:

Basic Format of the Cash Flow Statement

1. Cash flow from the profit-making activities, or operating activities, for the period. (Note: *Operating* means the profit-making transactions of the ALC.)
2. Cash inflows and outflows from investing activities for the period.
3. Cash inflows and outflows from the financing activities for the period. You determine the bottom-line net increase (or decrease) in cash during the period by adding the three types of cash flows shown in the preceding list.

Section one of the cash-flow statement explains why net cash flow from sales revenue and expenses—the business's profit-making operating activities—is are more or less than the amount of profit reported in the profit and loss account. The actual cash inflow from revenues and outflow for expenses run on a different timetable than the sales revenue and expenses. The sales revenues and expenses are recorded for determining profit. Imagine two different airplanes going to the same destination: the second plane (the cash-flow aircraft) runs on a later schedule than the first plane (the recording of sales revenue and expenses in the accounts of the business).

Section two of the cash-flow statement records the major long-term investments made by the business during the year, such as constructing a new assisted living building or replacing machinery and equipment. If the business sold any of its long-term assets, it reports the cash inflows from these divestments in this section of the cash-flow statement.

Section three records the financing activities of the business during the period, which concerns borrowing new money from lenders and raising new capital investment in the business from its owners. Cash outflows to pay off debt are reported in this section, as well as cash distributions from profit paid to the owners of the business.

The cash-flow statement reports the net increase or net decrease in cash during the year (or other time period), caused by the three types of cash flows. One might believe this increase or decrease in cash during the year is the bottom line; however, it should never be referred to as the *bottom line*. This important term is strictly limited to the last line of the profit-and-loss account, which reflects net income: the final profit after all expenses are deducted.

An illustration of a sample cash-flow statement for Kingsbridge Heights Assisted Living Community Corporation is shown in Table 10.5.

TABLE 10.5 KINGSBRIDGE HEIGHTS ASSISTED LIVING COMMUNITY CORPORATION CASH-FLOW STATEMENT

	WEEK 1	WEEK 2	WEEK 3	WEEK 4
Beginning cash balance	$330,000	$300,000	$294,000	$246,000
Cash inflow				
Commercial	570,000	510,000	540,000	660,000
Medicaid/DSS	345,000	345,000	345,000	345,000
Medicare Part B				35,000
Self-pay	195,000	150,000	165,000	195,000
VA				20,000
Workers' Compensation				5,000
Short-term investments	300,000		300,000	
Short-term loans			150,000	
Miscellaneous (gift shop, beauty salon, etc.)	90,000	75,000	60,000	90,000
TOTAL	1,500,000	1,080,000	1,560,000	1,350,000
Cash outflow				
Payroll	1,050,000		1,095,000	
Accounts payable	600,000	540,000	675,000	540,000
Delayed payments	(210,000)	210,000	(198,000)	198,000
Interest payable				50,000
Taxes	45,000			
Plant-in-progress payments				30,000
Purchase short-term investments		300,000		300,000
Pay short-term loans				100,000
Miscellaneous	36,000	45,000	36,000	48,000
TOTAL	1,530,000	1,086,000	1,608,000	1,266,000
Ending cash balance	300,000	294,000	246,000	330,000

DSS, Department of Social Services; VA, Veterans Affairs.

The Profit-and-Loss Statement (a.k.a. the *Income Statement*)

The purpose of the profit-and-loss (P&L) statement is to portray the results of the financial operations in terms of the amount of revenues the community has earned. This includes current assets (assets consumed in less than one year), such as cash, short-term investments (interest and dividends), patient accounts receivables, inventory, and the amount of expenses the community has incurred, which includes current liabilities (obligations to be paid in one year or less), such as accounts payables for vendors, and wages/salaries and taxes (e.g., Federal Insurance Contributions Act [FICA], Medicare) payable for employees in the given year. The P&L statement is sometimes known either as the "income statement" or the "statement of income and expenses," and is usually prepared monthly. The time periods reported by the P&L are monthly, quarterly, and annually. Furthermore, the statement of expenses should be departmentalized, thus enabling senior management to determine the actual income and expense of each department for proper analysis of efficiency (utilization of resources), profits (either a profit center or loss center), etc. It should be noted that the percentage of resident occupancy figure is significant because it helps senior management determine how many residents are required for the ALC to operate profitably or "in the black." As an industry benchmark, ALCs break even financially at about 70% to 75% resident occupancy and achieve financial stabilization (attain long-term economic viability) at approximately 93% occupancy. The profit and loss account is the all-important financial statement that summarizes the profit-making activities (or operations) of a business over a period of time. In very broad outline, the statement is reported like this:

Sales Revenue

Sales revenue is the sales of products and services to customers.

Less Expenses

Less expenses includes a wide variety of costs paid by the business, including the cost of products sold to customers, wages and benefits paid to employees, occupancy costs, administrative costs, and income tax.

Equals Net Income

Equals net income is referred to as the *bottom line* and is the final profit after all expenses are deducted from sales revenue; however, the P&L account gets the most attention from business managers and investors—not that they ignore the other two prior key financial statements. The very abbreviated versions of P&L accounts that you see in financial publications, such as *The Wall Street Journal* and *The Financial Times*, report only the top line (sales revenue) and the bottom line (net profit). In actual practice, the profit and loss account is more involved than the basic format shown here. Table 10.6 contains the income statement for the Kingsbridge Heights Assisted Living Community Corporation.

Other Financial Reports

In addition to the balance sheet, the cash-flow statement, and the P&L statement, a well-managed ALC will also use additional financial reports regarding supplies and expenses. Several of these reports that the fiscal administrator needs to successfully manage and grow the community's operations are: a daily report of cash receipts and disbursements, a resident accounts receivables report, and an accounts payable report.

TABLE 10.6 KINGSBRIDGE HEIGHTS ASSISTED LIVING COMMUNITY CORPORATION INCOME STATEMENT

REVENUES	JULY 20, 2010	YEAR TO DATE (YTD)
Operating revenues		
Healthcare	$1,072,809	$6,623,442
Total healthcare	$1,072,809	$6,623,442
Ancillary		
Physical therapy	29,922	185,517
Occupational therapy	29,670	178,020
Social services	8,598	50,727
Total ancillary	68,190	414,264
Gross operating revenues	1,140,999	7,037,706
Less deductions	136,920	844,524
Net operating revenues	1,004,079	6,193,182
Nonoperating revenues		
Miscellaneous		
Meals	1,290	7,482
Concession	4,074	26,073
Beauty shop	2,370	14,457
Total miscellaneous	7,734	48,012
Interest	7,920	45,936
Nonoperating revenues	15,654	93,948
Total revenues	1,019,733	6,287,130
Expenses		
Operating expenses		
Salaries		
Healthcare personnel	405,576	2,499,453
Food services	46,746	280,476
Administration	28,653	163,323
Laundry	10,227	61,362
Maintenance	15,861	96,435
Physical therapy	28,956	182,424
Occupational therapy	10,350	62,205
Social services —Admissions	6,438	39,915
Total salaries	552,807	3,385,593

(continued)

TABLE 10.6 KINGSBRIDGE HEIGHTS ASSISTED LIVING COMMUNITY CORPORATION INCOME STATEMENT (*CONTINUED*)

REVENUES	JULY 20, 2010	YEAR TO DATE
Supplies	$94,179	$569,784
Activity	6,195	37,170
Capital equipment	600	4,800
Utilities	26,292	157,752
Telephone/cellular/internet	489	3,129
Insurance	12,000	72,054
Taxes (real estate)	9,939	59,634
Capital costs		
Interest	83,448	500,688
Mortgage payment	72,087	432,522
Depreciation	118,881	713,286
Total capital costs	274,416	1,646,496
Total expenses	1,017,234	6,180,255
Net income (loss)	2,499	109,875
Income tax	1,125	48,093
Profit after taxes	1,374	58,782

Cash Report

The cash report (Table 10.7) provides the fiscal administrator a working knowledge of the amount of cash on hand. It is usually generated monthly and at the end of the month.

Resident Accounts Receivable Report

The resident accounts receivable report (Table 10.8) checks the ALC's fiscal operations from the income perspective. It includes only income from residents (cash) and third-party payers (state Medicaid, commercial long-term insurance). Furthermore, it indicates the effectiveness of the community's collection procedures, billings, and efforts to maintain positive cash flow. It is also generated monthly, at the end of the month.

TABLE 10.7 CASH REPORT

Cash on hand (3/31/2010)	$125,000.00
Plus cash receipts	+5,000.00
Total cash	130,000.00
Less cash disbursements	−10,000.00
Cash on hand (4/30/2010)	$120,000.00

TABLE 10.8 RESIDENT ACCOUNTS RECEIVABLE REPORT

Resident accounts receivable (1/31/2010)	$2,000,000.00
Plus resident charges	+500.000.00
Total accounts receivable outstanding balance	2,500,000.00
Less resident payments	−800,000.00
Resident accounts receivable (2/28/2010)	$1,700,000.00

TABLE 10.9 VENDOR ACCOUNTS PAYABLE REPORT

Communities' accounts payable (1/31/2010)	$500,000.00
Plus communities' purchases	+75,000.00
Total accounts payable outstanding balance	575,000.00
Less payments	−125,000.00
Communities' accounts payable (2/28/2010)	$450,000.00

Vendor Accounts Payable Report

The vendor accounts payable report (Table 10.9) also assists the fiscal administrator in keeping track of operating expenses (e.g., outstanding debts to vendors) in line with monthly cash flow. The operating expenses that are included in this report are only those payable within one year, such as short-term liabilities. Moreover, items that include employee salaries and benefits, mortgages, and loan interest payments are not included.

ACCOUNTING PROCEDURES

In order to operate successfully and profitably, an ALC must have tight departmental management controls in place. Four of the most essential financial standard operating procedures concern cash, accounts payable, resident accounts receivable, and credit and collections.

Cash Handling Procedure

The significance of cash in any kind of business is important because it finances the business operations. Cash transactions occur more than any other kind of transaction in an ALC. In addition, cash is the asset that is most susceptible to theft, fraud, and misappropriation. As part of financial management, it is important to have some type of internal control for cash receipts. A standard operating procedure (SOP) used as an internal control for the ALC's cash receipts includes the following five steps:

1. Incoming mail is opened by someone who does not have access to the accounting records and is not responsible for bank deposits.
2. Whoever opened the mail prepares a remittance list of all cash items received. One copy of the remittance slip is given to the person actually making the bank deposits.

3. All personnel who are handling cash are bonded (see Risk Management section);

4. A cash receipts slip is prepared for all cash received by the ALC; one copy of this is provided to the person paying the cash with a duplicate copy to the accountants. All cash receipts are recorded in the appropriate accounting records at the earliest time practicable. Separate staff personnel that do not handle cash or record cash transactions prepare the bank reconciliation. Cash receipts must be deposited in the bank daily. Immediately upon receipt of checks, endorsement is made by indicating on the back of the check "For Deposit Only to the Account of XYZ Assisted Living Communities"; and

5. Using copies of the cash receipts slips, the accountant then records all cash receipts in a cash receipts journal on a daily basis. Finally, the cash receipts are also posted to the resident's ledger.

Handling Accounts Payable Accounts

An accounts payable account is a creditor of the ALC. A standard operating procedure for handling this type of account is:

1. Start a file folder for each vendor/supplier/service contractor with which the ALC does business.

2. A PO number is issued or a purchase order written for all the ALC's purchases.

3. Have a central storeroom where all shipped vendor goods are received.

4. When supplies, equipment, or goods are received at the central storeroom, a receiving slip must accompany the items. Ensure that the number of cartons that is received corresponds to the items on the receiving slip. Document any item(s) that are backordered.

5. The receiving slip, after being checked by the storeroom (materials management) manager, is then sent to the bookkeeper in the accounting department.

6. When the ALCreceives the invoice from the vendor, the accountant or the accounts payable clerk: (a) reviews the invoice to determine that the purchase order is signed by the person authorized to order the item, (b) then checks it against the purchase order to determine whether the unit price and any extensions are correct, and (c) checks it against the receiving slip to determine whether all ordered goods were received.

The last step is that the information gathered in the preceding steps is given to the individual responsible for authorizing payment (typically either the CFO or controller). All approved hardcopy invoices are lastly filed away in accounts payable folders by alphabetical order of vendor names.

Handling Resident Accounts Receivable

This is the most important accounting procedure for the ALC because its survival depends on adequate cash flow from resident revenues. Therefore, the standard operating procedure to establish correct residential rates and to properly record resident revenue plays an essential role in the operation of the community. The bulk of all revenues received by the ALC come from resident revenues for room and board, routine preventive medical and housekeeping services, special rehabilitation, and private duty nursing services. The typical procedure for handling resident accounts receivable is:

1. Review and establish the proper rental rate structure for each residential unit, routine services, and special services at least on an annual basis.

2. At the time of resident acceptance into the ALC, set up a ledger card in the name for each resident, noting important data such as resident name, unit number, source of payment (i.e., private pay, commercial long-term care insurance, state-funded Medicaid), and any pertinent routine and special service charges.

3. At the end of each week and/or month, prepare a resident accounts receivable journal for each resident income. This would act as a check and balance on the ledger.

4. Gather all charge slips for any special services for each resident that are not included in the monthly rent. Keep a special service revenue journal to act as a check and balance. Residential charge receipts should also be summarized and reviewed on a daily basis.

5. At the end of each month, the totals in these resident accounts receivable journals should be posted to the general ledger and the resident's ledger card. Invoices for residential rent and board, routine services, and special services are prepared and submitted to the responsible financial parties.

Handling Credits and Collections

The accumulation of residential accounts receivable that are not collected can cause a major concern and financial crisis for an ALC. It might cause a severe cash-flow problem that would require the community to borrow funds at a high interest rate from a financial institution. For this particular reason, an effective credit and collection procedure must be implemented. A recommended procedure would be:

1. Financial information regarding the source of payment should be obtained from the resident upon acceptance into the ALC. If third-party payers are to pay for the resident's room and board and routine services, verify that these benefits are actually covered as soon as possible.

2. Determine whether the resident is eligible for state Medicaid or other governmental assistance (Medicare might pay for certain special services).

3. Explain to the resident the types of services and their respective charges at the time of their acceptance. Have them sign off on a written letter of agreement to these services and charges.

4. Furthermore, explain the ALC's billing and collection policies. Have the resident or third-party payer sign off on a written document of agreement to these billing and collection policies.

5. Prepare an accounts receivable aging schedule for each resident. If a resident account is over a month old, send the resident or third-party payer a notice of the past due account.

6. Further stringent and harsher collection efforts must be made if a resident account is more than 60 days past due. Instead of a gentle collection notice, a more personalized collection letter by senior management may be sent to remind the resident of their past due bill. In this situation, a great deal of tact and diplomacy must also be made by senior management in collecting past due accounts. The ALC must determine, as a matter of corporate policy, whether to utilize an outside collection agency or an attorney to collect unpaid resident bills.

ACCOUNT RECORDS

The ALC must maintain under federal and state laws and regulations specific account records for internal management controls and outside governmental regulatory audits. The most important accounts deal with human resources and staffing as employees are the major cost items in the ALC. The five essential account records are as follows

Payroll Records

Employee salaries/wages and benefits represent 50% to 60% of an ALC's operating expenses. Therefore, adequate, accurate, and up-to-date payroll records are critical.

Time and Earnings Records

A method of precise time keeping should be utilized for hourly and salaried full-time employees. In the past, a manual time clock and punch cards located at a central location were used to record employee hours worked. These days, electronic hand scanners at various locations are used at ALCs to clock in employees as they arrive for work and clock out when they finish their work. Some ALCs pay their lower salaried nonmanagement employees bi-weekly or weekly. Senior management and higher paid employees are usually paid monthly. The rationale in paying higher-level employees once per month is to conserve cash for the communities. For lower salaried employees, where for whom bi-weekly pay period is used, the following procedure is typically followed:

1. At the first day of the pay period, the employee's name and date of pay period are recorded on the employee time and earnings (T&E) record.
2. The T&E record is then given to the employee's supervisor.
3. At the end of each day (sometimes at the end of each week) the employee or supervisor enters the number of hours the employee worked in each department.
4. At the end of the pay period, the T&E record is returned to the accountant who calculates the employee hours worked, gross pay, and deductions.

Federal Payroll Taxes

Federal law requires that the employer make income tax withholdings from the employee's salaries and wages each pay period and remit these withholdings to the Internal Revenue Service. Most states and certain municipalities also require employers to withhold income taxes. The federal, state, and city withholding rates are determined from tax tables furnished by federal and state governments. Employers must also withhold FICA (Social Security = 6.2%) and Medicare (1.45%) taxes from employee wages. For both deductions, the amounts that are withheld are a percentage of the wages up to a certain amount. The employer must also match this amount paid by the employee to the IRS.

Payroll Journal

The employees T&E record serves as a basis for entries into the payroll journal. Two separate accounts are maintained as follows: "cash in bank—general checking" and "cash in bank—payroll checking." Accounts payable and wages/salaries should not be paid out of the same account as listed previously.

Once the total net payroll for the time period is determined from the payroll journal, a single check for the total net payroll is written out of the general account and place into the payroll checking account. When the payroll check clears at the bank, the payroll checking account should have a minimal balance. As an internal control, there should be different colored bank checks and different checking accounts (or have payroll and general checking from different banks) for the payroll checking and general checking accounts. Nowadays, most ALC's payroll is handled electronically and the payment is automatically deposited into the employee's bank at each pay period.

Employee Personnel File

An individual hardcopy folder and/or electronic file (scanned documents) should be maintained for each employee. The employee file should contain all personnel data such as résumé, reference checks, physical exam, drug testing results, salary increases, promotions, employee awards and reprimands, and payroll information (earnings records, W-2 form, citizenship verification, copy of social security card, etc.). Some older ALCs post from manual cards to employee's individual earnings records. Others prepare payroll checks in duplicate and file the duplicate copy to the employee's personnel folder.

BUDGET PREPARATION AND EXECUTION

The survival of any business is in direct correlation to its financial solvency. One of the most important tools for sound financial management is the budget, a planning and management control device. The budget is defined as the projection of financial data for a specific period of time; that period of time typically measures one year. A budget should not be completely restrictive and static. That is, after one or more administrative reviews of the budget throughout the year, it may be necessary to make several adjustments of the revenues and expenses, either upward or downward.

In managerial accounting, there are three basic kinds of budgets: operating, plant and equipment, and cash. Businesses that maintain all three are said to have comprehensive budgets.

The Operating Budget

The operating budget is a financial projection or forecast for 12 months of revenues, including the deductions from revenues and expenses. If the assisted living community's budget encompasses the 12 months from January 1, 2018 to December 31, 2018, the budget would be for the calendar year. Otherwise, the ALC's budget would be projected for the fiscal year (e.g., July 1, 2018 to June 30, 2019). In establishing the revenue budget, it is necessary to carefully review the monetary and statistical data concerning the income by each department in the assisted living community. Trends in the data should be considered carefully, established, analyzed, and then forecasted for the upcoming year. It may be necessary to review anticipated changes in the internal operations of the assisted living community which consists of the following items:

1.   Changes in the number of units (e.g., residents, employees),
2.   New services to be added (e.g., physical therapy, on-site pharmacy),
3.   New or amended corporate by-laws to be placed in effect,

4. New or amended federal and/or state and local government regulations that are imposed on the ALC,

5. A realistic projection of resident days (the more days the more resident revenue for the ALC),

6. A projection of the volume of service in each department for the entire budget period (assists in forecasting departmental revenues such as resident revenues, gift shop income, physical therapy [PT]/occupational therapy [OT], special services, and their contribution to overall company profitability).

To view revenues realistically, it is also necessary to budget deductions from resident revenue. The following budgetary steps will assist to project these deductions:

1. Relate the past ALC's experiences to the total budgeted resident service revenue.

2. Take into consideration the above changes in relationship to applicable government laws or new resident acceptances that relate to fiscal matters.

3. Develop a percentage of deductions to gross revenue that is classified by each type of deduction.

It is also important to establish a budget regarding expenses. Each year, senior management and each departmental administrator should sit down and discuss and review in detail the projected budget figures for expenses in their departments to remove unnecessary costs and/or over-ordered cost items. The participation by departmental heads in this level of detailed fiscal planning would encourage acceptance of responsibility by each middle-level manager and help provide managers with sufficient information and current up-to-date knowledge as to what is expected of their department. Steps in the budgeting expense process are as follows:

1. Use a master human resources staffing plan that contains the proper titles of all employee positions in the ALC.

2. Prepare salary projections for 12-month time period for each department.

3. Determine supplies for each department.

Plant and Equipment Budget (Capital Budget)

The following is a financial projection for 12 months of construction for new buildings costs, obtaining additional properties (e.g., adjacent land), and new or replacement equipment. The procedure for establishing a plant and equipment budget is as follows:

a. Each departmental administrator should submit proposals to senior management for anticipated purchases of equipment in his/her department.

b. The proposal should indicate what equipment is needed, why the equipment is needed, how many pieces are needed, the cost for each piece, any vendor discounts if applicable, and how the obtainment of the equipment would help either to generate additional revenues or minimize risks/liabilities.

Cash Budget

This reflects the projection of the cash balance at the beginning and end of each month. It forces senior management and even the company's board of directors to pay particular attention to the flow of cash in a given month. For example, the cash budget would help senior management anticipate the possible shortage of cash in the 6th and 7th months of a 12-month budget time period. The ALC can then make plans to either borrow monies from a bank loan to supplement this cash shortfall, or make adjustments such as raising resident rates and/or ancillary fees, cutting expenses, postponing capital equipment purchases, postponing new building capital construction, or delayed repairs. Most cash receipts for the ALC come from the following sources:

Resident's Accounts Receivable

A review of residents' accounts receivable would provide senior management with a guide to the budgeting of cash receipts from residents or third-party payers. For example, if past experience indicates that 85% of the current billings are collected in the month billed, 10% the following month, 4.9% the subsequent month, and 0.1% sent to collections, senior management would have a good idea of the monthly cash flow to pay expenses.

Interest (Money Market Funds, Certificates of Deposit) and Dividends (Bonds, Stocks)

If the ALC has excess cash for investment purposes, estimated income from these investments can then be based on information regarding the rate of interest, the probable yield of the investments and a determination of which month, quarter, or year end the dividends and interests are paid out. In addition, there may be potential capital gains from stock equities for ALCs, but this cannot be predicted.

Bank Loans

Bank loans are budgeted for periods when the cash flow is low. If the ALC needs to borrow monies from a bank, a cash budget would help. It is quite often that banks require the prospective borrower to submit a cash flow report as part of the loan application. This is to help the bank determine whether the borrower can repay the loan within the time period specified. Finally, in setting up a cash budget, it is also important to project cash disbursements from employee payroll, tax payments, and other ongoing expenses (e.g., insurance payments, maintenance contracts, equipment rentals, etc.).

FINANCIAL RATIO ANALYSIS

Liquidity ratios help indicate an ALC's ability to meet its short-term obligations and help financial analysts assess this aspect of a company's performance from the results of a financial model or financial statements. There are two common liquidity ratios that a financial modeler is likely to encounter: current ratio and quick ratio.

Current Ratio

Current assets are those assets that will be realized as cash within the next 12 months. Current liabilities are debts that are due for payment within the next 12 months. The current ratio gives an indication of whether the ALC will be able to pay its debts in the short term (i.e., the next 12 months). Clearly, this ratio should be as high as possible. A prudent ratio is 2:1.

$$\text{Current ratio} = \text{Current assets/current liabilities}$$

Quick Ratio

The quick ratio, or acid test, focuses on whether the assisted living community could pay its debts in the very short-term (i.e., tomorrow or next week). As company stock cannot always be sold quickly it is removed from the calculation of current assets. Again, this ratio should be as high as possible, and a prudent ratio is 1:1.

Quick ratio = Current assets less inventory/current liabilities

Both the current ratio and quick ratio give an indication of future solvency problems (i.e., whether the ALC will be unable to pay its debts).

Performance Ratios in Financial Modeling

There are four common types of financial ratios that a good financial analyst will use to assess the performance of a business or project in building or interpreting the results of a financial model. These four performance ratios are by no means exhaustive, but provide a good indication on the most important ratios of which to be aware.

Return on Assets

The return-on-assets ratio (ROA) provides an indication of how effectively a business is utilizing its investments as assets:

ROA = Net income/average assets

Operating Margin

A good high-level indicator of profitability and profit potential or "wiggle room" (robustness to competitive and external factors that may reduce profitability in the short term):

Operating margin = earnings before interest and taxes (EBIT)/sales

Asset Turnover

This ratio provides a further indication of the effectiveness of capital/asset utilization and relative "capital intensity" of a business:

Asset turnover = Sales/average assets

Return on Equity

Return on equity (ROE) is also known as the *return on average common equity* or *return on net worth*, and measures the rate of return on the ownership interest (shareholders' equity) of the common stock owners. ROE measures a firm's efficiency at generating profits from every dollar of net assets, and shows how well a company uses investment dollars to generate earnings growth.

Working Capital Ratios in Financial Modeling

Working capital ratios demonstrate a company's efficiency at managing its resources, with particular reference to cash flow, and allows a good financial analyst to quickly and efficiently assess this aspect of the company's performance in a financial modeling project. Some typical working capital ratios that a financial analyst will come across include:

Days Inventory

This tells us the amount of time on average each unit of stock is in the shop/warehouse before being sold. Clearly, the shorter this length of time, the better.

$$\text{Days inventory} = (\text{Average inventory/cost of goods sold}) \times 365 \text{ days}$$

Debtor Days

Days sales in receivables or debt collection period tells us the amount of time on average each debtor takes to settle their debt to the business. For the ALC, clearly, the shorter this length of time, the better. A very large debtor collection period might indicate that the business may be unable to collect its debts.

$$\text{Debtor days} = (\text{Average accounts receivable/sales}) \times 365 \text{ days}$$

Creditor Days

Creditor days refers to the day's accounts payable or credit period, and tells us how long on average the business takes to pay its creditors. The longer the length of this time, the better. However, a very large credit period may indicate that the business does not have the cash to pay its debts.

$$\text{Creditor days} = (\text{Average accounts payable/cost of sales}) \times 365 \text{ days})$$

Solvency Ratios in Financial Modeling

Solvency ratios indicate the risk inherent in the ALC as a result of its debt. A good financial analyst will use solvency ratios to keep tabs of the forecasts made in a financial modeling exercise on debt accumulation to ensure that they are realistic and prudent. A good financial analyst will also use solvency ratios to assess the debt profile of a company from its financial statements, and analyze whether the company needs to undergo debt restructuring exercises (such as mortgage refinancing, debt consolidation, etc.). There are two common solvency ratios that a financial analyst is likely to come across when building a financial model.

Leverage Ratios

The leverage ratio, or gearing level, effectively measures the fixed debt payment commitment. Too high a gearing level can imply a high risk upon the cash flow of a public assisted living community and its ability to pay dividends to shareholders.

$$\text{Leverage} = \text{Debt/[capital employed (i.e., equity + debt)]}$$

Interest Cover

This ratio measures the ability of an ALC to pay interest out of profits. Most banks would expect the cover to exceed 1.5 times.

$$\text{Interest cover} = \text{Profit before interest and tax/loan interest expense}$$

Limitations of Financial Ratios in Financial Modeling

Although financial ratio analysis can provide important insight into a company's performance, a good financial analyst will be aware that there are some important limitations that should be noted when using financial ratios as an analytical tool in financial modeling. These lmitations include:

- Ratio analysis is a retrospective, not prospective, examination.
- Ratio analysis is based on accounting, not economic data.
- Ratios do not capture significant off-balance-sheet items.
- Basic ratios can be manipulated through acceptable alterations of accounting policies (e.g., last in, first out [LIFO]/first in, first out [FIFO]).
- Financial statement accounts reflect historical cost, not necessarily current economic value.
- Cash-flow measures have been proven to be more closely correlated with stock price movement that income-based measures.

Table 10.10 illustrates how traditional accounting-based profitability financial ratios often yield ambiguous results.

RISK MANAGEMENT

Some of the potential hazards in an assisted living community relate to its employees. These hazards include injuries and illnesses suffered from helping residents, slipping and falling on wet floors while on the job, and having contact with residents with communicable diseases (e.g., tuberculosis, hepatitis). The federal government mandates that ALCs carry Workers' Compensation liability coverage and adhere to the applicable rules and regulations of the Occupational Standards of Health and Safety Act. A second area of possible liability is with the residents, their guests, and others (suppliers, repair and service personnel) who come onto the community's grounds in order to legally conduct business.

In addition to required commercial building insurance, it is also important that the ALC have an operational safety plan (major disaster, fire, and earthquake), safety committee, and periodic evacuation practice drills. Any community's accident and incident reports must be reviewed by senior management along with the safety committee on a regular basis to determine the causes, as well as to implement any remedial safety corrections. Furthermore, employee safety orientation and in-service training programs must also be scheduled for all staff members to emphasize safety precautions regarding residents, guests, and outside visitors.

TABLE 10.10 LIMITATIONS OF FINANCIAL RATIOS IN FINANCIAL MODELING

ISSUES	ROA	ROE	ROI	PROFIT MARGIN
Do not incorporate opportunity cost or risk.	x	x	x	x
Often mislead managers to slash assets rather than invest.	x	x	x	
Ignore cost of capital investments required to generate earnings.		x		x
Difficult to compare with other opportunities when used in isolation.	x	x	x	x
May be affected by financing decisions (e.g., tax implications of interest on debt, dividend policy).		x	x	

ROA, return on assets; ROE, return on equity; ROI, return on investments. (Owner's capital – shareholder's equity; profit margin–operating margin).

Commercial Insurance

The major risks that ALCs typically face can be broken down into two categories:

a.   Those liabilities risks for which the insured may be liable to others because of the insured's own actions, or those of staff members and invited guests and/or suppliers, outside contractors, and business service agents.

b.   Those liabilities involving property loss risks for which the insured may suffer loss or injury to property as a result of the insured's own actions or the actions of others.

Liability Insurance

Most liability insurances are divided into two separate categories: bodily injury and property damage. The ALC itself is also exposed to lawsuits for its own negligence and negligence of others. The most common liability insurance policy provides coverage only for amounts that the insured becomes legally obligated to pay as a result of accidents and does not provide coverage for incidents that are not considered accidents (such as illness that is caused by repeated exposure to unsanitary conditions, such as hepatitis and tuberculosis). Other incidents for which the insured is legally obligated to pay that are not covered in a basic insurance policy include the following: liabilities for which the insured is not obligated under negligence law until fault is proven, and liabilities where the insured voluntarily admits fault. Expanded insurance coverage can be obtained on basic policies for an additional premium, and by substituting such words as "occurrence" for "caused by accident." That is, comprehensive general liability and add-on insurance riders that would provide broader coverage can be obtained by the ALC to minimize its insurance risk. The ALC should be aware of the following basic liability insurances available in the marketplace.

Owners and Corporate Board of Directors Liability Coverage

The basic policy insures against claims that result from ownership and operation of the community. This is usually a scheduled policy in as much as it designates specific properties and risks assured against suit. The comprehensive general liability offers similar coverage via added optional insurance riders.

Workers' Compensation

All businesses are required by federal/state law to cover any employees who may be injured while working on the job.

Professional Liability

Also often known as *malpractice insurance*, in which the insured is covered under the areas of malpractice, error, negligence in rendering, or failure to render proper medical, nursing, and other professional treatment (e.g., resident OT/PT therapies, resident drug regiment), this insurance does not cover the liability of employees working in the ALC unless it is provided in a schedule within the insurance policy. In addition to paying insurance claimants, commercial liability insurance also provides a number of valuable services and benefits as follows:

Defense-of-Law Actions

The insurance company will defend, in the insured's name, all lawsuits or actions brought against the ALC's employees even if determined to be false or groundless. This insurance policy would pay all costs that include the investigation of the claim, in addition to procuring supporting witnesses and legal counsel. Furthermore, it also pays for bonds that may be required in appeal of any lawsuit, including bonds to release attachments.

Medical Payments Coverage

This is a rider that can be added to the liability policy for an additional premium. This rider would cover all reasonable medical, surgical, and funeral expenses incurred within one year of an accident to each person who sustains bodily injury, sickness, or disease caused by a workplace accident regardless of whether the insured is legally liable. Normally, without this rider, the insured or employees of the insured are not covered for these medical payments.

Property Insurance

The ALC must also consider insurance against direct loss to its tangible properties (e.g., the assisted living community's buildings, equipment, and supplies). These insurances and coverage include:

Fire Insurance

Fire insurance covers direct loss by fire and lighting. It also covers certain types of property damage (either insured separately or uninsured) caused by heavy smoke resulting from the fire. Smoke damage caused by defective heating devices is typically not covered by a basic fire insurance policy.

Extended Property Riders

Extended insurance coverage for other perils can be added to your basic fire insurance policy for additional premiums. The additional endorsements would insure against windstorm and hail (damage to the interior of a building and/or its contents resulting from water, rain, snow, or dust is covered but the actual building must be damaged itself by the force of wind and hail as well), heating oil/natural gas explosions (excludes steam boiler usually), riot or civil disobedience (includes direct loss due to theft, looting, etc.), and aircraft crash (includes objects falling from airplane/helicopter or actual strike by airplane/helicopter).

Additional Extended Property Coverage Endorsement

The extended coverage must be written for the same amount as the basic fire policy, whereby not increasing the face amount of the insurance policy. These endorsements merely extend the coverage to include additional perils, such as building collapse, explosion of steam or hot water boiler, vehicles owned or operated by the insured, falling trees, insect and rodent damage to building, equipment, or supplies, glass breakage, vandalism and water damage, ice, snow, and freezing, to community property and equipment.

Other Property Insurance Coverage

Additional endorsements to the basic fire insurance policy or separate coverage that the ALC might consider are earthquake insurance (especially in earthquake prone areas in California, Washington, and Oregon), federal flood insurance (especially in cities close to major rivers in the mid-west like the Mississippi and Missouri Rivers), automobile insurance (that includes all risks of damage and collision of vehicles owned by the ALC), war and military conflicts, and steam boiler and machinery insurance (two types: narrow form that limits coverage to damage caused by explosion, cracking, bulging, etc. to the boiler alone, and broad form that covers all damage caused by explosion, etc. to the boiler and surrounding properties).

Consequential Loss Insurance

A successful ALC must also consider the possibility of an indirect loss following destruction that prevens the use of all of or certain parts of its community. Three examples of consequential loss insurance are as follows:

a. Building interruption insurance: This provides a source of recovery for loss of resident income because of a reduction of business due to destruction or breakdown of the assisted living community or part thereof.

b. Extra- expense insurance: This insurance covers the costs of operations associated with emergencies.

c. Accounts receivable insurance: This insurance protects ALCs against physical destruction of the resident accounts receivable records. To determine the amount of coverage, beforehand, the insurer would perform an analysis of prior patterns of resident accounts receivable of the ALC.

Theft Insurance

The assisted living community should also review the need for theft insurance to protect itself. There are two broad categories of theft insurances as follows:

Burglary and Theft Insurance

Five types of policies are: (*a*) *open stock burglary policy* (insures against the loss by burglary of merchandise, furniture, fixtures, and equipment, and damage to the premises because of the burglary by all but the community's employees or agents. It does not cover the loss of cash, securities, records, or accounts); (*b*) *mercantile safe burglary policy* (covers loss of cash, securities, and other property, and damages that result from the burglary of the safe); (*c*) *money and securities broad-form policy* (comprehensive coverage for most mercantile risks that provides coverage for all risk for cash and securities); (*d*) *3D policy* (protects the ALC against comprehensive employee dishonesty, records disappearance, and employee destruction of property and equipment); and (*e*) *blanket crime policy* (similar to 3D policy, but provides a single fixed amount for all coverage, not open ended). There are also *fidelity bonds*, which the ALC can purchase to cover an employer against loss of any kind of property (cash, securities, raw materials or merchandise, and equipment) that results from dishonest acts by its employees. Such bonds insure only the named individuals (usually senior management); others may cover all employees at the ALC.

Multiple-Peril Coverage

This type of coverage is sometimes called *package policies* in which many different insurance policies are combined into one policy. The advantages of multiple-peril coverage are broader coverage, elimination of overlapping coverage and claims, and a lower cost. Some policies cover all risks, whereas others only insure specified perils.

MOST COMMON ACCOUNTING TERMS AND DEFINITIONS

Accounting, financial analysis, and financial modeling are integrated disciplines with which any good financial analyst is familiar. In particular, it is important to have a sound knowledge of fundamental accounting principles and accounting terms to ensure a common basis and language for understanding, interpreting, and analyzing financial statements and financial model results. Appendix A provides a useful list of the most common accounting terms that an assisted living accountant/analyst/financial administrator may encounter.

THE NATURE OF ENTITIES THAT OPERATE ALCs

Executive directors should have a working knowledge of the different kinds of entity structures or classifications under which ALCs may operate. When attempting to understand entities, there are three considerations that are helpful so decision-making can be consistent with form and requirements. First, which **legal form** should be used: corporation, partnership, limited liability corporation (LLC), or sole proprietorship? Second, is the ALC **publicly held or private**? Third, is it **for profit or nonprofit**?

Entity Form

Sole Proprietorship

This entity form is usually for smaller concerns, with a single owner, where the owner is not relying on a legal entity to shield them from liability exposure, and merely relies upon insurance for protection. They are also known as the *sole trader, individual entrepreneurship,* or *proprietorship*. They are owned and run by one person with no legal distinction between the owner and business. Do not be mistaken, however; as the enterprise grows, a sole trader can hire employees and engage other vendors to support their goals. This form is rarely used for ALCs, especially larger ones. Smaller, family-owned homes are more likely to utilize this form.

Partnerships (General and Limited)

A *general partnership* refers to two or more persons (or entities) who wish to work on a venture together in which the profits and losses are shared proportionally. In partnerships, the partnership agreement can specify various different aspects of the sharing of income, losses, write-offs, and return on capital; that is not as strict as outlined in corporations (discussed below).

If you study the history of business development, you will discover that a key breakthrough in commerce occurred with the creation of *limited partnerships*. This allowed for a framework of investors who didn't want to be personally liable (as with the sole proprietorship or General Partnership) for all activity of a business, but wanted to invest and be exposed only to the extent of their investment, and no more.

Corporations

A corporation is a group of individuals, using a legal structure provided by law, possessing a "life of its own" so to speak, and independent of the individual owners or investors. The powers and liabilities of the corporation are distinct from those of its members, *shareholders*, who own shares of the corporation's stock. Each state has variations on corporation law and their various shapes and attributes. Despite jurisdictional variations, however, the four main types of corporations are designated as: C, S, limited liability companies, and nonprofit organizations.

C corporation refers to any corporation that, under United States federal income tax law, is taxed separately from its owners. This means that each year the corporation pays a corporate tax rate and then later on, if distributions are made to shareholders, the shareholders are then taxed again on the dividends distributed. While this is often referred to as "double taxation" (corporation pays and individuals later pay again), there are many reasons why an organization may want to remain a C corporation, not the least of which is the stronger ability to reinvest in capital growth versus being pressured to make distributions for the shareholder's personal tax liabilities.

S corporations are corporations that elect to pass corporate income, losses, deductions, and credit through to their shareholders for federal tax purposes. In other words, electing with the IRS to be an S corporation can allow for lower taxes to the owners in the long run. However, S corporations, generally speaking, have more restrictions as to how many owners it can have and whom can even be an owner.

Limited liability corporations are a flexible form of enterprise that blends elements of partnership and corporate structures. Like corporations, the individual owners, usually called *members*, are not liable for the company's debts or liabilities. Furthermore, like partnerships, sole proprietorships, and S corporations, the income is not taxed at the LLC level, but "passed through" to the individual owners. The added benefit of an LLC is that in most states there are less restrictions as to who can be an owner, such as individuals, other corporations or LLCs, and foreign individuals or entities.

Nonprofit corporations: Most of the time when we think of corporations, we think of "for-profit" as a purpose or goal. That is not always the case. Indeed, many ALCs are owned and operated by *nonprofit corporations,* organizations that uses earnings ("profit") to reinvest and achieve the organization's goals rather than distributing profit or dividends to private individuals.

The confusion with such corporations is that there are two kinds of "nonprofits." Essentially, to summarize, there are the nonprofit *charities,* which generally obtain tax exempt status under IRS code 501c3. Then there are not-for-profit corporations that are not necessarily for charity, but are merely for the benefits of the customers or members. For example, just like a home-owners'association (HOA) is a nonprofit, it is not designed for "charitable" purposes. Rather, it is designed to reinvesting "profits" or excess earnings back into the entity to benefit the stakeholder/customers.

Publicly Traded Versus Privately Held Companies

A publicly traded company is a company whose ownership is made up of shares of stock that are publicly traded on one of several stock exchanges or "over-the-counter" markets. Privately held companies, to the contrary, are owned by fewer shareholders, and those stocks are not traded on the open market exchanges. As you can imagine, the financial reporting requirements of a publicly traded company is much more stringent than one that is privately held. There is much greater financial scrutiny on publicly traded companies, and to a certain extent, that scrutiny is more than just disclosure, but additional pressure for increased financial performance. Nevertheless, both publicly traded as well as privately held companies report financial data to the outside world and key stakeholders, not the least of which are banks and auditors. Officers and directors of ALCs should have a limited understanding of these various status requirements to stay in compliance with the government, investors, banks, etc.

RELATIONSHIP DYNAMICS OF REAL ESTATE, OPERATIONS, AND MANAGEMENT COMPANIES IN ALCs

One of the financial management topics executive directors of ALCs need to have a basic understanding of is the relationship between the real estate component and the operating component of the ALC, as well as the retention of a third-party management company.

Some organizations hold the real estate and the operations together in what is referred to as a *single-asset entity*. Holding the real estate and the operations together has both pros and cons. One significant pro is that it is simply easier to run everything through one entity than keeping separate records, especially when the ownership of the real estate and operations is identical. One big con is that combining the real estate and the operations all in "one basket," so to speak, offers more liability exposure in case of various liabilities that may ensue.

Other ALCs will—despite having the same ownership—kee the property and operations separate, in what is often referred to as the *"PropCo-OpCo" structure*. In this scenario, the owners will create one legal entity to hold the real estate and another legal entity to hold the operating company portion. In this scenario, there will be a lease agreement between the two entities to help preserve the legal separation. As alluded to previously, the benefit of this separation is that in case of a catastrophic loss (for example, jury verdict above insurance limits) the operating company can file for bankruptcy but the real estate has a much better chance of being protected from the loss. The owners can then lease the property to another operator and thus salvage or preserve the majority of their investment.

Often the separation of real estate and operations happens naturally due to the fact that the owner of the real estate is a separate owner other than the operator. In this case, some variation of a lease will be utilized to allow an operator to possess and utilize the property as an ALC.

In the senior housing industry, especially amongst the larger, national operators, a very large portion of the properties are held by various landlord entities, either through private or public equity investment funds. One very common segment of real estate ownership is through entities called *real estate investment trusts (REITs)*. REITs raise hundreds of millions of dollars and buy large portfolios of higher quality properties and then lease large portions of their portfolios to various larger operating companies. The pressure of leasing from REITs is not only that they expect the operator to pay the lease payment every month, but they also include covenants of performance on the part of the operator because even though the operating company owns their own operating company, the value of the underlying Real Estate is impacted by the profitability of the operator as well. Thus, even if the operator is able to make the monthly lease payments but they are not able to make as much operating profit as the REIT expected, then the REIT will lose "value" in their portfolio. Thus, it behooves a director of an ALC that is owned by a REIT or similar private equity firm to understand all the expectations and performance covenants so as to know what to expect.

Whether the ALC is structured as a single-asset entity, or if the real estate and the operations are separated into two entities, the operating company will often hire a professional, third-party *management company*. Hiring a third-party management company helps to provide yet one more layer of protection for the owners. The *management company* will often bear some—though often not all—of the liability exposure for operations. Besides providing some shield to liability, there are many other reasons why an operating company would retain the services of a management company. For one, sometimes a particular management company is more familiar with a particular market, or, for another, sometimes the operating company ownership is simply not in a position to run operations at that time.

COLLECTION AND UTILIZATION OF INDUSTRY FINANCIAL DATA

As with many industries, the senior housing industry collects financial data though various organizations and associations. Perhaps the largest such organization in the United States is The National Investment Center for Senior Housing (NIC), established in 1991 (https://www.nic.org/). NIC, as stated on their website, "enables access and choice in seniors housing and care by providing the data and analytics that investors and operators need to make informed decisions, and by facilitating the connections between these groups to benefit America's elders."

Process of Collecting Data on the Industry

The NIC is connected with most of the larger, professionally operated ALCs throughout the country, and through those connections, collects and reports timely quarterly and monthly data. Then, with the collected data, NIC collates the information and features data products such as market fundamentals time-series data on 140 metro markets, the seniors housing actual rates initiative, and the Skilled Nursing Data Report. NIC conducts two annual conferences each year, one in the spring and one in the fall, which are valuable networking opportunities of the seniors housing and care industry.

Importance of Market Data

It is important to have access to industry data so that ALCs and their management teams can make proper financial decisions. Decisions, such as budgeting income expectations, setting rates for services, or whether or not to expand the number of beds in a particular market, are all better informed when there is such industry data.

CONCLUSIONS

This chapter provides the reader with a comprehensive summary of information on financial management in ALCs. It is clear that knowledge about accounting systems, organization, financial reporting, department titles and staff, the use of accounting and financial software, standard accounting procedures, accounts records, budget preparation, financial ratio analysis, risk management, and common accounting terms and definitions help administrators and operators manage effectively and efficiently. In addition to management objectives, ALCs must also be concerned with fiscal objectives in order to have adequate funds to carry out the purposes and goals of the communities and meeting the needs of the residents.

REFERENCES

Crane, M. (2007). *How to run a senior living home: Technology.* Forbes.com. http://www.forbes.com/2007/02/28/yardi-assisted-living-ent-manage-cx_mc_0228assisttech.html

Jennings, R. (2001, May 1). *Cash or accrual?* https://www.journalofaccountancy.com/issues/2001/may/cashoraccrual.html

National Investment Center for Senior Housing. (2020). *Research and analytics.* https://www.nic.org

Oracle. (2016). *JD Edwards world contract billing guide.* https://docs.oracle.com/cd/E26228_01/doc.93/e21939/ww_gl_ent_rev.htm#WEACB531

FURTHER READING

Brealey, R. A., & Myers, S. C. (1988). *Principles of corporate finance* (3rd ed.). McGraw-Hill.

Brigham, E. F., & Gapenski, L. C. (1987). *Intermediate financial management* (2nd ed.). Dryden Press.

Davidson, S., Stickney, C. P., & Weil, R. L. (1985). *Financial accounting—An introduction to concepts, methods, and uses* (4th ed.). Dryden Press.

Gnanarajah, R. (2014). *Cash versus accrual basis accounting: An introduction.* https://fas.org/sgp/crs/misc/R43811.pdf

Gottlieb, M. (2015). Healthcare REITs and their operator partnerships. *Cornell Real Estate Review, 13*(1), 112–125. http://scholarship.sha.cornell.edu/crer/vol13/iss1/12

Motlagh, A. J. (2013). Accounting: Cash flow statement. *IOSR Journal of Business and Management, 7*, 4th ser., 109–116. http://www.iosrjournals.org/iosr-jbm/papers/Vol7-issue4/M074109116.pdf

Waqas, M., & Rehman, Z. (2016). Separate legal entity of corporation: The corporate veil. *International Journal of Social Sciences and Management, 3*(1), 1–4. https://doi.org/10.3126/ijssm.v3i1.13436

Weston, J. F., & Brigham, E. F. (1982). *Essentials of managerial finance* (6th ed.). Dryden Press.

Yardi. (n.d.). *Asset management & accounting software for assisted/senior living market.* https://www.yardi.com/markets-we-serve/assisted-living

LEGAL CONCEPTS AND ISSUES IN ASSISTED LIVING COMMUNITIES

WITH CONTRIBUTING AUTHOR ANTHONY M. CHICOTEL

LEARNING OBJECTIVES

Upon the completion of Chapter 11, the reader will be able to:

- Comprehend liability in relation to the administration of assisted living communities.
- Describe tort law in relation to personal injury lawsuits; negligence, corporate negligence, respondeat superior, governing body, elder abuse, and liability limits.
- Discuss the important elements of, and need for, contracts and admission agreements in assisted living communities.
- Understand the procedures for evictions and state-ordered relocations, appeals process, and readmission following a hospital stay.
- Comprehend elder law in relation to estate planning, including wills and trusts.
- Describe advance planning in relation to elder law with attention to financial and health-care management.
- Discuss surrogate decision-making, including powers of attorney, conservatorships, guardianships, and other forms of surrogacy.

INTRODUCTION

Some assisted living owners and operators may have a negative perception of legal issues. The law is often associated with burdensome regulations and costly lawsuits. However, the law can and should be an ally of assisted living providers. Laws and regulations that help establish an expected standard of care for residents can serve as helpful guides to owners and operators. Other laws clarify the relationship between assisted living communities and their residents, ensuring that both parties understand their roles with respect to one another. Finally, the law enables residents to plan for their incapacity, particularly with regard to their healthcare and finances, which accommodates and directs their care and reduces a provider's burdens.

TORT LAW

Tort Law and Personal Injury Lawsuits

Tort law is the law governing people's relationships with one another as general members of a civil society. A "tort" is committed any time a person or a business violates a basic expectation of a civil relationship. Examples of torts include battery, slander, and medical malpractice. Tort law is different from contract or criminal law. Contract law governs relationships between the participating parties only. Criminal law is similar to tort law in that it governs individual conduct within society, but violations are addressed by society as a whole, operating as a prosecuting agency, instead of by the victim. The key elements to tort law are: (a) a civil wrong against a person or property (b) prosecuted by the victim or their representative. Many torts are addressed by courts as "personal injury" lawsuits.

Common Law, Statutes, and Regulations

The law comes from many different sources which can create confusion even for seasoned lawyers. When most people think of laws, they think of statutes. Statutes are laws passed by a legislative body and codified in writing for all citizens to read and follow. Statutes come from federal, state, and local governments and usually vary considerably.

Another form of law is regulations. Regulations are similar to statutes in that they are written and created at the federal, state, and local levels. However, regulations are not passed by legislatures but by government agencies operating within the executive branch of the government. Agencies that address assisted living are often called *departments of health* or *departments of human services*. Regulations do not have the same force as statutes, so if they conflict in any way, the statute prevails.

One last form of law is the common law. Common law comes from judges, often dating back hundreds of years to fill voids caused by a lack of statutes and regulations. Common law developed as courts considered cases and rendered decisions based on principles of general fairness. As more and more cases were decided, the law was refined and became more stable. The common law is particularly prominent in tort law involving negligence. Although some tort law derives from statutes and regulations, it is predominantly grounded in common law.

PRACTICE TIP   Law comes from all three branches of the government. Statutes come from the legislature, regulations from the executive branch, and common law from the judicial branch.

Remedies

An important part of tort law is the remedies available to victims. There are many remedies available but they generally fall within one of two categories: monetary and equitable relief.

Monetary remedies are focused on compensation and making a victim whole. The money that is awarded to the victim is intended to return the victim to the position they were in prior to the commission of the tort. The computation of money damages begins with measuring the loss to the victim. For example, if the victim suffered a theft of $100, the perpetrator would be liable for $100. The victim is entitled to all reasonably foreseeable financial damages, including lost wages, medical expenses, and the replacement value of damaged property. These damages are often called *compensatories* as their purpose is to compensate victims for the harm they suffered.

Another form of monetary remedies is known as *general damages*, and is more difficult to precisely quantify. General damages cover an array of issues such as pain and suffering, loss of consortium, and loss of enjoyment. As these types of damages are not easily ascertainable, they are often controversial because they can lead to huge money awards based on mixed evidentiary support.

PRACTICE TIP   Elderly and disabled residents of assisted living facilities are often limited in recovering monetary damages because they often have very low incomes and do not suffer much in lost wages. In addition, they have shorter life expectancies which restrict the amount of compensable future damages.

Equitable relief is based on common law but is often supported by statutes as well. There are two main forms of equitable relief: injunctions and specific performance. Injunctions are court orders that typically prohibit a party from engaging in a particular action. Restraining orders are one well-known type of injunction. Specific performance is a court order requiring a party to complete its promises made in a contract. Orders for specific performance are rare.

Negligence

Negligence is perhaps the most significant tort for assisted living communities. The key to negligence is neglect: a failure to live up to the applicable standard of care. Negligence does not require a failure to act; positive actions can constitute negligence. The key to determining negligence is whether the action or inaction at issue violated the suitable range of reasonably expected action or inaction. Over the past 200 years, common law has established four elements of a negligence claim:

1. The allegedly negligent party must have a duty of exercising due care to the victim.
2. There must have been a breach of the standard of care.
3. The breach must have caused actual harm to the victim.
4. The harm must be measurable in damages.

Duty of Care

The most important element of negligence for assisted living communities is the duty of care. By law, all assisted living communities have important duties of care for their residents and even their visitors and family members. The critical issue is defining the standard of care that assisted living communities owe their residents. The applicable standard generally comes from two legal sources: state laws and professional standards. State laws vary, but a close examination yields generally applicable standards nationwide.

PRACTICE TIP   The laws regarding assisted living facilities are almost entirely state laws. There are minimal federal laws. The only noteworthy mention of assisted living facilities in federal law relates to the receipt of Supplemental Security Income (SSI) by residents (42 U.S. Code § 1382). The law allows states to reduce SSI payments to assisted living facilities that do not meet quality of care standards. The statute has had no meaningful impact on care as SSI reductions would actually discourage providers from serving SSI recipients (Carlson, 1999). The paucity of federal law reveals a national policy to leave assisted living matters to the state control.

Required Services

The first applicable standard of care expressed by state laws is required services. Required services are those mandated by state law to be provided in any facility that engages in assisted living services. The services consistently required, regardless of the state, are shelter, food, supervision, and assistance with activities of daily living. Room and board are staples of assisted living but the most salient feature is the provision of living assistance. Most states delineate the types of living assistance to be provided. Vermont, for example, requires certain assisted living communities to assist with "meals, dressing, movement, bathing, grooming, or other personal needs" (Vermont General Assembly, n.d.). North Carolina requires assisted living communities to provide transportation for residents to "necessary resources and activities" (North Carolina Assisted Living Regulations, n.d.). Most state laws simply mandate assisted living communities to provide oversight and assistance with the residents' personal care needs.

Care Plans

A second applicable standard for assisted living communities in many state laws is the formulation and revision of resident care plans (also called *service plans*). Alabama requires a care plan that documents each resident's personal care needs and required services, be updated whenever the resident's needs change, and be reviewed by a physician at least annually (AL Admin. Code § 420-5-4-.05 [3][d]). Care plans in Indiana and South Carolina must be updated at least semi-annually and after any change of condition (410 IN Admin. Code § 16.2-5-2[a]; SC Code Regs. § 61-84-703[A]). Regardless of state law requirements, professional standards of care seem to mandate a fair amount of care planning for residents. The elements of good care planning include a careful assessment of resident needs, a plan for addressing those needs, and continuous revision, especially after the resident has experienced a change in condition.

Although good care planning is definitely helpful to quality resident care, some providers may be wary of written documents that could ultimately be used against them in a lawsuit. If care planning is documented but not effectively implemented, it could serve as evidence of the care that was needed, but not provided. In that way, care planning becomes a liability. However, the advisable approach to care planning is not to abandon it, but to ensure that it is performed carefully and that implementation is routinely reviewed and updated. The care plan should be reviewed with the resident and the resident's representatives and, when possible, reviewed with the resident's physician. Most state laws and professional care standards require a fair amount of care planning and it cannot be avoided. Care planning should be viewed as an active, fluid process involving both assessment and implementation.

Staffing Levels

Another prominent care standard involves minimum staffing levels in assisted living communities. New Mexico is a typical state, requiring at least one staff person be on duty at all times in communities with 15 or fewer residents (7 NM Admin. Code § 8.2.18[A]). For communities with more residents, the staffing requirements increase. Florida uses a weekly standard of total staffing hours closely correlated to the number of residents (58 FL Admin. Code Ann. R. 58A-5.019[4] [a][1]). Other states, like Alabama, do not require a specific number of staff members but refer to "sufficient staff" necessary to provide "adequate care" to the residents (AL Admin. Code § 420-5-4-.04[1]). Regardless of whether the state sets a minimum number of staff or staffing hours, communities should always carefully monitor staffing levels and the care needs of the residents. Attorneys who litigate cases against assisted living communities will often target staffing levels whether or not staffing was initially an issue. If an attorney can demonstrate that the staffing was inadequate to satisfy the care needs of the residents, compliance with state prescribed staffing levels will not immunize the facility from legal action.

Medication Management

Medication management is a universal issue for assisted living communities; hence, the handling of medication is addressed by every state. Most states rely on an assumption that residents retain the mental capacity to give consent to the administration of medications, and the physical ability to take medications on their own. These states authorize facility employees to store and distribute medications to the hands of residents but usually prohibit actually placing the medication in the mouths of residents. The result is a fairly confusing process for medication administration where the law is inadequately matched to reality. Massachusetts provides for "self-administered medication management," limiting facility staff members to:

> reminding residents to take medication, opening containers for residents, opening prepackaged medication for residents, reading the medication label to residents, observing residents while they take medication, checking the self-administered dosage against the label of the container, and reassuring residents that they have obtained and are taking the dosage as prescribed. (The 191st General Court of the Commonwealth of Massachusetts, n.d.)

Illinois and Ohio allow staff members to place medications into containers and then place the containers into the mouths of residents with physical impairments provided they are mentally alert (77 IL Admin. Code § 330.1520[c][2]; OH Revised Code Ann. § 3721.011[B][2][c]). Similarly, Alaska law allows staff to guide medication in a resident's hand to the resident's mouth (AK Stat. Ann. § 47.33.020[c][7]). With laws that allow such leniency in the "self-administration" of medication, drawing a clear line between permissible and prohibited medication management is challenging.

A few states have addressed the problematic distinction between self and assisted administration of medication by allowing nurses to designate or train staff members in medication issues (TX Health & Safety Code Ann. § 247.026[g]; 6 CO Code of Regs. § 1011-1, chapter XXIV). In these instances, staff members may operate in a nursing capacity, provided the legal requirements are satisfied.

The issue of medication management, like that of care planning, poses a potentially significant legal dilemma for assisted living communities. In most states, where medication assistance is limited to helping with resident "self-administration," staff members must avoid conduct that is not expressly permitted. Residents with mental or physical incapacity therefore must have some ability to recognize medications and take them on their own. Assisted living communities face liability concerns whenever a medication mistake is made, particularly when residents are overdosed. If a resident is incapable of self-administration as defined within their state, the facility must be able to explain how the resident nonetheless continued to receive medication. In states where nursing duties can be delegated, communities have to ensure that all staff designations and training requirements are completely satisfied. If assisted living communities employ nurses, they should carefully supervise the nursing performance, as the appropriate care standard may be higher than a customary assisted living standard.

Resident Falls

Risks of resident falls present another interesting dilemma to assisted living communities that is often found when dealing with the legal issues of elderly people or people with disabilities. On one side of the dilemma is resident autonomy, allowing residents to make their own decisions regarding risk and benefits, and choosing when and how they would like to walk or ambulate. On the other side of the dilemma is resident safety, which suggests that facility staff have a duty to prevent residents from falling. Falls, after all, can be a catastrophic event for residents, often leading to severe injuries and permanent declines in functioning or death. About 20% to 30% of falls result in moderate to severe injuries that affect mobility, independence, and increase risk of premature death (Sterling et al., 2001). Therefore, falls often lead to personal injury lawsuits against assisted living communities. However, the only way to truly prevent falls is to restrain the resident. State laws usually prohibit restraining residents but do not set any care standards for preventing falls.

Common law standards do impose a duty to prevent falls on assisted living communities. Resident care plans should assess a resident's fall risk and the staff should implement appropriate measures to limit that risk as much as possible, including assistance to and from the bathroom, consensual use of modest restraints such as wheelchair lap belts, and even facilitating the acquisition of ambulatory aids such as walkers, wheelchairs, or mobility carts. Assisted living communities should carefully document its resident fall care plans and be sure to note residents' acceptance or refusal of recommended fall prevention techniques. In addition to resident-centered approaches, communities should also be cognizant of simple environmental issues such as carpeting, grab bars, lighting, and spill cleanup. The law does not require that falls be prevented; it rather expects reasonable measures will be undertaken to minimize them at all times.

Aside from preventing falls, communities should be sure to have a detailed postfall procedure that, at a minimum, assesses the resident for a physician visit, documents the incident, and triggers additional care plan revision. Seemingly insignificant falls can cause significant latent injuries and even falls resulting in no injury at all can be evidence that more falls may be imminent. Postfall procedures will be scrutinized by attorneys whenever a fall leads to significant injury.

Resident Wandering and Supervision

Preventing resident wandering is much like preventing falls in that it sometimes pits resident autonomy against resident safety, and state laws provide very little direction and cannot be relied upon as setting a specific standard of care. Again, as with falls, staff should be vigilant regarding resident wandering and plan care accordingly. Wandering is rarely purposeless. Even residents with impaired capacity move for a reason: e.g., to avoid a loud or stressful environment, unfamiliarity with their surroundings, or boredom. Good care practices and avoiding legal liability require staff to try to identify why a resident may be moving (wandering) and ways to ameliorate those triggers.

The law requires that communities allow residents to move freely about their environment and prevents the use of physical restraints barring an emergency medical situation. However, communities are also expected to provide significant supervision to residents, particularly those with dementia, by ensuring they do not leave the facility unless they are supervised or have a safety plan in place. Communities must be careful to balance the rights of residents to be free from restraints with the expectation that they will be supervised and safe. In terms of legal liability, residents who wander and suffer injury are likely more problematic than overuse of restraints. Nonetheless, liability can be incurred whenever a facility fails to properly balance the two competing interests.

Conclusion on Duty of Care

The standard of care means different things for assisted living communities in different states. Although certain national standards are discernible, state laws that specifically set forth minimal care standards are exceptionally important to facility owners and providers. Even in instances where there is no state statutory or regulatory guidance, communities should be aware of common law standards set forth in case law, and understand that appreciably specific standards can exist outside of what is stated in state code books. The requisite standard of care is of paramount importance in assisted living and tort law liability.

Breach of Duty

Once the appropriate standard of care has been identified, the next step in assessing a facility's liability for negligence is determining whether or not the standard was breached. A breach is simply a failure to satisfy the duty of reasonable care. An old-time U.S. Appellate Court Judge, Learned Hand, devised a simple method for determining whether a breach of reasonable care had occurred by comparing the cost of an untaken precaution versus the expected benefit such precaution would have had. If the cost outweighs the potential benefit, there is no breach. Few states use the Learned Hand "formula" for determining breach of duty, but the efficiency of actions taken or not, does play a role in evaluating whether a breach has occurred. Providers should carefully document efforts made and costs considered whenever a resident's care needs are being evaluated.

Causation

The third element of a negligence claim is causation. The alleged injuries of the victim must have been caused, at least in part, by the breach of the duty of care that occurred. The perpetrator or the tort is only liable if the tort was the primary reason for the victim's damages. Causation is usually broken down into two elements: (a) factual causation and (b) legal causation.

Factual causation is concerned with whether the action or nonaction at issue caused the victim's damages. One rule of thumb for establishing factual causation is to use a "but-for" test: Would the victim's damages have occurred but for the perpetrator's action or nonaction? If the answer is no, then factual causation likely exists.

Legal causation, also known as *proximate causation*, is concerned with the chain of events between the perpetrator's actions or nonactions and the damages at issue. The perpetrator is held liable for all of the reasonably expected consequences of negligence. If a subsequent act causes additional damages, the chain of causation is broken and the initial negligent actor is not liable for those additional damages.

Related to the causation issue in a negligence claim are the defenses of contributory and comparative negligence. Contributory negligence is a doctrine by which an alleged tortfeasor (a person who has committed, or allegedly committed, a tort) can avoid any liability for damages if the victim's own conduct contributed in any way to the causation of the damages. Contributory negligence is used in a handful of states, including Alabama, Maryland, North Carolina, and Virginia, as well as Washington, DC. Most states instead use a related concept of comparative negligence. Under comparative negligence, the alleged tortfeasor's liability is limited to the proportion to which their conduct caused the damages. If the tortfeasor's negligence was 75% responsible for the damages suffered, their liability is limited to 75%. Contributory and comparative negligence can be powerful tools in a lawsuit. Assisted living owners and providers should therefore have an even greater incentive to carefully document all instances where a resident's risk of injury was assessed and communicated to the resident or their legal decision maker.

Damages

The fourth and final element of a negligence claim is quantifying the damages. Damages are the amount of money the tortfeasor will owe for the negligence. Damages were briefly discussed previously in the review of remedies. Compensatory damages are the money needed to make the victim "whole," including lost wages, medical expenses, replacement property, and compensation for pain and suffering. In addition to compensatories, many states allow for punitive damages: Money that is not meant to compensate the victim, but rather to punish the tortfeasor to send a clear public message that such behavior will not be tolerated. Punitive damages are usually not available unless the tortfeasor has acted recklessly or intentionally; thus, negligence does not usually generate punitive damages. Some states, like California, allow for damages to be multiplied in cases where the victim is an elder or adult with disabilities to provide further protection to such populations.

Corporate Negligence

Corporate negligence is a relatively recent concept, holding corporate healthcare providers liable for negligence that occurs from a flawed system as opposed to a single identifiable incident. Although corporate negligence is most often associated with hospitals, its principles can easily be extended to assisted living communities. Corporate negligence assigns healthcare systems a duty to oversee the general quality of their care as provided by individual members whether they are "staff" or not. The system manager, in this case the facility owner or operator, is to remain alert for patterns of incompetent behavior and to address those issues in a timely manner. For assisted living communities, corporate negligence may impose additional duties to carefully supervise staff members, and terminate those who provide inadequate care, as well as to constantly review its overall delivery of care and identify and address problem areas.

Governing Body

Assisted living facility owners must also be cognizant of potential personal liability for personal injury claims of residents. Owners or corporate directors may be liable under various legal theories, including *piercing the corporate veil* and *governing body*. If alleged resident injuries are the result of particularly egregious conduct that was known or should have been known by any reasonably diligent owner or director, they may be personally liable. As with corporate negligence, the issue is oversight of the entire care system at issue, especially the quality and performance of the direct-care staff members. In healthcare settings, this oversight must be particularly focused as life or death outcomes may be at stake. The law presumes that owners and corporate directors are immune from liability and piercing corporate veils and governing body liability are rarely realized; however, corporate providers should be careful to exercise diligent oversight and must take action whenever they are informed of significant problems within an assisted living facility.

Respondeat Superior

Respondeat superior is a Latin term that means *let the master answer*. For legal purposes, the doctrine of *respondeat superior* is used to hold employers liable for the actions of their employees. The liability in such situations is often called *vicarious liability* because the actual wrongdoing is performed by one person (the employee) but may be answered by another (the employer). Generally, *respondeat superior* does not exist unless the employee was acting within the scope of employment at the time the alleged wrongful conduct occurred. If an employee who is not "on the clock" takes a resident to the movies and the resident chokes on some popcorn, the employer facility would not generally be liable. However, the resident or his family may allege the facility had inadequate policies regarding staff member outings with residents, or that the resident did not have capacity to decide about outings at all. The facility may also be liable if it knew that this staff member was engaging in risky activities with residents after hours. Communities can reduce their liability by having detailed policies governing the actions of its employees regarding all aspects of a resident's care. Some states have "strict liability" provisions whereby certain actions create liability for employers even if employees were acting outside of the scope of their employment.

Elder Abuse

Most states treat elders and disabled adults together as protected classes in abuse prevention statutes. For simplicity's sake, this chapter will use the term *elder abuse* to cover both elder and disabled adult abuse. Elder abuse is a special tort in some states, whereas in others it is merely a method of enhancing the penalties for conduct that is some other form of tort. For assisted living communities, there are two concerns regarding elder abuse liability: perpetrating elder abuse and failure to report elder abuse.

Elder abuse occurs in assisted living communities. Often, the perpetrator is a staff member of the facility itself. Abuse can be overt and obvious, including the hitting or emotional harming of residents, but it also covers instances of neglect, where the facility's inaction is the problem. Assisted living providers are at particular risk of elder abuse tort actions because they have legally assumed the responsibility of caring for the elder; thus, any failure to provide reasonably expected care could be treated as both negligence and elder abuse. Most elder abuse statutes require that the neglect be significant, including reckless or intentional conduct, and more than simple negligence. Facility owners and operators can be liable for elder abuse perpetrated by their employees.

The second issue regarding elder abuse in assisted living communities is compliance with mandatory reporting requirements. Every state has statutes that require certain professionals that are expected to regularly assist elders and disabled adults to report any suspected incidents of abuse or neglect to a state agency for investigation. The list of "mandated reporters" varies from state to state but usually includes law enforcement officers, nurses, and social workers. Assisted living facility staff members and administrators are often named mandated reporters (e.g., VA Code Ann. 63.2-1606[A][1]). States may issue civil fines to mandated reporters for failing to report suspected elder abuse, but failure to report could also subject the facility to tort litigation, particularly if proper reporting would have prevented potential harm from occurring.

Limiting Liability

Medical Injury Compensation Reform Act (MICRA) caps. Many states have instituted laws to limit the liability of healthcare providers in personal injury lawsuits to counter what they perceive as the deleterious effects of excessive money judgments against them. California was the first state to address this issue when it passed the Medical Injury Compensation Reform Act in 1975. MICRA placed a $250,000 limit on awards for noneconomic damages, the main target of which was pain and suffering. Many states have followed California's lead, including Florida, Maryland, Massachusetts, Michigan, Oregon, and Wisconsin, by also limiting the recovery of noneconomic damages in cases of medical malpractice. The application of MICRA caps for assisted living communities depends on whether or not they are considered healthcare providers in their particular state.

Tort Reform

Tort reform is the name given to efforts that aim to reduce both the number of personal injury lawsuits filed, and the awards given to victorious claimants. Well-publicized cases of million-dollar judgments for seemingly insignificant torts, such as the McDonald's coffee burning case (where a woman was awarded nearly three million dollars by a jury), have precipitated various movements for tort reform in states and in the federal government.

As previously discussed, one of the primary methods of tort reform is capping noneconomic damages. Texas has caps in place to limit the maximum amount plaintiffs may receive in noneconomic damages in medical malpractice cases. This cap is stipulated in the Medical Malpractice and Tort Reform Act of 2003 also known as *House Bill 4 (HB 4)*. One cannot recover more than $250,000 from each healthcare facility that was involved, and noneconomic damages may not exceed $500,000 among all of the medical facilities involved. Consequently, the maximum amount one may receive for noneconomic damages in a medical malpractice lawsuit is $750,000. Several times in recent years, Congress has considered imposing damages caps nationwide, although without success. Another type of tort reform targets punitive damages, which can often far exceed the actual damages suffered by the victim. Several state courts and even the U.S. Supreme Court have weighed in on punitive damages, finding that the amount of punitive damages must bear some relation to the actual damages, often expressed as a ratio. For example, an award of punitive damages that is more than 10 times that of the actual damages may be considered unconstitutional. Other efforts have focused on limiting class action lawsuits and attorneys' fees. One proposal, yet to be adopted in any state, is to create a "loser pays" system in which the loser of a lawsuit has to pay the attorney fees and court costs of the winning side. Such a proposal would likely reduce the number of lawsuits dramatically because the plaintiff would risk significant costs if the lawsuit ultimately fails.

Licensing Reports' Admissibility

Another issue concerning legal liability is the admissibility of reports generated by state licensing agencies during their investigations of complaints or during annual inspections. The reports, if admitted in court, could be influential with judges and juries as a definitive opinion on whether a facility was in compliance with state standards of care. The admissibility of these reports varies from state to state but the possibility should remind providers to be especially responsive to visits from licensing. Licensing reports not only publicly reflect on a facility's performance, they also serve as ammunition for savvy plaintiffs' lawyers.

CONTRACTS

The General Law of Contracts

For assisted living providers, contract law may be nearly as important as state laws that establish basic care standards. The contract between providers and residents establishes many of the rules that will govern their relationship. The contract, usually known as the *admission agreement*, is critically important.

Elements of a Valid Contract

Although there are differences among states regarding contract law, most share consistency in identifying the basic elements of a contract. The four most important elements of a valid contract are:

- Offer and acceptance,
- Consideration,
- Capacity, and
- Writing.

The first element of a valid contract is offer and acceptance. An offer must be made by one party that is accepted, in full, by the other. An offer and acceptance do not need to be formal steps, one right after the other; rather they must simply reflect a "meeting of the minds." Both parties to the contract must have a mutual understanding of what is being agreed, and intend to be bound by it. A counteroffer made in response to an offer is not the same as acceptance and does not create a contract unless the counteroffer itself is accepted.

PRACTICE TIP   The law regarding offer and acceptance should encourage assisted living facilities to scrutinize their marketing materials used to promote the sale of their services. Marketing materials are often considered by courts in lawsuits to convey promises that go beyond the legal standard of care. Marketing materials often describe services to be provided, creating expectations and becoming part of the offer that is implicitly extended to prospective residents.

The second element of a valid contract in many states is consideration. Consideration is a term for the exchange of something of value. In other words, a valid contract requires that each side give something up in the agreement. The value of the consideration can be minimal (i.e., one penny). Consideration can be particularly important for assisted living communities, where relatives or other third parties often sign the admission agreement as financial guarantors. If consideration is required for a valid contract, third-party agreements to undertake financial responsibility for the resident may be unenforceable. Third parties can claim that they did not receive anything of value in a resident admission agreement and thus have no obligation to pay for services provided to another person. Assisted living communities should check with a local attorney if it uses a third-party financial responsibility clause in its admission agreements.

The third element of a valid contract is capacity of the signing parties. This is a key issue in assisted living communities where residents often have questionable capacity to make their own decisions. If a proposed agreement is signed by a person without capacity, it is unenforceable. Providers should demand that a legally authorized surrogate, along with the resident, sign an admission agreement if the resident has questionable capacity. Signing issues will be discussed further below.

The fourth element of a valid contract is that it be committed to writing. The law does not require that all contracts be in writing but all states have a "statute of frauds" that requires some types of agreements be in writing. Usually, contracts with duration of more than 1 year and those involving a fair amount of money ($500 or more in many states) must be in writing. Other states require that all leases involving residential use of property be in writing. Regardless of whether a written agreement is required or not, good practice dictates that providers reduce their agreements with residents to writing. Assisted living communities should also ensure that all residents have a written agreement *prior to* move-in, because once a resident has moved in, they potentially receive the protection of landlord–tenant laws and might have a residency claim without having signed anything.

Unconscionability

Sometimes, a contract that meets all of the above elements is nonetheless legally unenforceable because it is considered unconscionable. Unconscionability is a concept of fairness whereby a contract that is manifestly unfair to one of the parties can be declared void by a court of law. Unconscionability has two elements that must be satisfied to void a contract: an absence of meaningful choice by one of the parties, and contract terms that are unreasonably favorable to the other party. The absence of meaningful choice is always a potential problem when both sides of a contract are perceived to have drastically unequal bargaining positions. The formation of a contract is supposed to be an interactive process. The more one side dictates the terms, the more likely an absence of choice is to be found.

Assisted living providers have to be extra watchful for unconscionability because residents are often elderly or disabled, need placement right away, do not have much time to meaningfully shop for alternatives, and receive written contracts that are offered on a take it or leave it basis. Communities may enjoy disproportionate bargaining power, making the contract process one-dimensional. In order to avoid satisfying the first step of unconscionability, assisted living communities should make extra efforts to engage residents in the bargaining process, allowing them to choose services from a menu of options and explaining their rights to seek services at other assisted living communities.

PRACTICE TIP   A "contract of adhesion" is a contract that is standardized and does not permit the signing party to alter the terms. Adhesion contracts usually include boilerplate language and are offered as take it or leave it agreements. Adhesion contracts are legal but sometimes receive special scrutiny by courts when considering a contract's unconscionability.

The second element of unconscionability involves contract terms that are unreasonably favorable to one party. This element is difficult to satisfy as virtually every term of the contract must somehow favor one party. Contracts are not substantively unconscionable unless they are grossly unfair for one party.

A concept somewhat related to unconscionability is when contracts are unenforceable because they violate public policy. For example, a contract in which someone agreed to be another person's slave would be void as against public policy. For assisted living communities, contractual waivers of individual rights could be void against public policy. Such waivers are often found in mandatory arbitration agreements or other forms of limiting a person's right to sue that are discussed later in the chapter.

Two other fairness concepts that may void a contract are duress and undue influence. Duress allows a party to void a contract if entering into the agreement was involuntary due to an inordinate amount of pressure. Undue influence happens when a party enters into a contract because a person with extraordinary ability to persuade the party took advantage of their mental incapacity in forcing them to sign the agreement.

Admission Agreements

Admission agreements are the contractual foundation of the assisted living resident relationship. States have different laws about assisted living admissions, but nearly all limit the type of residents a facility may take. State laws also vary on what admission agreements must contain and what is prohibited.

PRACTICE TIP   Facilities are wise to require residents or their legal representatives to sign an admission agreement prior to admission. If a resident moves in before signing the agreement, they may refuse to sign the agreement or some of its provisions and the facility would likely have to use a burdensome eviction process to remove the resident. Admission agreement issues should be resolved before the resident moves in.

Who May Be Admitted

Nearly all states require that potential residents be formally assessed before they are admitted into an assisted living facility. New York law requires all residents have a health examination performed by a physician within 30 days prior to admission (NY Soc. Serv. Law § 461-c[7][a]). Other states, such as Ohio, Pennsylvania, and South Carolina, require that residents be physically assessed at least annually (OH Admin. Code § 3701-17-58[D]; 62 PA Stat. § 1057.3[a][2]; SC Code Regs. R. 61-84-1101[A]). Maryland, New Mexico, and a few other states use standardized forms for assessments. Even if state law does not require an assessment, providers should require them. Aside from assisting in care planning and provision, such physician assessments can give providers a useful tool in identifying a resident's potential problems, as well as a baseline for judging changes in condition.

Prohibited Conditions and Waivers

State laws invariably limit the type of resident to whom assisted living communities may provide care. Communities must be especially careful in ensuring that residents with prohibited conditions are not admitted or allowed to remain if they have developed a prohibited condition. Admitting or keeping a resident with a prohibited condition can lead not only to trouble with the state licensing authority, but could impose significant liability exposure to a facility.

Generally, assisted living communities are considered nonmedical communities. Residents with significant medical or nursing needs usually cannot reside in assisted living. Prohibited (restricted) conditions vary from state to state but some common conditions include:

- Intravenous therapy (IVs), including feeding tubes;
- Ventilator assisted breathing;
- Stage III or IV bed sores;
- Bed bound;
- Catheter care;
- Not oriented to person and place;
- Nonambulatory; and
- Danger to self or others.

Many states that list prohibited health conditions also include waivers allowing assisted living communities to care for residents with the foregoing conditions or needs. Waivers are typically allowed to enable a current resident to remain in the facility despite the development of a serious medical condition. They are not often available for admitting new residents who already have such conditions. In waiver cases, the facility or resident must actively request permission from the state licensing agency. Waivers are more likely to be granted if the facility has made arrangements with suitable medical professionals to provide the necessary care at issue, usually in the form of a staff nurse or home healthcare providers. Some states allow assisted living communities to obtain hospice waivers in order to care for terminally ill residents using a hospice care agency (e.g., CA Health and Safety Code § 1569.73[a]; FL Stat. Ann. § 429.26[9]).

Admission Agreement Elements

Like most other things, state laws vary on what may and may not be included in assisted living admission agreements. Many of the common requirements are listed below. Even if certain elements discussed below are not required in your state, providers should nonetheless consider including them to protect against possible contractual disputes.

Fees

Some states mandate that certain elements be included in assisted living admission agreements. Nearly all state laws on the subject require that the contracts carefully specify the nature and costs of the services that will be provided to the resident. The base monthly rate should be explicit, along with the costs of any additional services the facility provides. The listing of services and costs must often include details about the charging, usage, and refunding of preadmission fees or resident deposits. Admission agreements should also detail third-party payments if such payments are contemplated at the time of admission. Remember, from the previous discussion of contracts and considerations, the contract should specify the benefits that third parties receive by the provision of care and supervision of the resident. Third-party payment agreements may be subject to special state laws, as in Maine, where an admission agreement "may not require or encourage anyone other than the [resident] to obligate himself/herself for the payment of the [resident's] expenses" (Department of the Secretary of State (Maine), n.d.). Maine does allow voluntary third-party payment agreements if they are raised by the third party and are written in a separate agreement.

The admission agreement might also need to explain exactly how rate increases will be conducted, stating how the amount of a rate increase will be calculated, and what the resident can expect to receive in terms of advance notice. Some states, like Alabama and Utah, require that all assisted living fee increases be preceded by at least 30 days' notice to the resident (AL Admin. Code § 420-5-4-.05[3][g][19]; UT Admin. Code R. 432-270-10[8][b]). Even if a state does not require advance notice specific to assisted living, general landlord–tenant laws almost always require notice in advance of an eviction, ranging from 3 to 60 days, depending on the circumstances. Providers should not ignore their state landlord–tenant laws as they may be more stringent than those for assisted living communities. State law may also limit the circumstances under which fees can be increased. New York, for example, limits additional charges in some circumstances to when the facility has experienced "increased cost of maintenance and operation" (N.Y. Soc. Serv. Law § 461-c[2]).

Termination

Many states require that the grounds and procedures for termination of the admission agreement be specified in the contract. The termination provisions should explain the process for facility-initiated terminations as well as resident-initiated terminations. State landlord–tenant laws may be applicable. Assisted living communities should also include a careful discussion of refunds and returns of prorated rent and security deposits. Some states, like California, also require the contract to detail what the resident can expect if the facility has to close (CA Health and Safety Code §§ 1569.884, 1569.886).

Negotiated Risk

In an effort to minimize liability to lawsuits and enforcement actions and to retain residents with exceptional care needs, some assisted living communities are using "negotiated risk" agreements. Negotiated risk is a relatively new concept and is not universally understood. From a facility's perspective, negotiated risk allows residents to waive the provision of care to remain in the facility when their care needs would otherwise require they move out. The waiver allows residents to exercise their personal choice for their own level of care and accept the risks of doing so, just as they might acknowledge the inherent dangers of skiing or hang-gliding. Negotiated risk agreements are used for potentially problematic care issues such as resident falls, diabetes management and dietary needs, bedsores, and wandering.

Negotiated risk agreements are quite controversial and their legality is dubious. The agreements purport to allow the assisted living standard of care to be set by contract, foregoing state legal minimums in some cases. Courts may be skeptical of negotiated risk agreements and may void them as contrary to public policy. Voluntarily agreeing to inadequate care is inapposite to the nature of assisted living. People go to assisted living communities to receive care and supervision. Negotiated risk agreements undercut this arrangement.

At this time, there is no definitive legal treatment of negotiated risk agreements. Some states, such as Illinois, have explicitly outlawed the use of negotiated risk that purports to waive a facility's regulatory requirements (77 IL Admin. Code § 295.2070[e]). Other states, like Kansas and Ohio, require assisted living communities to document any necessary services the resident has refused, including an explanation of the potential risks of the refusal, and express acceptance by the resident (KN Admin. Regs. § 26-41-202[f]; OH Revised Code Ann. § 3721.012). Assisted living communities can certainly consider using negotiated risk agreements, but they should be sure to avoid any agreements that attempt to lower the standard of care below state minimums. The agreements should also not be used to retain residents who have obvious care needs that necessitate greater care than is provided in assisted living. Even when the agreements are used appropriately, providers should be prepared for the possibility that negotiated risk may be found unenforceable by a local court.

Arbitration Clauses

Another controversial contract clause in admission agreements call for mandatory arbitration of legal disputes between the facility and residents. A mandatory arbitration clause holds that any legal dispute between the facility and the resident will be submitted to a private arbitrator instead of a court. Arbitration is a less formal and often less costly method of resolving legal disputes. Arbitration clauses are fairly standard in many service contracts but are subject to some important rules in assisted living.

No states currently prohibit the use of mandatory arbitration agreements in assisted living facility admission agreements, but some states do impose limitations on their use. Some states may require a mandatory arbitration agreement to be presented as a separate document, whereas others may require the agreement not be required as a condition of admission to the facility. Signatures on arbitration agreements are often carefully scrutinized if a dispute arises between a resident and a facility so it is important to make sure that representatives who are asked to sign actually have the authority to commit the resident to arbitration. Arbitration agreements remain a controversial topic. Several bills have been introduced in Congress to prohibit their use in various contexts, including in nursing home admission agreements.

PRACTICE TIP   In order to increase the enforceability of an arbitration agreement, facilities should use clear language explaining that residents are waiving their right to go to court. Facilities may also want to consider including the agreement to arbitrate in a document separate from the admission agreement, and make clear that the agreement is completely voluntary and not a condition of admission.

For assisted living communities that use mandatory arbitration clauses, the signature of the resident or legal representative should be scrutinized. If the resident has any possible capacity problems, the facility should insist on the signature of a legal representative. Legal representatives may not have the ability to waive a person's right to sue by signing a mandatory arbitration agreement. For that reason, assisted living communities should carefully review the document that conveys the representative's legal authority. Spouses and relatives typically do not have the authority to bind residents to arbitration without a document like a power of attorney specifically authorizing them to do so.

Mobility Devices

A burgeoning problem with assisted living management is the control of resident mobility devices such as wheelchairs and electric scooters. Many assisted living communities are imposing rules that limit the use of mobility devices, but these rules are likely illegal.

Several federal laws, such as the Americans with Disabilities Act, Fair Housing Act, and Section 504 of the Rehabilitation Act of 1973, all prohibit discrimination in housing on the basis of disability. State laws may also prohibit such discrimination. If a resident can demonstrate that the resident suffers from a disability and uses a mobility device to have equal use and enjoyment of the residence, the facility may not unilaterally prohibit the use of a mobility device.

Many assisted living communities have issued rules that are intended to limit the use of mobility devices in their facilities. Some of these limiting rules require residents to:

- Obtain special permission to use a mobility device.
- Obtain a doctor's note or evaluation of safety.
- Obtain liability insurance to operate a mobility device.
- Sign a waiver releasing the provider of any liability for use of the device.
- Pass an operating test.
- Transfer into dining chairs during meals.

Generally, rules that limit the use of mobility devices are not legal unless the devices truly pose a threat to others (i.e., violent acts committed toward/against others with a wheelchair). The reason for such a high standard is that the mobility device provides the resident with their only way of maintaining their independence.

The Fair Housing Act does not allow any discriminatory terms to be imposed on residents due to their disability. However, one federal court found that requiring liability insurance for the use of a mobility device could be legitimate if there is a valid business purpose, and the restrictions are narrowly tailored and based on individual inquiries of actual threats posed by specific individuals. A facility may not impose a blanket restriction, however, based on a broad stereotype that assumes the general dangerousness of mobility devices. A facility also may not impose restrictions on device use if the resident does not pose a risk to anyone other than themselves.

Signing Authority

The issue of who signs the admission agreement is frequently overlooked to the detriment of assisted living communities. Residents, regardless of their capacity, should always be asked to sign the admission agreement. If they do not sign the agreement and are later determined to have had capacity, the agreement may not be enforceable. There is no harm in asking a resident with questionable capacity to sign the agreement. The key is to make sure that a legally authorized surrogate also signs the agreement. Surrogates are discussed below. Assisted living communities can rely on the signatures of relatives, but ideally would obtain the signature of a court-appointed guardian or agent under a power of attorney with the ability to contract for services on behalf of the resident.

For residents who have no capacity to sign an admission agreement and no surrogates, assisted living communities should be exceptionally cautious. Such a resident may not be bound to pay rent, comply with facility rules, or other issues that are covered in an admission agreement. The plight of unrepresented residents is discussed at the end of this chapter.

Locked-Door Care

Assisted living communities that use secured perimeters or locked doors to prevent residents from leaving their building must be particularly careful about contracts and resident autonomy. In short, locking residents into a facility requires legal authority to do so. Legal authority must come from a court or other legally authorized surrogate. Generally, the law does not provide surrogates with the power to lock up the principal. Court-appointed guardians may have such power, but agents under powers of attorney usually do not. Even if a power of attorney purports to give the agent the ability to lock the principal in a facility, it may not be enforceable. This limitation on the power of surrogates is widely misunderstood and rarely talked about among providers, attorneys, and lawmakers. In California, state law explains that only conservators or residents themselves may sign for an admission to a locked-door facility (CA Health and Safety Code § 1569.698[f]). Despite this explicit policy, providers throughout the state permit agents or family members to sign locked-door admission agreements. Assisted living communities that do so are rarely reprimanded but are risking significant liability for false imprisonment at some point in the future.

New Admission Agreements

Some assisted living communities require residents to sign new admission agreements following a temporary hospitalization, an ownership change, or some other change in residency. Providers are legally free to seek new admission agreements at any time provided the elements of a valid contract are satisfied. However, they should be careful about insisting. Many states limit the reasons for evicting a resident, and failing to sign a new admission agreement is not one of them. Providers should check with an attorney about their local laws before undertaking any punitive action against residents who refuse (or whose representatives refuse) to sign a new admission agreement following some change in residency.

EVICTIONS

Evicting residents from assisted living communities is a common problem and is fraught with legal concerns. Almost all states have laws that limit the reasons for evicting a resident and prescribe a series of procedures that must be followed. In addition, general landlord–tenant laws may apply. Providers must be wary of many laws when pursuing an eviction of a resident.

Grounds for Eviction

Most states limit the grounds for legally evicting a resident. Some common reasons include the following:

- The resident's medical needs exceed what can be provided by the facility.
- The resident engages in conduct that is harmful to the resident, other residents, staff members, or facility property.
- The resident violates the terms of the admission agreement or other documented rules of the facility.
- The resident violates state or local law.
- The resident can no longer pay for services.
- The state or a physician orders the resident be transferred.
- The facility is closing.

PRACTICE TIP   If a resident is unable to pay for services, the facility should warn the resident, in writing, that eviction proceedings may be commenced. The facility should *never* withdraw services that jeopardize the health or welfare of the resident.

The mere satisfaction of one of the foregoing eviction reasons may not be sufficient to justify an eviction. Many state laws, regulations, and eviction oversight processes require that the proposed eviction be the absolute last resort for resolving the problem at hand. Therefore, assisted living communities should carefully document every attempt at resolving the problem and efforts to avoid eviction. Physician assessments should be used whenever possible. The facility should give plenty of warning to a resident who is violating the admission agreement or rules. A resident who has failed to pay should be given ample advance notice of the impending consequences. The facility's documentation should not only illustrate that the resident eviction is merited but also that it has exhausted every other method for resolving the issue.

State-Ordered Relocations

Some states have a process by which residents can be ordered to move into a higher level of care by the assisted living oversight agency. In such situations, the state usually has a fairly detailed procedure by which it will ensure the resident is transferred; however, assisted living communities may also be required to undertake action, especially if the resident refuses to leave. The state relocation orders are often directed to the facility, not to the resident, so the facility may have the burden of physically sending the resident to another home. Providers should learn their local laws and have policies and procedures in place for dealing with state-ordered relocations.

Eviction Procedures

Aside from having satisfied the reasons for eviction, assisted living communities must also comply with any required procedures. The initial procedure for an eviction is usually providing legally sufficient notice to residents that they are being evicted. The notice usually has two components: the format and the timing. Some states prescribe one or the other or both.

The format of the notice is actually specified in a handful of states. New York is one such state (18 NY Compilation of Codes, Rules and Regs. § 487.5[f][3]). Even if the form of notice is not mandated, many states require that certain information be included. Many states require the proposed date and reasons for the eviction to be set forth. California requires that details, such as facts and witnesses, be included so that the resident has a fair ability to oppose the proposed eviction (22 CA Code of Regs. § 87224[d]). Many states also require residents to be told of their right to appeal the proposed eviction through a state appellate process.

The required timing of an eviction notice varies from state to state, but is generally 14 to 30 days. Some states, like Texas, allow the timing of the notice to be accelerated if there is an emergency situation requiring immediate action for the safety of the resident or other residents (TX Health and Safety Code § 247.065[b][P3]). Although the law may allow for relatively short notice of eviction, providers should be aware that residents may have a difficult time finding alternative housing and should consider working closely with residents to assist them as best they can.

No states explicitly require an assisted living facility to help a resident find a new home. Assisted living communities can proceed with evictions regardless of whether a resident has found new housing or not, but explicit legal requirements and pragmatic liability concerns are often separate notions. Any facility that evicts a resident with no place to go by casting them into the streets or to a homeless shelter with nothing but bus fare is risking significant legal problems if the resident suffers an adverse outcome. Again, assisted living communities should be very careful about the posteviction plans of residents. Providers are certainly not responsible for finding the best alternative housing possible, but the level of resident dependence coupled with the care services universally offered in assisted living seem to suggest that communities do have more responsibility to evicted residents than standard landlords.

Appeals

A few states augment their eviction laws with an administrative appeal process to weigh the merits of proposed evictions that are opposed by residents. State processes are all that is available to residents as there is no federal constitutional right to a hearing to contest an eviction from an assisted living facility. Missouri, North Carolina, and Ohio have administrative hearing processes for resident appeals. Rhode Island also offers administrative hearings but prior to the eviction the facility is required to make "a good faith effort to counsel the resident if the resident shows indications of no longer meeting residence criteria, or if service with a termination notice is anticipated" (RI Gen. Laws § 23-17.4-16[a][2][xviii][E]). New Jersey and Utah specify methods for appeal but they are most likely not very meaningful. New Jersey allows individual communities to establish their own appeal procedures and directs residents to appeal a proposed eviction to the facility administrator (8 NJ Admin. Code § 8:36-4.1[a][40]). Utah limits residents to an informal conference with facility representatives (UT Admin. Code R. 432-270-11[5]). Appeals decided by facility administrators or staff are doubtlessly difficult for residents to win.

Landlord–Tenant Requirements

Besides laws that are specific to assisted living eviction procedures, facility operators may have to be watchful of landlord-tenant laws as well. Landlord–tenant laws do not typically make explicit exemptions for assisted living communities. Therefore, an argument can be made that landlord–tenant laws apply to assisted living communities. Wisconsin assisted living laws use the term *tenant* to refer to residents, whereas Iowa law explicitly applies the state's landlord–tenant law to assisted living (WI Admin. Code § DHS 89.24; IA Admin. Code R. 321-25.42[231C]).

State landlord–tenant laws and even local ordinances may limit the reasons for discharge to a small number of "just cause" reasons that are more narrow than those found in assisted living laws. The landlord-tenant laws may also mandate additional procedures for evicting residents, prescribing more information that must be in the notice and longer periods of time for providing it.

Even if general landlord–tenant laws do not apply to assisted living communities in a particular state, evicting residents almost certainly requires a court order if the resident refuses to leave past the period of time provided in the notice. Physically removing a resident is patently illegal in all circumstances, unless a court order has been obtained and is executed by an authorized law enforcement representative. If residents remain past the time given in the eviction notice and administrative appeals have been exhausted, providers should seek the counsel of an attorney to learn about landlord–tenant evictions. The judges involved may be unfamiliar with assisted living communities and the laws governing their operations.

Housing Discrimination Laws

Resident evictions may also be subject to federal and state housing anti-discrimination laws. Such housing laws may be unfamiliar to the average provider but recent academic focus has been placed on evictions as a form of disability-based discrimination. Many of the legal theories involved are untested, but there is some likelihood that future evictions may be scrutinized for discrimination.

If a facility allows a resident with a prohibited health condition to stay by obtaining a waiver, it may have some explaining to do if it chooses not to seek a waiver for the next resident with that condition. Federal and state disability discrimination and housing law may preclude assisted living communities from refusing a resident's admission based on a disability. In such a case, the resident may elect to file a lawsuit seeking an order to compel admission, or may file a complaint with the federal Department of Housing and Urban Development or a state housing agency.

Requests for Reasonable Accommodations

Federal and various state housing disability discrimination laws require housing providers to make "reasonable accommodations" for persons with disabilities. A reasonable accommodation requires providers to give special assistance or waive the enforcement of a particular rule or practice, so that a person with a disability can obtain or maintain residence. So long as the accommodation does not entail unreasonable expense or impose an "undue hardship," providers are required to make modifications to give persons with disabilities an equal opportunity to have assisted living housing and services. Reasonable accommodations can range from wheelchair access to rooms and showers to relaxing house rules for residents with cognitive impairments.

Readmission Following a Hospital Stay

Assisted living communities frequently contemplate resident evictions after a resident has been hospitalized. Hospitalizations often indicate a significant change of condition in a resident that may necessitate additional care that either the resident cannot afford or the facility cannot provide. Medically clearing a hospitalized resident to leave the hospital does not necessarily mean that the resident's needs may be managed in assisted living. A facility's reaction in such situations may be to refuse to readmit the resident until their condition has improved. State laws, however, usually do not permit communities to lock residents out of their homes, regardless of whether they have been hospitalized or not. A few states permit quick evictions in emergency situations, but even those states may require advance notice be provided to those residents, and they may have legal rights to appeal the move. In addition, a state's landlord–tenant laws likely strongly discourage landlords from locking residents out.

Returning residents pose a legal dilemma for communities. On one side, the law usually directs communities to allow residents to return to their home at the time of their choosing. Landlords simply cannot lock tenants out of their homes. On the other side, however, communities have a limited range of services that may not meet the care needs of a resident returning from a hospital. If a facility were to accept the return of such a resident, it risks liability if the resident suffers neglect or another form of harm. One possible compromise is to allow the resident to return to the facility, engage the legal eviction process immediately, and write a letter to the resident or their representative explaining the facility's reservations in detail. That way, the facility has complied with the law while also undertaking everything it can do to warn the resident of the risks of returning.

ESTATE PLANNING

Estate planning means different things to different people, but it always includes advance planning for the disposition of a person's property at the time of their death. Estate planning can be accomplished in a few different ways: through wills, trusts, or by operation of law in the absence of any formal documents.

Wills

Wills are written documents that specify the division of a person's property at the time of their death. The formalities of wills varies from state to state but usually require the maker of the will (the testator) to sign the document in front of witnesses and make a formal declaration that the document is intended to be a last will and testament. Wills may also include the testator's wishes regarding the disposition of their remains and a designation of an executor, the person(s) in charge of ultimately distributing the testator's property according to the division directed in the will.

PRACTICE TIP   In most states, when a person dies without having executed an estate planning document, the distribution of their property is governed by state law. This process is known as *intestate succession*. Intestate succession usually distributes property to spouses and close relatives first, and then moves out to more distant relatives. The beneficiary of last resort, in the absence of any family, is usually the state itself.

As an estate planning device, wills have several advantages, but also a couple of important disadvantages. One, they are well known among all people as perhaps the primary method for distributing property after death. Two, they are relatively easy to draft and execute, often costing modest amounts for preparation by an attorney, and can even be done using a computer program or simple form found on the internet. Another advantage to wills is that they are relatively easy to change or terminate, as long as the testator retains the mental capacity to do so. The only disadvantages of wills are that they do not provide any mechanism for handling an estate prior to the testator's death, even if they become incapacitated, and they do not help an estate avoid probate. *Probate* is the generic term for the process by which the distribution of an estate via a will is supervised by a court. Each state is different, but states often require that estates of a certain size ($250,000 or more in California) require court supervision of the property distribution to ensure no fraud occurs. The probate process is often cumbersome and costly, reducing the value of an estate by up to 10% after paying state fees and court costs.

Trusts

Trusts are another form of written estate planning. Much like wills, trusts allow the person creating the trust (trustor) to direct the distribution of their property at the time of their death. A trust is a legal entity, apart from the trustor, so only property that is actually placed in the trust is distributed at the time of the trustor's death. The trustor's valuable property, such as houses, cars, and large financial accounts, must be formally re-titled into the name of the trust. Although the trustor is alive, the property in the trust is usually at their disposal just as if it were not in a trust. At the time of the trustor's death, however, the trust terminates, and the property is distributed to beneficiaries as it would be in a will.

The primary advantage of a trust is that it usually allows the property in trust to avoid the state's probate process. Since the property in the trust does not technically belong to the trustor at the time of death, the trustor's "countable" property is below the probate threshold. Another significant advantage of trusts is that they almost always include a financial management component, whereby the property in trust can be managed by a substitute "trustee" if the trustor ever becomes incapacitated. The disadvantage of trusts is that they are often fairly complicated—even simple trusts run over 20 pages—and thus require an attorney's assistance, which can be costly. The complexity of trusts also increases the difficulty of amending or terminating the documents.

PRACTICE TIP   Trusts fall into one of two categories: irrevocable or revocable trusts. Irrevocable trusts are permanent and cannot be changed once they are executed. Irrevocable trusts are often created for tax purposes or to exert control over property after the trustor's death. Setting up a college fund for a grandchild is a popular goal of irrevocable trusts, for example. Revocable trusts, as their name suggests, may be altered or terminated by the trustor at any time as long as they retain capacity. Because revocable trusts may be changed as long as the trustor is alive, they are often called *living trusts.*

Totten Trusts

Totten trusts are an older name for an arrangement in which a particular account is paid to a beneficiary at the time of death of the original owner. Under Totten trusts, while the bank depositor is still alive, the beneficiary does not have the ability to access the bank funds. Such arrangements are also called *payable on death (POD)* or *transferrable on death (TOD)* accounts, and supersedes a contrary designation in a will or trust. POD or TOD accounts are not included in a person's probate estate and can be a simple method for estate planning.

Rep Payee

For incapacitated beneficiaries of Social Security or SSI benefits, a representative payee or "rep payee" may be appointed to manage the money that is paid out each month. State laws do not prohibit assisted living providers from becoming rep payees but assisted living communities should be cautioned against such an appointment. Providers acting as rep payees create an obvious financial conflict of interest. Many states have local agencies that will act as rep payees for incapacitated beneficiaries for free or for a minimal cost.

Providers as Beneficiaries or Executors

Assisted living communities should be aware that the law frowns on providers acting as beneficiaries in wills and trusts. Most states do not expressly prohibit providers as beneficiaries or executors, but all states do consider "undue influence" when the validity of a will or trust is contested. Providers usually have a relationship of limited duration but exceptional intensity with residents. If providers are named as beneficiaries in a resident's will or trust the presumption may be that the designation must be the product of undue influence exerted on the testator. Providers should be particularly wary of being named or having staff named in wills or trusts, particularly if the resident's family members do not know that such a designation has been made. Providers may want to consider personnel policies that prohibit staff from being named as beneficiaries, as well as discussing such matters with residents at the time of admission.

ADVANCE PLANNING

Aside from estate planning, people may also engage in other forms of advance planning that allow them to account for the management of their estates or healthcare while they are alive but incapacitated. There are many methods for creating such advance planning, and they are quite important to residents of assisted living communities.

Trusts

As previously mentioned, trusts almost always include estate management provisions that allow a substitute trustee to handle all property that is in the trust if the trustor loses the capacity to do so. Property that is not in the trust may only be managed by a substitute decisionmaker if there are other forms of estate management in place.

Powers of Attorney

Powers of attorney are documents that designate a substitute financial decisionmaker (agent) to serve if the creator of the power of attorney (principal) loses the capacity to do so. Powers of attorney must be in writing, signed by the principal, and witnessed or notarized. Powers of attorney can be very broad or extremely limited; the breadth of the document can be tailored according to the principal's needs. The power that can be granted ranges from control over financial accounts and insurance policies, to retirement and government benefits, lawsuits, and real property. Usually, the principal may grant or withhold powers from a menu of options.

The agent's ability to manage the various granted powers usually do not begin until the principal loses capacity. In these circumstances, the power of attorney is said to be "springing" because the powers are dormant at the time of execution and then "spring" into effect if capacity is lost. The loss of capacity is typically determined as specified in the power of attorney form, but usually requires a doctor to state the principal has lost capacity to manage their financial affairs. Other power of attorney forms become effective immediately, as soon as the principal signs them. These forms are riskier to the principal because it allows the agent to immediately begin handling their financial affairs, with or without the principal's knowledge.

PRACTICE TIP   Powers of attorney are often called *durable powers of attorney*. Long ago, powers of attorney had very limited usage and would expire at the time a person lost capacity to manage their affairs. Now, powers of attorney are completed specifically to cover periods of incapacity. For that reason, the powers granted continue despite incapacity, making the form durable.

Employees of assisted living communities should be wary of acting as agents under a power of attorney. Oregon, for example, explicitly prohibits any facility staff members from acting as a resident's guardian, trustee, or agent (OR Admin.Code § 411-054-0027[2]). Other states' laws may not prohibit such a relationship, but it could create substantial conflicts of interest that subject the facility to allegations of fraud, undue influence, or elder abuse.

Joint Ownership

Another method of providing for financial management is adding a joint owner to property or a financial account. This method, less formal than a power of attorney, allows the joint owner to undertake property management. However, joint owners have full access to the property and are not bound to exercise fiduciary responsibility, meaning they may sell, withdraw, or spend any funds just as any owner would. For that reason, joint ownership is a risky form of advance planning, and not recommended in most situations.

Healthcare Planning and Decision-Making

Informed Consent

Any understanding of healthcare decision-making begins with the legal and ethical principle of informed consent. Informed consent doctrine holds that every person has the right to determine what healthcare treatment they receive or not. Unsurprisingly, there are only two elements of informed consent: (a) information provided to the patients, and (b) consent. The right to give or withhold informed consent is grounded in constitutional principles of privacy and self-determination. If the patient does not have capacity to make healthcare decisions, state laws allow surrogate decisionmakers to provide or withhold consent. When a patient lacks capacity and a surrogate decision-maker, state laws vary on how informed consent requirements are satisfied.

The information necessary to obtain informed consent varies from state to state, but prominent state law cases have set a functional baseline. Before consent can be considered "informed" the healthcare provider must tell the patient or surrogate decision maker the following:

- Diagnosis,
- Nature and purpose of the proposed treatment and the desired outcome,
- Risks and benefits of the proposed treatment,
- Alternative treatments and their relative benefits and risks (including the likely results of doing nothing).

Right to Refuse Treatment

A corollary to the right to informed consent is the right to withhold consent, or the right to refuse proposed treatment. The right to refuse proposed treatment is extensive, recognized by the U.S. Supreme Court to include the ability to refuse life-sustaining treatment. If the patient does not have capacity, surrogates may generally refuse treatment, although the refusal of life support sometimes requires procedural safeguards be satisfied. Patients, or their surrogates, may also refuse proposed medications at any time and may refuse placement in long-term care communities, including assisted living. Treatment and placements may be forcibly applied at times, although the circumstances are rare and court intervention is almost always required.

One legal issue that is often intertwined with a patient's right to refuse treatment is physician-assisted suicide. Active measures undertaken by a patient or physician to end a life (i.e., euthanasia) are treated much differently under the law than the withdrawal of life-sustaining treatment. The U.S. Supreme Court has addressed physician-assisted suicide, and held that a state law ban was constitutional. In doing so, the Court found that the right to assisted suicide is neither fundamental nor traditional. Since that case, California, Colorado, Hawaii, Maine, Montana, New Jersey, Oregon, Vermont, Washington, and the District of Columbia have legally authorized physician-assisted suicide effective during 2019. These states use a highly detailed process for limiting suicides to people who are terminally ill and have decision-making capacity.

Advance Directives

All states provide legal mechanisms by which people can express their wishes regarding healthcare treatments in advance. These efforts were reinforced by Congress when it passed the Patient Self-Determination Act of 1990. The idea of an advance directive is to allow any adult to declare their preferences regarding certain healthcare treatments, particularly regarding the provision of artificial life support, to guide healthcare decisions if the person ever becomes unable to make decisions. Advance directive laws were in direct response to well-publicized medical cases where young people were victims of terrible accidents that left them in persistent vegetative states. In these cases, courts were asked to authorize the withdrawal of artificial life support, often receiving great resistance from religious groups and state officials. In an effort to avoid such controversy, state lawmakers adopted advance directives to clear up confusion about the decision-making preferences of the person lacking capacity and to allow them to exercise their constitutional right to refuse treatment in advance.

Every state authorizes advance directives by using a written form. An advanced directive created in one state is valid in all states. Some states have the forms written into the law, other states simply list some requirements and let lawyers or healthcare providers draft the forms. The forms almost always include an expression of preferences regarding the provision of artificial life support in situations where the principal is in a persistent vegetative state, or has a terminal condition that is likely to result in their death in a short period of time. Some forms allow the principal to state other preferences, including anatomical gifts, placement in a long-term care facility, and disposition of remains. The forms must be signed by the principal and often have very specific witnessing requirements. Assisted living providers should learn the basic requirements for advance directives in their states and consider stocking some forms for residents to execute while residing in their communities. Advance directives can make a critical difference in healthcare provision, particularly for elderly people, yet they remain largely underutilized.

PRACTICE TIP   Advance directives are often called *living wills,* which can be confusing to people who have also heard of wills and living trusts. A living will is an advance directive, limited to advance healthcare decision-making. Wills and living trusts, on the other hand, deal exclusively with property, primarily to designate a distribution of property at the time of death. Living wills deal exclusively with healthcare and have nothing to do with property.

Other Forms of Advance Healthcare Planning

Besides advance directives or living wills, many states allow people to designate their healthcare preferences in advance in other formats, often after a person has been diagnosed with a terminal condition. Physician orders regarding life-sustaining treatment (POLST) are methods for a doctor and patient to address specific types of life-sustaining care, including the administration of CPR, artificial nutrition and hydration, and ventilators. A similar document, known as a *do-not-resuscitate order (DNR)*, also allows advance declarations about life-sustaining treatment, although they tend to be more narrow in scope than POLSTs.

Whenever a person has failed to make advance written expressions of their wishes regarding healthcare, courts will nonetheless allow evidence of a person's verbal expressions in cases to determine whether treatment should be initiated or terminated. Even seemingly unimportant conversations about artificial life support can serve as evidence to assist a court in deciding what a currently incapacitated person would want in their current situation.

SURROGATE DECISION-MAKING

As medical science continually improves, life can be preserved even after a person has lost decision-making capacity, thereby increasing the need for surrogate decisionmakers. States have devised several methods for allowing surrogates to make healthcare decisions for incapacitated people.

Powers of Attorney

Much like financial powers of attorney, state laws enable surrogate decision-makers (agents) to handle healthcare whenever a person loses the capacity to do so. The designation of the agent must be performed in writing on a document that must be signed by the principal and comply with witnessing requirements. The principal may designate a surrogate and substitute surrogates in case the first person cannot serve. Healthcare powers of attorney are often combined with advance directive forms so that an agent is designated and instructed on the principal's wishes regarding specific healthcare treatments. The extent of the agent's authority over the principal's healthcare is as broad or limited as the document states.

Guardianships and Conservatorships

For people who have not named an agent in advance, the courts can be asked to name a surrogate decision-maker. This process is known as *guardianship* in most states, conservatorship in California. Petitioning for guardianship is often a complicated and time-consuming process, engaging piles of paperwork, attorneys, and court hearings. Once a guardianship is awarded, many states require constant court reviews. Since the process is so burdensome, many people treat it as a last resort only, to be used only after every other form of surrogate decision-making has been exhausted. If a person in need of guardianship does not have a relative or other person willing to act as guardian, states have public guardians whose job is to act as guardian in such cases. In some states, public guardians are required to go through licensure, training, and supervision before the decision-making. In other states, the decisions a public guardian can make are limited.

Guardianship law was designed mainly to name surrogates for people who did not nominate a surrogate in advance of losing capacity. Since that time, some states have created new laws that permit family and others to circumvent guardianship. These far less formal devices are legal when state law has expressly permitted them; however, many states have not addressed informal surrogacy. In these states, guardianship is still legally necessary. In reality, however, illegal surrogates are often allowed to make healthcare decisions for a person who has allegedly lost capacity.

Some states have created a formal mechanism for healthcare decision-making under court supervision that does not require the appointment of a guardian. These methods are used to make a one-time healthcare decision and thus do not require the same number of procedures that guardianship does. This alternative court process is often used to make critical healthcare decisions regarding such things as surgery and the withdrawal of artificial life support when the proposed patient has not made an advance directive.

Informal Forms of Surrogacy

A few forward-looking states have passed laws allowing people to designate healthcare surrogates in advance without having to execute a written document. These oral surrogacy designations must usually be made to a healthcare provider who is instructed to document the designation. The oral designation may be of limited duration and scope but is a practical alternative in an emergency situation.

Another informal method for assigning healthcare surrogacy status is based on simply having a close relationship with the person who has lost capacity. Most states allow spouses and domestic partners, by mere existence of their relationship, to act as surrogates when one has not been designated formally. These states also often include family members as informal surrogates if the person who has lost capacity has no spouse or partner.

Unrepresented Residents

One national study estimated that 3% to 4% of nursing home residents have lost capacity, have no formal or informal surrogates, and have not executed any advance directive (Karp & Wood, 2003). These residents are sometimes called *unrepresented residents*. Assisted living communities are also sites where unrepresented residents can be found. The provision of healthcare to such residents is nearly impossible to figure legally in most states as their laws are silent regarding an applicable informed consent process. Iowa, New York, and Texas have state-authorized deci-sion-making committees to provide informed consent for unrepresented people. These states are the exception, however, as most states are left with a completely unregulated process by which healthcare providers are left to their own internal policies and procedures or to seek the assistance of the local public guardian.

PRACTICE TIP   Careful assisted living facilities will not have unrepresented residents because they will require someone with legal authority to sign the admission agreement. Providers should not admit any residents who have neither capacity to sign an admission agreement nor a legally authorized surrogate. Providers cannot contract with unrepresented residents.

Assisted living communities should adamantly avoid acting as healthcare surrogates for their unrepresented residents. The law is clear that informed consent is required before any healthcare can be provided. Most states have a hierarchy of potential surrogates to provide consent if a person has lost mental capacity. If a resident does not have capacity or a surro-gate, no consent can be legally given and any provider who does so may be guilty of battery, false imprisonment, or other crimes and torts. The local public guardian should be engaged for unrepresented residents.

PRACTICE TIP   A recent study performed in San Francisco revealed that informed consent laws are often violated for unrepresented patients of healthcare services (White et al., 2007). Doctors routinely make healthcare decisions unilaterally for their unrepresented patients despite state law and professional guidelines requiring much more process. And these decisions have fatal consequences: one third of the studied physicians have withdrawn life support for at least one unrepresented patient. In the study, 37 unrepresented patients required life support decisions. For 30 of the 37 patients, physicians and other direct-care clinicians made the life support decisions without formal court or even internal hospital review. In some cases, the clinicians did not even follow their own hospital's internal policies. Hospital policies provide guidelines designed by organizations, such as the American Medical Association, and state laws were not followed despite a supposed belief by physicians that they are in legal jeopardy when they make life support decisions for unrepresented patients. Any concern about legal liability was not enough to dissuade physicians from ignoring state law and recommended best practices.

CONCLUSIONS

This chapter provides the reader with a comprehensive overview of legal concepts and issues pertaining to assisted living communities. It is evident that elder law and liability are important concerns for assisted living administrators. This chapter illustrates the need for assisted living administrators to be well informed about tort law, contracts, estate planning, advance planning, and surrogate decision-making. It is important to be mindful that the law can, and should, be an ally of assisted living administrators in their pursuit to address the concerns and needs of both residents and staff.

REFERENCES

Carlson, E. (1999). *Long-term care advocacy*. Mathew Bender & Co.
Department of the Secretary of State (Maine). (n.d.). *Chapter 113: Regulations governing the licensing and functioning of assisted housing programs*. https://www.maine.gov/sos/cec/rules/10/ch113.htm

Karp, N., & Wood, E. (2003). *Incapacitated and alone: Healthcare decision making for unbefriended older people*. ABA Commission on Law and Aging.

North Carolina Assisted Living Regulations. (n.d.). *Subchapter 13F Licensing of homes for the aged and infirm*. http://www.hpm.umn.edu/nhregsplus/ALF%20by%20State/North%20Carolina%20ALF.pdf

The 191st General Court of the Commonwealth of Massachusetts. (n.d.). *Chapter 19D: Assisted living*. https://malegislature.gov/laws/generallaws/parti/titleii/chapter19d

Sterling, D. A., O'Connor, J. A., & Bonadies, J. (2001). Geriatric falls: Injury severity is high and disproportionate to mechanism. *Journal of Trauma, 50*, 116–119.

Vermont General Assembly. (n.d.). *The Vermont statutes online*. https://legislature.vermont.gov/statutes/section/33/071/07102

White, D., Curtis, J. R., Wolf, L. E., Prendergast, T. J., Taichman, D. B., Kuniyoshi, G., Acerra, F., Lo, B., & Luce, J. M. (2007). Life support for patients without a surrogate decision maker: Who decides? *Annals of Internal Medicine, 147*(1), 34–41. https://doi.org/10.7326/0003-4819-147-1-200707030-00006

FURTHER READING

Carder, P., O'Keeffe, J., & O'Keeffe, C. (2015). *Compendium of residential care and assisted living regulations and policy: 2015 edition*. U.S. Department of Health and Human Services, Office of the Assistant Secretary for Planning and Evaluation, Office of Disability, Aging and Long-Term Care Policy and Research Triangle Institute. https://aspe.hhs.gov/basic-report/compendium-residential-care-and-assisted-living-regulations-and-policy-2015-edition

Carlson, E. (2005). *Critical issues in assisted living: Who's in, who's out and who's providing the care*. National Senior Citizen's Law Center. http://nsclcarchives.org/index.php/critical-issues-in-assisted-living-whos-in-whos-out-and-whos-providing-the-care

Mollica, R. (2006). *Residential care and assisted living: State oversight practices and state information available to consumers* (AHRQ Publication No. 06-M051-EF).

National Center for Assisted Living. (2019). *2019 Assisted living state regulatory review*. Author. https://www.ahcancal.org/Assisted-Living/Policy/Documents/2019_reg_review.pdf

Polzer, K. (2009). *Assisted living state regulatory review 2009*. National Center for Assisted Living. http://www.ahcancal.org/ncal/ resources/Documents/2009_reg_review.pdf

Radigan, C. R., & Gobes, F. J. Trusts and estates law the transfer-on-death security registration act. *Ruskin Moscou Faltischek, P.C.* rmfpc.com/trusts-and-estates-law-the-transfer-on-death-security-registration-act

IV

ENVIRONMENTAL MANAGEMENT

ACCESSIBILITY, FIRE SAFETY, AND DISASTER PREPAREDNESS

LEARNING OBJECTIVES

Upon the completion of Chapter 12, the reader will be able to:

- Describe selected federal regulations, laws, and statutes related to accessibility, and disaster preparedness.

- Describe the National Fire Protection Association (NFPA), the International Code Council, and the NFPA Life Safety Codes.

- Identify accessibility issues relevant for assisted living administrators.

- Identify fire safety issues relevant for assisted living administrators, including current life safety codes.

- Identify selected workplace safety issues relevant for assisted living administrators.

- Discuss disaster preparedness issues relevant for assisted living administrators.

- Discuss strategies for disaster preparedness, including disaster preparations, disaster protection, and recovery from disasters.

- Describe selected best practices in fire safety and disaster preparedness.

INTRODUCTION

Assisted living administrators must have a comprehensive understanding of current federal, state, and local laws and regulations that relate to accessibility, fire safety, and disaster preparedness within assisted living facilities. Awareness of landmark federal laws and agencies are an important first step in this process. Federal legislation, which includes the Americans with Disabilities Act of 1990 as amended by the Americans with Disabilities Amendment Act of 2008, the Occupational Safety and Health Act of 1970, and the creation of the Federal Emergency Manpower Agency, is presented and briefly discussed in this chapter. Also identified are important national fire safety codes. Selected issues related to accessibility, fire safety, and disaster preparedness are discussed and presented as important components of the work of administrators. Best practices in selected areas associated with fire safety and disaster preparedness will be presented at the conclusion of this chapter.

REGULATIONS, LAWS, AND STATUTES

Although there are numerous laws, regulations, and statutes that administrators must address on a daily basis, administrators should be able to identify landmark federal legislation. In addition, administrators should have an understanding of national fire and safety codes. Both federal laws, along with national fire and safety codes, are briefly reviewed and discussed.

Americans With Disabilities Act of 1990

Signed into legislation by President Bush in 1990 and amended in 2008, this wide ranging civil rights law was designed to protect Americans with disabilities from discrimination in any setting. Disability is defined in this legislation as "physical or mental impairment that substantially limits major life activity" (Americans with Disabilities Act, 2009). Title I of the legislation notes that discrimination should not occur against any qualified individuals with disabilities, and applies to job applications, hiring, advancement, and the discharge of employees. Discrimination is defined here to include limiting or classifying job applicants in adverse ways, denial of employment to qualified applicants, failure to make reasonable accommodations to address physical or mental limitations of disabled employees, failure to provide training accommodations, and failure to advance employees with disabilities. Title II of the legislation covers in part access to all programs offered by specific entities. Physical access to facilities is more fully described in the Uniform Federal Accessibility Standards and the Americans with Disabilities Act Standards for Accessible Design and Access. Title III of this legislation states that no individual may be discriminated against based on disability, and is entitled to full and equal enjoyment of all services, facilities, and accommodations of any place of public accommodation. Public accommodations are defined to include most places of lodging, transportation, recreation, dining, stores, and care providers. Of special note is the application of Title III to existing facilities. One definition of discrimination in this area is the "failure to remove" architectural barriers in existing facilities.

Awareness of this important legislation is important because assisted living facility administrators will need to provide services to elders residing in assisted living facilities that are nondiscriminatory. Administrators must also be prepared to create work environments that prevent employee discrimination and will thus benefit from review of the disability laws.

Occupational Safety and Health Act of 1970

The Occupational Safety and Health Act of 1970 (as amended in 2004) was authorized by the United States legislature to ensure safe and healthful working conditions for working men and women, to assist states in assurance of safe and healthful working conditions, and to provide information, education, training, and research in the field of occupational health. Additionally, this legislation is designed to encourage employers and employees to reduce the number of occupational safety and health hazards, as well as to improve and institute new existing programs for safe and healthful working conditions, and for the development and dissemination of occupational and health safety standards.

Administrators working in assisted living facilities must have an awareness and understanding of current health and safety legislation as it serves to protect both employers and employees from a number of potential problems that may occur in settings designed for elder care.

Federal Emergency Management Agency

The Federal Emergency Management Agency (FEMA) was initially created by Presidential Order in 1979. As an agency of the United States Department of Homeland Security, FEMA has been designed to coordinate disaster responses that are not controlled by local or state agencies. This new federal agency included services from a number of federal departments, including the National Fire and Prevention Control Administration, the Federal Disaster Assistance Administration, and the Department of Defense Civil Preparedness Agency. FEMA currently offers a number of emergency response services as well as training programs for emergency personnel in the United States.

Administrators in assisted living facilities should be aware of FEMA and the role that this agency plays in local, state, and federal emergencies and disasters. While most administrators will hopefully not have to utilize these resources, awareness of what is available before emergencies or disasters occur is an essential component of comprehensive emergency preparedness.

National Fire Safety Code

Assisted living facility administrators must adhere to a number of fire safety codes, many of which are determined by state laws and regulations. Administrators can benefit, however, from an understanding of two national associations dedicated to national fire protection.

National Fire Protection Association

The NFPA is a U.S. organization developed in 1896 to standardize the new market of fire sprinkler systems. Originally composed of insurance underwriting firms, the NFPA now consists of fire departments, insurance companies, unions, trade organizations, and manufacturing organizations. The current work of this organization involves the development and maintenance of over 300 fire safety codes and standards. Many state and local governments incorporate these standards and codes into legislation. The association standards and codes are accepted by many courts and exist as the standards currently in use in the United States. Evidentiary use of these codes can be found in the "life safety regulations" sections of assisted living facilities in a number of states. The Assisted Living Workgroup Report to the U.S. Senate Special Committee on Aging (2003) Topic Group Recommendations on Operations noted that assisted living facilities should comply with the most current versions of the NFPA Life Safety Code. The codes are created by groups of experts in fire safety and are regularly updated to reflect current standards of fire safety professionals (Wolf, 2002).

International Code Council

The International Code Council (ICC) was established in 1994 in the United States and focuses on building safety and fire prevention. This association develops codes used for residential and commercial building construction, and are adopted in many U.S. cities, counties, and states. The International Codes or I-Codes are designed to provide minimum safeguards for individuals in homes, schools, and institutions, and include coordinated building safety and fire prevention codes. All 50 states have adopted the use of I-Codes at either the state or local level. The Assisted Living Workgroup Report to the U.S. Senate Special Committee on Aging (2003) Topic Group Recommendations on Operations noted that assisted living facilities should comply with applicable state and local building codes. States, however, should in part adopt the most current national versions of building codes to ensure that the most current perspectives on building safety are incorporated into state requirements.

ISSUES RELATED TO ACCESSIBILITY, FIRE SAFETY, AND DISASTER PREPAREDNESS

There are a number of issues related to accessibility, fire safety, and disaster preparedness that are of relevance for assisted living facility administrators. Selected issues in each of these areas will be presented and further discussed.

Accessibility Issues

Each state has individual regulations and codes that govern many aspects of accessibility within assisted living facilities. Administrators should be familiar with their state-specific requirements. In addition, administrators should note that accessibility is also legally mandated throughout the Americans with Disabilities Act of 1990. The construction and design of new facilities must ensure that buildings are readily accessible for disabled individuals. Regulations and codes are also applicable to older facilities. Existing facilities undergoing alterations must be designed whenever possible to ensure access to altered areas by individuals with disabilities, including wheelchair access. Paths of travel through such altered areas should ensure access to bathrooms, telephones, and drinking fountains whenever possible for individuals with disabilities (Americans with Disabilities Act, 1990).

The Assisted Living Report to the U.S. Senate Special Committee on Aging (2003) recommends that environmental management in assisted living facilities should include the maintenance of safe conditions for all residents, staff, and visitors in compliance with all applicable federal, state, and local laws. Resident needs should be accommodated, and common areas should be accessible to residents using a variety of assistive devices. Administrators need to assess their use of environmental management to ensure that all residents have access to accommodations within the assisted living facility.

The Assisted Living State Regulatory Review of 2019 (National Center for Assisted Living, 2019) describes assisted living regulations in each state as well as the District of Columbia. Information is provided for regulations detailing physical plant requirements, including a summary of the square foot requirements for residential units, the maximum number of residents allowed per residential unit, and bathroom requirements, including the number of toilets, lavatories, and facilities required for each resident. As administrators review and adhere to the regulations for their state, accessibility issues should also be addressed. For example, in California, physical plant requirements allow for private or semi-private resident rooms that must be of sufficient size to allow for easy passage of wheelchairs, walkers, and any required equipment such as oxygen (National Center for Assisted Living, 2019). In Hawaii, physical plant requirements state that residents must be provided with an apartment unit that includes in part a refrigerator and cooking capacity, along with a separate and complete bathroom with a sink, shower, and toilet. This would include accommodations for the physically challenged and wheelchair bound persons as needed. (National Center for Assisted Living, 2019).

Administrators working in states where regulations do not specify accessibility requirements will need to review and implement resources required to accommodate residents with disabilities. Assisted living facility administrators should refer to the regulations, codes, and laws that are relevant to their state, as they work to ensure that all residents in their facility are provided with accessible accommodations.

Fire Safety Issues

Administrators in assisted living facilities are responsible for ensuring that their facilities are safe from fire hazards and workplace fire safety issues. As previously noted, the National Fire and Safety Codes and the National Fire Protection Association provide information and regulations on a national level for fire and safety protection. Administrators are responsible for adhering to state and local fire safety regulations and codes that vary within each state and the District of Columbia. The Assisted Living State Regulatory Review (National Center for Assisted Living, 2019) described the regulatory category of life safety to summarize fire safety requirements and other standards to ensure residents' physical safety. Variation is noted among each of the state regulations in the area of life safety. For example, life safety regulations for the state of Delaware are comprehensive, noting that assisted living facilities must comply with all applicable state and local fire codes, and must implement fire safety plans through staff training and drills. These plans must be approved by the jurisdictional fire marshal and must include an evacuation route posted on each floor and unit. At minimum, fire drills must be conducted annually. Additionally, the Delaware regulations require that specified incidents must be reported within an 8-hour period to the Division of Long-Term Care Residents Protection, including in part, any fire or resident burns greater than first degree. This regulation exists in contrast to states such as Iowa, where life safety regulations require the use of sprinkler systems and smoke detectors that comply with the National Fire Protection Association (NFPA) 101, 2003 Edition, and NFPA 72, National Fire Alarm Code. Additionally, sprinkler systems must comply with the NFPA 13 or 13R standards (National Center for Assisted Living, 2019). As demonstrated, state regulations differ widely, and administrators should clearly understand and implement their states' regulations to protect assisted living residents from fire and safety problems.

The importance of understanding and implementing life safety regulations is underscored by reports from the National Fire Protection Association (NFPA) regarding board and care facilities, with senior assisted living facilities falling under the designation of board and care facilities according to the Life Safety Code (Wolf, 2002). United States fire departments responded to around 1,830 fires in residential board and care or similar facilities annually from 2009 through 2013 (Ahrens, 2016). Additionally, the NFPA documented annual averages of six civilian deaths and 46 civilian injuries in board and care facilities from 2009 to 2013 (Ahrens, 2016). NFPA analysis of the fires revealed that major contributing factors to fire deaths included a lack of automatic sprinklers, unprotected vertical openings, doors open in the room of fire origin, and an insufficient staff and resident training response to disasters.

Updated Life Safety Codes (2006) address two main concepts: (a) larger buildings are more difficult to evacuate than smaller buildings, and thus require more fire protection; and (b) occupants who are more difficult to move and evacuate will require more built-in fire protection than individuals who require less assistance during evacuations (Kaspar, 2008). The 2006 codes stress a "defend in place" approach through the use of fire and smoke barriers in combination with automatic sprinkler systems. These strategies allow for the evacuation of residents to safe locations within the building's structure. Fire sprinkler systems are required in new assisted living facilities and should be either quick response or residential sprinklers.

Assisted living administrators must maintain a safely engineered environment for all residents. All floor surfaces, hallways, doorways, stairs, and ramps must be accessible for residents with decreased mobility (Kaspar, 2008). Assisted living facilities have specific means of egress requirements as determined by NFPA 101. Hallways must accommodate equipment such as oxygen tanks, and a minimum of 60 inches of clearance must be maintained in all hallways (Kaspar, 2008). Residents must also have an appropriate amount of time to respond to emergencies. Newer assisted living facilities should be designed with travel distances from corridor doors to building exits no more than 100 feet, and overall maximum travel distances should not exceed 200 feet (Kaspar, 2008).

Best Practices in Fire Safety

Assisted living administrators can also benefit from understanding best practices in fire safety. The use of fire safety measures in assisted living includes not only smoke detectors, fire alarms, and sprinkler systems, but also the institution of training drills for residents. The institution of these combined measures saves the lives of residents.

Workplace Safety Issues

Issues related to workplace safety in addition to fire safety, must also be addressed by assisted living administrators. Regulations governing life safety for residents of facilities are identified in state regulations. Many states have regulations regarding the number of staff required on a per shift basis in assisted living facilities. In addition to work hours, many states regulate the training and education required for all staff members to ensure workplace safety. For example, Arkansas addresses staffing requirements for their level-one and level-two facilities, and also requires staff education and training in the areas of building safety, appropriate responses to emergencies, communicable diseases, along with food and sanitation safety (NCAL, 2019). Administrators should also follow all state and local regulations designed to provide staff members with safe and effective working environments.

Disaster Preparedness Issues

Administrators in assisted living facilities must be prepared for any number of potential disasters and emergencies, natural as well as man-made. Disaster preparedness begins with preparations for disaster and emergency plans, protection during the actual emergency or disaster, assessment and treatment of problems during an emergency or disaster, and efforts toward recovery and rebuilding. The information discussed will be of benefit to administrators running assisted living facilities.

Preparations for Disaster or Emergency

Administrators in assisted living facilities must be prepared for any number of disasters and emergencies, including hurricanes, tornadoes, floods, fires, earthquakes, epidemics, pandemics, and acts of bioterrorism. The initial step in disaster preparedness involves risk assessment. As noted by Robertson (2017), good plans begin with an understanding of the risks associated with the area in which the facility is located. Natural risks include storms, earthquakes, high winds, heat waves, and severe weather. Technological risks include electrical fires, toxic spills, and computer and power failures. Security risks include theft, fraud, sabotage, and vandalism. Finally, proximity risks need to be considered. These are risks from problems such as fires, toxic spills, explosions, and accidents that occur outside of assisted living facilities in neighborhoods or nearby communities. Such risks have the potential to create an emergency situation for residents and staff of facilities as a result of close geographic proximity to emergencies or problems (Robertson, 2017).

Once administrators have assessed and determined potential risks, the next step is to ensure that both residents and staff in assisted living facilities have the resources to care for themselves in the initial phase following a disaster or emergency, and also to build on existing relationships and reduce or minimize risks (Grachek, 2006). The disaster plan should include the following: (a) plans for sheltering in place and for evacuation; (b) plans for coordination with community, city, county, and state agencies and emergency management services; (c) discussion of emergency plans with staff and residents; and (d) plans and communication strategies for family members and friends of assisted living residents and staff, including out-of-town phone numbers for emergency family contacts.

The U.S. Department of Health and Human Services Center for Medicare and Medicaid Services has developed an emergency planning checklist for persons in long-term care facilities (2007). This extensive checklist begins with an understanding of the location of emergency exits, and the need for emergency evacuation plans for residents, staff, and family members. Also included are plans for long-term care ombudsmen working with assisted living administrators, staff, and residents.

Emergency disaster plans must include evacuation plans for residents and staff. Plans should include verification of emergency evacuation shelters, and strategies in place to transport staff and residents to emergency shelters. Written contracts for bus or transportation services should be prepared in advance, along with emergency supplies and kits prepared to accompany staff and residents as they are evacuated to emergency shelters. Back-up electronic pharmacy records should be kept in a separate geographic location to ensure access to this important information during a disaster (Cefalu, 2006).

Effective communication of disaster plans is essential to successful plan implementation. Communication will impact the establishment and maintenance of effective plans, and can in fact mean the difference of life, death, injury, or health for both residents and staff. Everyone involved in the disaster plan must understand the plan, and easily access the plan information (U.S. Department of Labor, n.d.). This includes administrators, staff, and residents of assisted living facilities. It is important to note that all communication strategies must be effective for staff and residents with disabilities as the Rehabilitation Act of 1973 and the Americans with Disabilities Act of 1990 do not specifically require emergency preparedness plans. Equal access for people with disabilities is required, however, and emergency plans must include provisions for individuals with disabilities (U.S. Department of Labor, n.d.). Effective communication systems should include accessible signage, emergency telephone and TTY numbers, lobby posters, occupant emergency plans, and fire alarm evaluations to ensure that alarm sounds are adequate to warn both staff and residents (U.S. Department of Labor, n.d.).

Protection During Disasters

Once a disaster or emergency occurs, administrators will need to implement established disaster plans. If plans have been made to evacuate staff and residents to alternative emergency shelters, triage of residents is an essential first step. Ambulatory residents should be evacuated first, followed by residents in wheelchairs, and finally those residents requiring additional assistance and support. Having roommates or close friends evacuate together will help to reduce stress and anxiety for residents. Staff should also plan to carefully check the facility (including bathrooms) to ensure that all residents have been evacuated (Cefalu, 2006). Administrators should plan to maintain facility security during a disaster. Security is needed to prevent the theft of drugs, personal possessions, and food from evacuated facilities, and administrators should also consider business interruption insurance to cover costs of facility mortgages, payroll, and other expenses during a facility evacuation (Cefalu, 2006).

Administrators who develop disaster plans which have residents and staff shelter in place, rather than evacuate the facility, should have arrangements to ensure the health and safety of both residents and staff members. Frequently, power outages accompany disasters resulting in loss of heating or air conditioning, leaving residents at risk for dehydration, heat stroke, or hypothermia. A lack of electricity also means a loss of electronic alarms, door locks, and equipment for cooking and laundry. Administrators should plan to have generators available to power refrigerators, and provide residents with ice (Cefalu, 2006). In addition, emergency equipment, including chain saws, hand tools, extraction equipment, and tarps, should be available at the facility. Emergency transportation should also be available for staff members who need alternative transportation methods (Cefalu, 2006).

Assessment and Treatment During Disasters

Administrators must be prepared to assess and treat residents for problems that may result from disasters or emergencies. Incontinence can be a major problem for residents who must evacuate their facility. Preparations should include appropriate incontinence and hygiene supplies (Cefalu, 2006). Administrators should also have information available to address hazards that may result from pandemic or man-made disasters, including biological and chemical attacks.

Recovery

Administrators must develop disaster plans that also focus on recovery from the disaster. Adequate emergency preparations that include adequate supply of resident medications and supplies will enhance recovery following the disaster. Technology and the use of back-up computer systems will also serve to provide essential medical information that will serve to facilitate recovery efforts following a disaster. Residents in assisted living communities can improve their recovery from a disaster or emergency by maintaining a healthy state of mind prior to the disaster. Mental and emotional preparation serve as an effective strategy to counteract the stresses associated with disasters and terrorist acts. Commonly used strategies that elders can implement to deal with emotions following a disaster include the following: (a) talking about the disaster; (b) sharing feelings with others who have been through the same events or are trustworthy; (c) taking care of physical needs, including adequate nutrition, adequate sleep, and regular use of medications; (d) gathering information about resources that may help with disaster-related needs; and (e) returning to normal routines as soon as possible. Additionally, elders can enhance their ability to stay healthy and to recover from disasters through connections with family members, friends, significant others; adherence to regular exercise programs; use of stress management programs; and asking for any help and service that might be needed. It is also important to note that assisted living administrators can enhance disaster recovery resilience among older adults through information sharing, assessment and planning, and improved overall communication (Shih et.al., 2018).

Resources for Administrators

As administrators develop disaster plans, their work can be facilitated by using a number of available resources. The American Red Cross, the Federal Emergency Management Agency, and the Occupational Health and Safety Agency all have websites with information on disaster preparedness. Administrators may also access a number of resources to assist in the planning of emergency and disaster plans. As earlier noted, the U.S. Department of Health and Human Services (2007) serves as an excellent resource to ensure that disaster plans address necessary emergency services. Administrators must also investigate resources made available by state agencies addressing disaster preparedness and emergency service availability.

Administrators can additionally benefit from review of best practices in disaster preparedness. The Florida Department of Elder Affairs serves to promote best practices in disaster preparedness for elders in Florida and throughout the United States. In his testimony to the U.S. Senate Special Committee on Aging, Douglas Beach, Secretary of the Florida Department of Elder Affairs, identified emergency preparedness plans for Florida elders (2009). This disaster plan is comprehensive and encourages the coordination and integration of federal, state, and local emergency response plans specifically designed for elders. Hallmarks of this plan, important for all elders, including those residing in assisted living facilities, include preparations prior to the onset of emergencies, a focus on the nutritional needs of elders in the development of shelf-stable meals that are specific for elders, development of evacuation plans designed to protect elders, and recovery plans that additionally address the care needs of seniors.

CASE STUDY

CK is a new assisted living administrator of a medium-sized facility in the eastern United States. Disaster preparedness is an important consideration for CK, who understands that preparations for disasters begin with an understanding of the risks associated with the area in which the facility is located. Geographically, CK's facility is in a low-lying area about 3 miles from a small river that floods during seasons with heavy rain or snow falls. This puts the facility at risk for flood-related disasters. As CK begins the development of a comprehensive disaster plan, he identifies the importance of communication about emergency evacuation plans if river flooding should occur.

The staff plan a number of information sessions with the assisted living facility residents. The information sessions include a discussion of how residents can inform family members and friends if they are evacuated from their assisted living facility. Although all of the residents have contact phone numbers for family and friends, and some of the residents use text messaging for ongoing communication, CK decided to use social-networking sites, such as Facebook and Twitter, to enhance communication during potential emergencies. His decision was based in part on the reported successful use of these strategies in a number of disasters, including the recent Haitian earthquake.

Interested residents were invited to participate in the social-networking emergency preparedness communication project. CK purchased a cell phone with text-messaging and social-networking capabilities for each of the resident participants. The phones were adapted to ensure that residents with hearing and visual problems as well as arthritis or motor problems were able to use them. Facility staff members assisted residents in learning how to use the phones successfully as well as in creating a social-networking site. Residents then contacted family members and friends and developed emergency communication networks.

One outcome of this project was an overall increase in resident communication with family members and friends as residents reported the use of the cell phones and the social networking sites to be both easy and enjoyable. Although CK has not experienced a flood-related emergency to date, he is confident that if a disaster occurs, communication among residents, their families, and friends will be both effective and enhanced due to the use of cell phones and social networking sites. CK has also now started to discuss the benefits of social networking communication in disaster preparedness with other assisted living administrators.

CONCLUSIONS

This chapter highlights the importance of protecting disabled elders and other individuals by adhering to federal legislation designed to promote access to facilities and services. Protecting elders from residential fires through a focus on fire safety and prevention is discussed, and current life safety codes are reviewed. Issues related to the engineering of residential environments to promote fire safety, from the installation of sprinkler systems to the numbers of staff on duty during evening and night shifts, are introduced, along with the protection of elders through disaster preparedness. Issues associated with disaster preparedness, along with additional resources for assisted living administrators during disasters and disaster recovery, are also presented. Assisted living administrators can potentially benefit from ideas discussed in the best practices case study regarding the use of social-networking sites to enhance communication during potential disasters.

REFERENCES

Ahrens, M. (2016). *Structural fires in residential board and care facilities* (pp. 1–38). National Fire Protection Association.

Americans with Disabilities Act. (2008). Americans with Disabilities Act of 1990 as amended by the ADA Amendments Act of 2008 (Pub.L. No,110-325).

Assisted Living Workgroup. (2003). *U.S. Senate Special Committee on Aging. Final report.* U.S. Government Printing Office.

Cefalu, C. A. (2006). Disaster preparedness for long-term care facilities. *Annals of Long-Term Care, 14*(9), 31–33.

Grachek, M. K. (2006). *Community-wide emergency planning involving long-term care: The Joint Commission approach to enhancing community support of long-term care during disasters.* http://findarticles.com/p/articles/mi_m.3830/is_5_55/ai_nl6485900

Kaspar, J. (2008, February 1). *Protecting a vulnerable population.* http://www.csemag.com/articles/protecting-a-vulnerable-population.org

National Center for Assisted Living. (2019). *Assisted living state regulatory review.* Author.

Robertson, G. (2017). *Surviving the worst: Emergency planning for long-term-care facilities.* http://scitechconnect.elsevier.com/ emergency planning-longterm-care-facilities

Shih, R. A., Acosta, J. D., Chen, E. K., Carbone, E. G., Xenakis, L., Adamson, D. M., & Chandra, A. (2018). Improving disaster resilience among older adults. *Rand Health Quarterly, 8*(1), 3.

U.S. Department of Health and Human Services. (2007). *Emergency planning checklist.* http://www.hhs.gov

U.S. Department of Labor. (n.d.). *Preparing the workplace for everyone: Implementation, communicating about and distributing the plan.* https://www.dol.gov/agencies/odep/publications/ reports/preparing-the-workplace-for-everyone

U.S. Senate Special Committee on Aging. (2009). *Department of Elder Affairs state of Florida. Florida Elder Affairs Secretary testifies to Senate committee on emergency preparedness for seniors.* http://elderaffairs.state.fl.us/english/News/PressReleases/2009

Wolf, A. (2002). NFPA standards guide life safety for many assisted living facilities. *NFPA Journal,* 39–42.

FURTHER READING

Federal Emergency Management Agency. (n.d.). *Department of Homeland Security.* http://www.fema.gov

International Code Council. (n.d.). *About the ICC: Introduction to the ICC.* https://www.iccsafe.org/about/who-we-are

13

MODELS OF CARE

LEARNING OBJECTIVES

Upon the completion of Chapter 13, the reader will be able to:

- Discuss the philosophy of service delivery in assisted living communities.
- Identify the Medical Model of Care in assisted living communities and discuss the roles of staff, administrators, residents, families, and communities within this care model.
- Describe the concept of culture change in assisted living communities.
- Discuss the Green House Model of Care, including the roles of staff, administrators, elders, families, and communities within this care model.
- Describe the Eden Alternative as a care delivery model in assisted living communities and discuss the roles of staff, administrators, elders, families, and settings within this care model.
- Identify benefits and challenges associated with the Medical Model of Care.
- Identify benefits and challenges associated with the Green House Model of Care.
- Identify benefits and challenges associated with the Eden Alternative.
- Describe selected best practices associated with the use of the Green House Model of Care and the Eden Alternative.

INTRODUCTION

Many assisted living communities continue to use the traditional medical model to govern resident care, facility administration, and organizational functions. Assisted living administrators can benefit from an understanding of the benefits and challenges of newer care models including the Pioneer Network, Green Houses, and the Eden Alternative. Information about traditional approaches to service delivery and current alternative care approaches, including potential benefits and possible challenges associated with each approach, can be of benefit to assisted living administrators and will be discussed further.

MODELS OF CARE IN ASSISTED LIVING COMMUNITIES

Current definitions and philosophies of assisted living are applicable to both the traditional and newer alternative care models. The Assisted Living Workgroup Report to the U.S. Senate Special Committee on Aging (2003) Topic Group Recommendations defines *assisted living* in part, although no state or federal mandated definition exists. This definition notes that assisted living is a state-regulated and monitored residential long-term care option. Services that are required by state law or regulation include the following: (a) 24-hour awake staff to provide scheduled and unscheduled elder needs; (b) health related services; (c) social services; (d) assistance with activities of daily living and instrumental activities of daily living; (e) meals; (f) housekeeping; and (g) transportation. Elders in these assisted living communities have the right to receive these services in ways that promote their dignity, autonomy, independence, and quality of life.

The Assisted Living Workgroup Report to the U.S. Senate Special Committee on Aging Topic Group Recommendations (2003) also provided additional information on assisted living communities. A philosophy of service delivery was articulated and designed to maximize individual choices, independence, autonomy, dignity, and quality of life. In addition, core principles of assisted living are identified and should be reflected in a setting's mission statement, culture, policies, and procedures. The core principles include: (a) creating a residential environment that is supportive of each resident's right to privacy, choice, dignity, independence, quality of life, and privacy rights as defined by each resident; (b) offering quality supportive services that are collaboratively developed and individualized for each resident; (c) providingf resident-focused services emphasizing individual needs and incorporating creativity, innovation, and variety: (d) supporting an individual's decision-making control whenever possible; (e) fostering a social climate that allows individuals to develop and maintain social relationships; (f) providing consumers with full disclosure of service provision and cost prior to and during the elder's stay in the facility; (g) minimizing the need to move; and (h) creating a culture that provides a quality environment for elders, staff, administrators, families, volunteers, and the larger community.

MEDICAL MODEL OF CARE

The Medical Model of Care is a traditional approach to care delivery in many facilities throughout the United States and is recognized by most assisted living administrators. In this model, the medical problems experienced by elders serve as a focus for service care and delivery. Aging is viewed in terms of a series of changes to both physiological and psychological processes, as well as in changes in functional capabilities, and abilities to perform activities of daily living. Diseases are identified as alterations in physiological or psychological functioning with the goal of treatment and management to improve elder functioning. The Assisted Living State Regulatory Review (National Center for Assisted Living, 2019) identifies the services provided in assisted living communities in each of the 50 states and the District of Columbia. While facility definitions are variable, many are focused on care delivery from a traditional perspective. For example, the assisted living community definition used in the state of Illinois notes in part that assisted living establishments provide community-based residential care for residents who need assistance with activities of daily living, including personal, supportive, and intermittent health related services available 24-hours daily to meet both scheduled and unscheduled resident needs (National Center for Assisted Living, 2019). Other states have similar definitions of assisted living care that remain centered on a traditional medical care model.

Philosophy of the Medical Model of Care

The focus of care in this traditional model is to promote health, maintain functioning, and improve outcomes and quality of life for older adults. Because aging is viewed in part as involving physiologic and psychological changes, the goals of care involve management are intended to improve existing problems and prevent future problems.

Elements of the Medical Model of Care

As noted, the Medical Model of Care is focused upon a traditional disease and treatment approach to problems associated with aging. As elders enter into assisted living communities, initial assessments include information obtained from standardized medical and functional histories, as well as physical examinations. Care plans for elders are determined in part from data obtained from medical evaluations. Frequently, indicators of effective care delivery and effective functioning within the assisted living facility are determined from these initial assessments.

Roles of Staff and Administrators in the Medical Model of Care

Staff and administrative roles are traditional in the Medical Model of Care. Staff provide services to elders and work in roles that support care for existing physical, psychological, and functional problems, as well as potential problems in each of these areas. Staff and administrative roles are congruent with the state regulations governing assisted living communities in the United States. The National Center for Assisted Living State Regulatory Review (2019) identifies information from applicable state statutes and regulations in a series of categories that delineate the roles of staff and administrators. The scope of care in assisted living communities encompasses the nursing and personal care services provided in individual facilities. Resident assessment indicates in part the assessments conducted by staff on residents. Medication management indicates whether medication administration is permitted in assisted living communities and the staff who may be eligible to provide this service. Staffing requirements are based on the number of residents, and staff education summarizes qualifications for different staff positions (National Center for Assisted Living, 2019). Although care in assisted living communities should be focused on resident choices and resident dignity, roles within traditional medical models of care adhere closely to state regulations and statutes. This has the potential to present confusion or a conflict of interest when staff and administrative roles that adhere to regulations conflict with individualized resident care.

Roles of Residents and Families in the Medical Model of Care

Residents in assisted living communities select their facilities in part to reflect care that is individually centered and designed to promote healthy aging, well-being, and improved quality of life. Family members of assisted living residents expect to be included in the care process. Assisted living communities that focus on traditional care delivery are designed to provide residents with these services within a structure that emphasizes medical care delivery and the prevention of physical and psychosocial problems. Administrators and staff members also work with family members to provide services that include caring for the well-being of the resident within a framework of medical service provision.

Roles of Community in the Medical Model of Care

The role of the community in a traditional or medical model is often formalized. Although connections with members of local communities are encouraged, and in fact desired, many of these interactions occur in more formal programs, such as volunteer programs, or those which connect school children with elders in facilities.

CULTURE CHANGES IN LONG-TERM CARE DELIVERY AND ASSISTED LIVING COMMUNITIES

Administrators working in assisted living communities should have an awareness of changes being proposed within long-term care settings, especially nursing homes. Understanding new ways of conceptualizing care for older adults and the culture changes that accompany proposed changes is beneficial to administrators in assisted living communities. Most cultural changes are designed to improve quality of life and well-being for elders, and therefore have relevance and applicability in a number of settings including assisted living communities.

According to the Pioneer Network (2019), culture change is a common name for a national movement designed to transform services for elders. Culture change is focused on person-directedOMP: C values and practices with a goal of having older adults and caregivers provide input into care that is respected and valued. The core person-directed values include dignity, respect, choice, self-determination, relationship, and a sense of purposeful living (Pioneer Network, 2019). Culture change is also viewed as a regenerative model designed to increase resident's sense of control and autonomy in what can be identified as a resident-centered care model (Touhy & Jett, 2018). Additionally, culture change refers to a progressive view of aging and reformulating the essential meaning of growing older in the United States (Brawley, 2007). As noted by Misiorski (2003), culture change transforms an institutional approach to care into a person-centered approach to care. Culture is seen as a community where individual capabilities are affirmed and developed. Additionally, Farrell and Elliot (2008) identify culture change as person-directed care developed as an alternative to traditional institutional frameworks used in many settings. The goals of culture change are centered in increased resident autonomy, control, and life choices; improved quality of life for residents; as well as enhanced community with a continuity of individual social life and individual interests (Touhy & Jett, 2018).

Much of the literature describes the concept of culture change within nursing homes. In these settings, culture change refers to a transformation of nursing homes as models of acute medical care to models more towards the person or consumer. Quality of care, quality of life, and positive financial benefits for nursing home administrators are goals associated with the implementation of culture change in nursing homes (Baker, 2007). The National Citizen's Coalition for Nursing Home Reform (2006) describes culture change in nursing homes as a rethinking of practices, and values that involve changes in working relationships among administrators, staff, residents, and families to create a humane environment supporting resident rights, dignity, and freedom. In essence, culture change involves the de-institutionalization of nursing homes, and supports individualized resident care.

Pioneer Network

The Pioneer Network, based in Rochester, New York, was established in 2000 as an umbrella organization for the nursing home culture change movement. Designed as a loose association of providers, regulators, advocates, and elders who advocate for improvement in the quality of life for institutionalized elders, this network advocates for a process of culture change that brings a sense of community into nursing home settings (Pioneer Network, 2019). The Pioneer Network has also been designed in part to: (a) create communication and networking opportunities; (b) participate in community building; (c) identify and advocate for transformation in practice and research; (d) serve an advocacy role in public policy; and (e) develop resources and leadership (Pioneer Network, 2019).

The Pioneer Network works with the National Citizen's Coalition for Nursing Home Reform to disseminate a number of culture change principles and practices. There are a number of key principles that have been framed by the Pioneer Network for use in culture change. As noted in a publication on culture change in nursing homes (National Citizen's Coalition for Nursing Home Reform, 2006), the principles used by the network include the following: (a) know individuals in the institutional setting; (b) recognize that each individual makes a difference; (c) recognize that relationships are the fundamental building blocks of cultures that are transformed; (d) note that responses should be to mind, body, and spirit; (e) identify risk taking as a normal part of life; (f) recognize that individuals and their needs should be put ahead of tasks; (g) recognize that all elders are entitled to self-determination; (h) note that communities can be considered as an antidote to institutionalization; (i) encourage growth and development for all individuals; (j) recognize environmental potential to be used in all aspects including physical, organizational, psychosocial, and spiritual aspects; and (k) recognize that culture change and transformation are a journey rather than a destination, and are always a work in progress.

Green House Model

The Green House Model is an alternative care model of nursing home care developed by William Thomas, a geriatrician, to deinstitutionalize the traditional nursing home environment. In 1999, Thomas determined that long-term care facility reform could best be achieved by a major redesign of nursing home architecture and organization. Thomas named his concept "Green House" to signify life and continued growth. Rather than one large building, Thomas' Green House was conceptualized as a community of small homes with a total of six to eight elders living in each home (Robert Wood Johnson Foundation, 2007). The model creates a small and intentional community of elders and staff with a focus on fostering relationships among the groups. Radically different from the traditional medical model of care, the Green House Model was designed to serve elders with assistance and support in activities of daily living with residence care remaining the focal point of all activities.

Philosophy of the Green House Model

The Green House Model operates on the concept that a community of small homes housing a total of six to ten elders and staff will provide an environment of support and growth for both residents and staff. Clinical services are provided in Green Homes but are de-emphasized in favor of a quality of life focus. The underlying philosophy of the Green House Model is focused on habituation and improved quality of life for elders in a normal and home-like environment, rather than a medical or clinical environment. The focus is on "person-centered care" emphasizing autonomy, dignity, and well-being (Larsen, 2019). (Rabig et al., 2006). The model emphasizes quality of life outcomes without ignoring clinical or therapeutic issues. Quality of life outcomes include a sense of security, meaningful activity, physical comfort, relationships, dignity, functional competence, privacy, individuality, and spiritual well-being.

Elements of the Green House Model

The elements of this alternative model of care are centered upon architectural changes to the traditional long-term care facility. As noted, the Green House Model promotes the use of small houses with a small number of residents and staff. The units are designed so that each resident has a private room and bathroom. Rooms are designed to receive increased levels of sunlight, and all are situated around an open area containing a hearth, an open kitchen, and an open dining area

(NCB Capital Impact, 2009). Easy access to all areas of the house, outdoor gardens, and patios are provided for elders who can also access laundry and kitchen facilities. Green Houses are designed to blend into existing neighborhoods. Architectural designs eliminate long hallways, institutional furnishings, overhead calling systems, nursing stations, and medication, as well as other carts (Rabig et al., 2006). The Green Houses are designed not to resemble medical or nursing home units commonly found in traditional medical model facilities.

Roles of Staff and Administrators in the Green House Model

Roles of staff in the Green House Model are significantly different from traditional medical models. Certified nursing assistants are considered to be the key staff members in the Green House Model. Provided with 120 hours of additional training, the nursing assistants have additional work responsibilities. They work in self-managed work teams and assume responsibility for cooking, cleaning, and managing the house, as well as working with and nurturing residents (Robert Wood Johnson Foundation [RWJF], 2007).

Reporting structures are different in the Green House Model. Staff is not supervised by nursing service personnel as is customary in traditional models; staff members report to an administrator who is labeled a guide. Clinical support teams provide services to elders that are required by regulations in long-term care settings. Clinical teams consist of physicians, nurses, social workers, dieticians, and therapists. Although the services that team members perform are similar to services in traditional medical model settings, they are expected to behave as guests in the elders' homes, and have no direct supervisory authority over other staff members (Rabig et al., 2006).

The language that is used to describe staff is different as well. Certified nursing assistants are called by a different title, *shabaz*, which is a Persian term meaning *royal falcon*. Residents are referred to as elders, administrators are called guides, and members of the community who provide assistance to the elders are known as sages. Convivium is a term used to describe food preparation and dining (Rabig et al., 2006). The rationale for these changes in language is to further delineate Green House operations from those found in traditional medical model facilities.

Role of Elders and Families in the Green House Model

The roles of elders and families are redesigned in the Green House Model. Decision-making is given to elders who do not adhere to fixed schedules. Elders make choices about meal times, sleep and rest times, and the types of activities they wish to participate in during the day. Elders and caregivers have close and informal relationships. Elders are encouraged to interact with staff members in daily activities, household activities such as gardening, cleaning, laundry, and pet care (Rabig et al., 2006).

Family members are also considered to be active participants in the Green House Model. Because elders have control over their daily schedules and do not adhere to fixed times for meals, activities of daily living, or other activities, family members can be encouraged to fully participate in these more flexibly organized living arrangements.

Role of Community in the Green House Model

The role of the community is viewed differently in the Green House Model. As noted earlier, houses are designed to be integrated into the surrounding community so that elders and staff become part of the neighborhood in general. Open relationships with community members are encouraged, and visitors are also welcomed to work with elders and staff informally, rather than in the more formal volunteer programs seen in traditional settings.

Eden Alternative

The Eden Alternative was developed by William Thomas, a geriatrician, in 1991 in the reformation of the long-term care industry. The goal of this approach to long-term care delivery was culture change, including the improvement of quality of life for older adults through the introduction of pets, plants, and children into traditional long-term settings. These changes were designed to improve and create meaningful relationships among long-term care residents through improvements in social and physical environments (RWJF, 2007). The addition of pets, families with children, plants and gardening were designed to create an environment that was more normal and less institutional in nature.

Philosophy of the Eden Alternative

The Eden Alternative was designed to create significant culture change in long-term care facilities. Thomas noted that long-term care facilities created a number of problems for elders, including boredom, helplessness, and loneliness. The Eden Alternative was designed to eliminate these problems through the encouragement of meaningful relationships. The addition of pets, plants, gardens, and families with children was included in the culture change to provide elders with the opportunity to provide care to others, as opposed to only being passive care recipients. The Eden Alternative was also conceptualized to promote a more meaningful life for elders in long-term facilities through re-distribution of both power and energy (Rabig et al., 2006).

Elements of the Eden Alternative

As noted earlier, the Eden Alternative was designed to create culture change in long-term care facilities. While the Green House Model focused on architectural changes to effect culture change for elders, the Eden Alternative focuses on social and environmental changes to effect culture change.

The addition of nontraditional elements, such as pets, to what are otherwise traditional long-term care settings was developed to provide elders with more control over their environment, as well as to promote an enhanced sense of well-being and improved quality of life. The introduction of pets was designed to help elders deal with issues of loneliness through companionship with a variety of birds, dogs, and cats. The introduction of staff members' children, as well as family members into the long-term care facility, was designed to provide elders with the opportunity to care for others, and thus alleviate loneliness. Pets and children have been noted to help elders deal with feelings of helplessness. As elders provide care for others, they in fact are making empowering decisions, and lack of engagement may be less of an issue for elders who live in an environment that is engaging, constantly changing, and filled with a number of unanticipated events.

Role of Staff and Administration in an Eden Model

Although the roles of staff members and administrators are more traditional in an Eden Model, staff members are encouraged to work with elders in nontraditional activities focused around pets, children, plants, and gardening. This is designed to empower staff and to enhance opportunities for staff to engage with elders and family members in ways that have meaning for both groups. Although administrative roles are also more like roles in traditional medical model settings, there are opportunities for administrators to work in interdisciplinary teams. Eden Alternative settings have staff working in nursing care teams. Each team is responsible for a small number of residents and the operation of work units. Eden teams consist of all workers who provide services to residents including certified nursing assistants, nurses, rehabilitation specialists, housekeepers, laundry workers, and maintenance staff members. The focus is on the creation of a vibrant atmosphere to promote a sense of purpose in elders (Burgess, 2015).

Role of Elders and Families in an Eden Alternative

As noted earlier, the roles of elders in an Eden Alternative are designed to be more participatory, more engaged, and more empowered than the roles played by elders in more traditional settings. Elders are encouraged to provide care to pets and to children, to participate in the care of plants and gardens, and to enhance their control and decision-making opportunities in a number of areas. Planning in an Eden Alternative facility is focused on the person or individual, as opposed to more central organizational planning in traditional care models. Elders are encouraged to flexibly plan meals, choose the times they sleep, wake, and perform daily activities in an effort to promote decision-making, and ultimately improve quality of life.

Role of the Community in an Eden Alternative

In an Eden Alternative setting, the community is considered to be a part of the long-term facility. Community volunteers are encouraged to participate in a number of Eden related projects, and to work directly with residents in the care of pets and gardens.

Issues Related to the Medical Model of Care in Assisted Living Communities

Many assisted living communities use the traditional Medical Model of Care. The benefits of using this model are underscored by the state statutes and regulations that govern assisted living community operations. Most state regulations require assisted living communities to comply with standards that are congruent with traditional care models. Definitions in state regulations include definitions of care, facility scope of care, resident assessments, medication management, physical plant requirements, staffing requirements, and staff education and training, and are traditional in scope (National Center for Assisted Living, 2019). Administrators have a responsibility to adhere to standards and regulations. The development and design of assisted living communities in compliance with existing regulations offer a number of administrative, economic, and staffing benefits that are not present in settings using alternative care models.

Resident well-being and quality of life are the primary challenges of traditional models. Elders who reside in traditional assisted living facilities have less control over their environment, schedules, and interactions with family and friends. This has the potential to impact quality of life and well-being for these elders.

Issues Related to the Green House Model of Care in Assisted Living Communities

Although the Green House Model of Care has been developed for use in long-term facilities, many of the benefits of this model can be applied to assisted living communities. The idea behind this project is to change institutions to improve the lives and health of elders (Larsen, 2019). Designed to promote culture change, this care model was initially designed to promote improved quality of life, social involvement, and enhanced well-being for residents. Elders are more involved and engaged in activities within their homes. Families are more involved with elders because they have more opportunities to interact with them, and both groups have more opportunities to interact with members of the community.

Research applying the Green House Model in Tupelo, Mississippi, in 2006 (Rabig et al., 2006) revealed positive outcomes and experiences for residents, staff members, and family members participating in this project. A two-year, longitudinal quasi-experimental study was conducted comparing residents in Green Housing to residents in two traditional comparison sites. The study findings revealed statistically significant differences in self-reported quality of life with residents in the Green House Model. These residents reported improved quality of life over residents in more traditional settings. Additionally, residents in the Green House Model experienced improved functional status and quality of care as compared to residents living in more traditional facilities. This study provided data to indicate that the Green House Model can impact and improve quality of life and well-being for elders. This model has implications for services provided in assisted living communities.

Challenges associated with the implementation of the Green House Model in assisted living communities are fiscal and regulatory in nature. Building and staffing the environment that is required for implementation of a Green House Model is expensive, and may be beyond the resources of many administrators. Because assisted living communities must be in compliance with state statutes and regulations, conversion of traditional facilities into a Green House Model can involve many challenges and problems that must be addressed by administrators.

Best Practices in Implementation of Green House Approach

Best practices in the implementation of the Green House approach to elder services demonstrate and illustrate how resident-focused cultural changes improve life for elders. The Green House approach also supports benefits not seen in the traditional medical care models found in many assisted living communities.

Issues Related to the Eden Alternative in Assisted Living Communities

The Eden Alternative has been designed to create culture changes in long-term facilities. This model of care is elder controlled and focused and can be applied to assisted living communities as well. Benefits from this model include improvements in elder well-being and quality of life. Principles of the Eden Alternative (Burgess, 2015) include: life revolving around plants, animals, and children; easy access to loving companionship; living in an elder-centered community that does not separate human growth from human life; and daily life imbued with variety to prevent boredom. Administrators in assisted living facilities may wish to consider these findings as they consider implementation of the Eden Alternative in their settings.

Challenges to implementation of the Eden Alternative are focused primarily on the fiscal costs of implementation and maintenance of this model. Changes to the social structure of assisted living communities, the addition of pets, children, plants, and gardens are costly, requiring additional staff resources and funding. Administrators who consider implementation of the Eden Alternative must also make sure they remain in compliance with all state regulations and statutes.

Research conducted in 2016 by McAllister and Beaty demonstrated the effectiveness of person-directed care model delivery in many nursing homes over a 5-year time period with high occupancy rates, lower return to hospital percentages, and higher Centers for Medicare & Medicaid Services (CMS) ratings.

Best practices have been identified in the integration of assisted living facilities and local communities, an integral component of the Eden Alternative approach to elder-care service delivery. Data from the Europe Study (Eden Alternative Data, 2017) revealed in part that social capital within elder communities was strengthened, and the health and well-being of residents was considered to be a strong investment

CASE STUDY

YHY is a 90-year-old female who has recently moved into an assisted living community from the home she lived in for 50 years. Although YHY was able to initially transition without many problems, she has recently become more withdrawn from the other residents, spending most of her time alone in her room. During a recent evaluation for depression, YHY notes that she "lost her will to live" with the move to the assisted living facility and stated that she missed sitting in her kitchen where she could watch the neighborhood cat climb the maple trees in her backyard, and also watch different birds eat from the birdfeeders that her husband crafted prior to his death 10 years ago. YHY's physician recommended medication to treat her depression, but the facility staff noted that the medication served to make YHY sleepy and confused and did not resolve her depression.

The administrator of YHY's facility has been interested in the implementation of culture change to improve the quality of life for elders as noted in work done by the Pioneer Network (2019). The administrator has been working to transform the assisted living community from an institution based exclusively on the medical model to one with a focus on individual values and needs. The administrator worked with the facility staff to identify strategies for decreasing YHY's depression. Although the staff were unable to move YHY to another room or change the view from her windows, the staff were able to obtain several photographs of the maple trees in her former backyard. YHY was able to hang the photographs where she could view them on a daily basis. The staff were also able to obtain birdfeeders similar to those crafted by YHY's husband and placed the feeders in the facility garden. YHY was then able to sit or walk in the garden at different times of the day to observe both the birds and bird feeders. YHY was also encouraged to make recommendations to the staff regarding the types and amount of bird seed that would be best used in the bird feeders.

The assisted living community also participated in a pet therapy program with a local animal shelter. YHY was encouraged to attend regularly scheduled sessions, especially during times when cats were brought into the facility. YHY enjoyed the opportunities to spend time with the animals in the pet therapy program, stating that she even enjoyed the opportunity to pet the hamster who accompanied the animal therapist at one of the visits. Both the administrator and facility staff noted that YHY was less depressed with the implementation of simple environmental changes. YHY was able to discontinue the medications for depression and she became less confused and more outgoing, more engaged in facility activities, indicating that she was "happier in her new home."

CONCLUSIONS

As stated in this chapter, administrators in assisted living communities must adhere to state regulations in the operation of their facilities. Regulations that are parallel with traditional operations seen in the medical model are identified. This approach is discussed as a more cost-efficient method that is better aligned with existing regulations. The challenges associated with the use of the medical model are focused in part on the provision of elder-centered and individualized care within a traditional structure. The use of culture-changing models as identified in the Pioneer Movement include the Green House Model and the Eden Alternative. Culture-changing models propose to improve quality of life and well-being outcomes for elders, and are designed to provide elders with additional control over daily activities and service provision within residential settings. The benefits of these models were noted and included a focus on improvements for elderly individuals. Challenges associated with culture-changing models are discussed, and included increased costs of service provision in nontraditional residential settings. Adherence to regulations in settings that are not traditionally structured, and difficulties in care delivery and provider roles within altered new and different care models are also discussed. The best practices and case study provided assisted living facility administrators with examples of culture change implementation in a variety of settings. Administrators can then reflect on some of the potential advantages associated with individualized, person-focused care delivery.

REFERENCES

Assisted Living Workgroup. (2003). *U.S. Senate Special Committee on Aging. Final report.* U.S. Government Printing Office.

Baker, B. (2007). *Old age in a New Age: The promise of transformative nursing homes.* Vanderbilt University Press.

Brawley, E.C. (2007). What culture change is and why an aging nation cares. *Aging Today, 28*(9) 9–11.

Burgess, J. (2015). Improving dementia care with the eden alternative. *Nursing Times, 111*(12), 24–25.

Eden Alternative Data. (2017). *The eden alternative: Culture change in eldercare.* https://seniorcareadvice .com/wp-content/uploads/2017/05/eden_alternative_data_4.09.pdf

Farrell, D., & Elliot, A. E. (2008). Investing in culture change. *Provider,* 18–30.

Larsen, D. (2019). The greenhouse project: The next big thing in long-term care. *Senior Living Blog.* https:// aplaceformom.com/blog/green-house-project-next-big-thing-in-long-term-care

McAllister, A., & Beaty, J. A. (2016). Aging well: Promoting person-directed care. *Journal of Aging Science, 4*(3), 1000164. https://doi.org/10.4172/2329-8847.1000164

Misiorski, S. (2003). *Pioneering culture change.* http://www.ltlmagazine.com/ME2/dirmod.asp?sid=&nm= &type=Publishing& Mod=Public

National Center for Assisted Living. (2019). *Assisted living state regulatory review.* Author.

National Citizens' Coalition for Nursing Home Reform. (2006). *Culture change in nursing homes.* U.S. Government Printing Office.

NCB Capital Impact. (2009). *The green house concept.* https://senate.texas.gov/cmtes/82/c802/0322-Jenkins-GreenHousePrroject.pdf

Pioneer Network. (2019). *Defining culture change.* https://www.pioneernetwork.net/culture-change/what-is-culture-change

Rabig, J., Thomas, W., Kane, R. A., Cutler, L. J., & McAlilly, S. (2006). Radical redesign of nursing homes: Applying the Green House concept in Tupelo, Mississippi. *The Gerontologist, 46*(4), 533–539. https://doi .org/10.1093/geront/46.4.533

Robert Wood Johnson Foundation. (2007). *"Green Houses" provide a small group setting alternative to nursing homes and a positive effect on residents' quality of life.* Author.

Touhy, T. A., & Jett, K. (2018). *Ebersole & Hess' gerontological nursing and healthy aging* (5th ed). Elsevier.

FURTHER READING

Coleman, M. T., Looney, S., O'Brien, J., Ziegler, C., Pastorino, C. A., & Turner, C. (2002). The Eden alternative: Findings after 1 year of implementation. *The Journals of Gerontology Series A: Biological Sciences and Medical Sciences, 57,* 422–427. https://doi.org/10.1093/gerona/57.7.M422

Pioneer Network. (2009). *Pioneer Network.* http://www.pioneernetwork.net

Redding, W. (2009). Best of the best. *Assisted Living Executive,* 11–19.

UNIVERSAL DESIGN AND AGING IN PLACE

Upon the completion of Chapter 14, the reader will be able to:

- Identify definitions and philosophy of universal design.
- Describe key principles of universal design.
- Identify strategies for connecting universal design elements to assisted living communities.
- Identify definitions and philosophy of aging in place.
- Describe selected elements of successful aging in place programs.
- Identify the roles of administrators, staff, residents, and families within aging-in-place programs.
- Describe selected benefits and challenges related to universal design.
- Describe selected benefits and challenges related to aging in place.
- Describe selected best practices related to aging n place.

INTRODUCTION

Assisted living administrators can best serve the residents and staff of their communities through an understanding and awareness of universal design as well as the importance of assisting elders to age in place whenever possible. These two concepts are presented in this chapter, along with selected issues, benefits, and challenges associated with the use of universal design and aging in place in assisted living communities. Best practices in selected areas associated with universal design and with aging in place will also be briefly discussed throughout this chapter.

UNIVERSAL DESIGN IN ASSISTED LIVING COMMUNITIES

Assisted living administrators need to have an understanding of the definitions, philosophy, and history of universal design. Strategies for connecting key principles of universal design to the structure of assisted living communities are also important for administrator consideration.

Definitions and Philosophy of *Universal Design*

Universal design is defined as the development of buildings, housing, and products that can be used by all people in the most effective way possible. The goal of universal design is the creation of buildings, building interiors, and products that can be used by most individuals, including those with disabilities. Designers balance artistic integrity with human needs and environment, which include recent technological design innovations and also address the need for accessible and adaptable environments (Mace et al., 1991). Adaptable environments are designed with a number of universal features that can later be modified for the needs of specific users or user groups. Adaptable designs frequently include all of the elements required for users in wheelchairs, but in a universal design approach, fixed accessible features are combined with adjustable, and optional or removable elements. This results in the creation of an environment that will be used by many individuals, but can also be tailored to the functional limitations of specific individuals (Mace et al., 1991).

The philosophy of universal design is to simplify life for everyone through the creation of housing that is more accessible at little or no additional cost to users. The universal design concept is focused on environments used by individuals with varied needs and requirements. This contrasts with building codes, regulations, and standards developed to address needs (primarily mobility needs) for selected groups of individuals, usually those with disabilities or those in specialized settings such as assisted living facilities. Universal design also requires the use of universal features, or elements within facilities that can be used by everyone regardless of their abilities, representing standard products that are placed differently or carefully selected. Examples of universal design include: door handles that do not require gripping or twisting to operate; alarm systems that are both audible and visible; and storage space that is accessible to individuals with height differences (Center for Inclusive Design and Environmental Access, 2012).

History of Universal Design

The movement toward universal design was formed in response to many of the changes experienced by older adults and those with disabilities in the United States. Demographic shifts now show more Americans to be living longer lives. According to Vespa (2018), the U.S. Census Bureau projects that people aged 65 and older in the United States will number 78 million by 2035, a trend that is followed in Europe, Japan, and Eastern Europe. The numbers of individuals with disabilities also continue to increase as those with disabilities live longer and more productive lives. Many of these individuals either live or will plan to move to assisted living or long-term care facilities, prompting the need for improvements in the design of these settings.

A number of federal legislative changes have influenced the universal design movement in the United States. The Civil Rights Act of 1964 provided a starting point for subsequent legislation to improve the lives of older adults and those with disabilities. The Center for Universal Design (2000) identified a number of these legislative efforts. The Architectural Barriers Act of 1968 required that all buildings constructed, leased, designed, or altered with the use of federal funding be made accessible to those with disabilities. The Rehabilitation Act of 1973 (specifically section 504 of the act) made discrimination illegal on the basis of disabilities, and was applicable to any agency receiving federal funding, including federal contractors, federal agencies, and public universities. The Fair Housing Amendments Act of 1988 served to expand the Civil Rights Act of 1968 to include people with disabilities. This act required that all housing built after 1988 include accessible units in buildings with four or more units. The act is applied to both public and private housing, and is applicable to newly constructed assisted living facilities. Finally, the

Americans with Disabilities Act (ADA) of 1990 required the removal of physical barriers that had the potential to impede access, and banned discrimination in access to public accommodations, programs, services, public transportation, and telecommunications. The ADA Standards for Accessible Design were further developed as a result of work done by the Architectural and Transportation Barriers Compliance Board in 1991. This work serves as the federal standard for accessible design in the United States (Center for Universal Design, 1997).

Universal design was influenced in part by the barrier-free movement that began in the 1950s as a response to individuals with disabilities demanding services that would increase their employment and educational opportunities, rather than institutionalize them for their differences. These individuals recognized that physical and environmental barriers created significant problems, especially for individuals with mobility challenges, including a number of older adults. As a result of the barrier-free movement, architects noted that changes to building and space design for those with disabilities would also benefit others without disabilities. The recognition that many design features could be provided in ways that were attractive, marketable, and less expensive was considered by many to be the beginning of the universal design movement. Again, the concept behind universal design was the creation of designs that would address the needs of all individuals with and without disabilities (Center for Universal Design, 2008). The applicability of this design approach in assisted living facilities with older adults is readily apparent.

Key Principles of Universal Design

There are seven principles of universal design. They were developed by a group of engineers, architects, environmental design researchers, and product designers to serve as a guide for members of design disciplines. The principles may also serve to evaluate existing designs, guide the implementation of new designs, and also educate consumers and designers about more usable environments and products (Center for Universal Design, 2008). Each of these principles, with applicability to those working and residing in assisted living facilities, will be briefly addressed. Information about each of the seven principles is obtained from the work done through the North Carolina State University Center for Universal Design (2008). The first principle involves equitable use, with designs that are useful and marketable to individuals with diverse abilities. Guidelines for this principle include development of the same or equivalent means of use for all users to eliminate stigma or segregation of users. Additionally, equitable use must include provisions for security, privacy, and safety for all users. One example of equitable use in assisted living facilities is the use of power entrance doors with movement sensors that are convenient for all users.

The second principle of universal design involves flexibility in use. The goal here is to develop designs that accommodate a wide number of individual abilities and preferences. Adaptability to user pace, accuracy, and precision are important components of this principle. An example of flexibility in use in assisted living facilities includes the use of scissors that can be used by either right or left-handed older adults.

The third principle of universal design is focused on use that is both simple and intuitive. Here the goal is to design products and environmental factors that are simple to use and easy to understand despite the users' knowledge level, experience, language skills, or cognitive abilities. The goal of the simple and intuitive use principle is to accommodate individuals with a wide range of language and literacy skills, arrange information that is consistent with the importance of the information, and eliminate unneeded and unnecessary complexity. One example of simple and intuitive design is the development of emergency plans and guidelines in a manual with drawings and no text, for use by a wide range of residents in assisted living facilities.

The fourth principle of universal design centers onperceptible information. Here, objects are designed to effectively communicate necessary information to users, regardless of the environment, or the user's sensory capabilities. The goals of perceptible information are to provide information that is redundant using different strategies (verbal, visual, or tactile), to make instructions easy to understand, and to be compatible with other devices that may be in use for sensory problems. For example, residents in assisted living facilities who can access a thermostat using verbal, visual, and tactile instructions are utilizing designs with perceptual information.

The fifth principle of universal design involves a tolerance for error with designs that minimize hazards and the consequences of either accidents or unanticipated actions. The design goals of this principle are to provide warnings of potential hazards, provide failsafe features for the designs, and minimize hazards or errors. Providing elders in assisted living facilities with double-cut room keys that have been designed for insertion into door keyholes in either of two ways serve to create a tolerance for error.

The sixth principle of universal design is low physical effort, or the minimization of fatigue, in which products can be used both efficiently and comfortably with a minimum of fatigue. The goals here are for users to maintain neutral body positions, use reasonable operating forces, minimize repetitive actions, and minimize sustained physical efforts. Those residing in assisted living facilities who use loop or lever handles on faucets or door handles, or use lamps that are operated by touch rather than by a switch, are using products with low physical effort.

The seventh principle of universal design involves both size and space for approach and use. The appropriate size and space are provided for reach, approach, manipulation, and use independently of each user's size or mobility. The goals here are to make reach comfortable for all users whether standing or sitting in a wheelchair, provide space for those individuals using a number of assistive devices, accommodate variations in handgrip size and strength, and provide clear visibility for individuals who are either standing or sitting. Assisted living community residents who have clear space around mailboxes, appliances in their homes, and other elements of their environment will have easy access for approach and use of these items.

The Center for Inclusive Design and Environmental Access at the University at Buffalo added social participation and health and wellness to the existing design principles in 2012 (Center for Inclusive Design & Environmental Access, 2012). The Center also developed eight goals, including: (a) body fit, (b) comfort, (c) awareness, (d) understanding, (e) wellness, (f) social integration, (g) personalization, and (h) cultural appropriateness (Center for Inclusive Design & Environmental Access, 2012).

Strategies for Connecting Universal Design to Assisted Living Communities

Universal design strategies can be used to improve both living conditions and quality of life for both residents and staff in assisted living facilities. As administrators consider the use of existing space or the renovation or building of new spaces, universal design can be employed in all settings. The use of lever handles on room doors can improve entry, especially for elders with arthritis or mobility limitations in their hands and arms. The costs of replacing traditional doorknobs with levers are considered to be reasonable, as the materials for this change are found in a number of hardware stores and equipment centers (Steinfeld, 1988).

Universal design solutions to bathrooms can enhance life for residents in assisted living communities. Changes to the walls above bathtubs that reinforce the walls with blocking, will allow for the placement of grab bars to facilitate balance and improve mobility as needed. Placement of bathtub faucets close to the outer rim of the tub provides for easy access, especially for elders in wheelchairs or those experiencing mobility problems. The design of new bathroom facilities large enough to accommodate wheelchairs and more than one person at a time can also serve to improve function and provide a universal feature to such an important living space (Steinfeld, 1988).

There are a number of fixed accessible design features that should be elements of an assisted living community's design. These elements include: (a) doorways that provide a minimum of 32 inches of clear opening space; (b) clear pathways at least 36 inches wide that are connections between all accessible living spaces, and the avoidance of stairs and steps at all building entrances; (c) living facilities that are all on the same level unless all levels are connected by ramps, elevators, or lifts; (d) clear floor spaces, especially around appliances, fixtures, toilets, tubs, showers, and sinks; (e) controls, including light switches, faucets, and thermostats that are mounted between 9 to 54 inches above the floor, and are also operable with only one hand; (f) operable windows that have controls that are easy to reach and operate; (g) visual alarms with smoke and fire detectors providing both visual and auditory warnings; (h) tub seats that are built into the tub; (i) showers that are either a 3 foot by 3 foot size, or bathroom that have the provision of a roll in shower space to provide accommodations for individuals in wheelchairs; and (j) reinforced walls or wood blocking for the addition of grab bars around tubs, toilets, and showers as needed (Mace et al., 1991).

Administrators may also wish to consider the use of adaptable designs in assisted living communities. Here, a number of basic and universal features in a number of living spaces can be easily changed or adapted to the requirements of specific users. Adaptable design includes features that are required for wheelchair access. These features can be hidden from sight, added as needed, and adjustable to accommodate users of different heights, sizes, and abilities. Countertop segments that can be raised or lowered; adjustable height closet rods and cabinet shelving; adjustable toilets, tubs, and shower grab bars; and attachable tub seats are all examples of adjustable design elements that can be installed as needed in assisted living facilities (Mace et al., 1991).

AGING IN PLACE

Universal design serves to improve the quality of life and well-being for elders in assisted living communities through a careful process of environmental change created primarily through space and product redesign. Aging in place also serves to improve life quality and well-being for elders in assisted living communities through the process of policy and regulatory adjustments, care delivery, along with environmental and space changes that allow individuals to live in an assisted living community for as long as possible. Definitions of *aging in place*, as well as the philosophy and elements of this approach to living arrangements for older adults, are briefly discussed. In addition, space allocation and the roles of administrators, staff, residents, and families will be reviewed.

Definitions and Philosophy of *Aging in Place*

Aging in place has been defined as the ability of older adults to age in their own homes or in assisted living facilities, to live safely, comfortably, and independently regardless of ability level, age, or income (Centers for Disease Control and Prevention, 2013). Many reports indicate that many adults would prefer to age in place in a home of their choice for as long as possible. Estimates are that 90% of adults over the age of 65 would prefer to remain in their current residence as they grow older. Research on aging in place reveals that a majority of elders want to grow older without moving from their homes and express concerns about their ability to age in place (Guide to Retirement Living Sourcebook, 2018).

Aging in place requires modifications of the living environment to include changes that allow elders to compensate for disabilities and limitations, and thus prevent or slow down admission from home or assisted living facilities into long-term care facilities. Interventions to maintain independence include home modifications and universal design changes to reduce barriers (Touhy & Jett, 2018). Many elders assume that as they age and become increasingly frail they will need to move from their homes to a facility setting. Modifications in living environments can allow elders to remain in their home setting for longer time periods.

Successful aging-in-place strategies create healthcare and housing options that are flexible and designed to allow individuals with the personal desire to live independently to do so for as long as possible. It is important to note that aging in place works best when it is a component of a comprehensive and holistic approach, including support for personal care, healthcare, meals, household chores, and money management. Technology in the form of smartphones and tablets can also enhance aging-in-place when elders implement new technologies (Peek et.al., 2014). Emerging technologies such as robotic technology are in development and are expected to be used to assist elder care in the future (Touhy & Jett, 2018).

The philosophy of aging in place within assisted living facilities involves resident control over service delivery, including the types of services and ways in which those services are delivered. This is a consumer-oriented model in which the setting and delivery of services are organized around the resident as opposed to the assisted living community. In contrast to a medical model of care delivery, in which residents are patients cared for in institutional settings, residents are active participants and consumers of healthcare services (Chapin & Dobbs-Kepper, 2001). The key to an aging-in-place philosophy is for facilities to adjust service provisions and level of care criteria to address the needs of residents, as well as avoid premature discharge to higher-level care facilities. Provision of nursing care services and medication management are also elements of aging in place (Chapin & Dobbs-Kepper, 2001).

Chapin and Dobbs-Kepper (2001) conducted research to examine the aging-in-place philosophy in the midwestern state of Kansas. The researchers conducted a survey of assisted living and residential care facilities in Kansas, collecting data from 141 facilities, on their admission and retention policies, reasons for resident discharge, discharge destinations, and average length of resident stay in their facilities. The study findings note that some of the Kansas facilities had admission and retention policies that supported aging in place. Study residents who were able to age in place for longer time periods were not ambulatory, had self-managed incontinence, mild forms of dementia, or a number of special nursing care needs, including medication administration, medication monitoring, oxygen administration, catheterization, or ostomy care (Chapin & Dobbs-Kepper, 2001). Many administrators used facility policies to limit admission and retention. Residents with severe cognitive impairments, an inability to work with staff to manage incontinence, and residents at risk for running away from the facility found their options for aging in place to be very limited. Thus, the researchers found that resident's ability to age in place to be determined by facility policies that were more stringent than state assisted living regulations, and noted that full implementation of aging in place in Kansas assisted living communities would require additional funding and concomitant staffing, as well as more inclusive admission and discharge criteria (Chapin & Dobbs-Kepper, 2001).

There are a number of elements associated with successful aging-in-place programs. One element includes choice, or the provision of both housing and healthcare options designed to meet the diverse needs of aging individuals. These options should be both available and affordable so that elders as well as their caregivers can make appropriate care delivery choices (Lawler, 2001). A second component of successful aging in place involves flexibility, or the provision of care services that can be applied in a variety of contexts. The levels of healthcare services and housing or living options must be adjustable for elders (Lawler, 2001).

A third component of successful aging in place involves the maintenance of mixed generation communities. Here, elders' enhance their ability for self-help through contributions to the community. For example, these contributions can take the form of tutoring, and the provision of day care services for young children. Children, in turn, can provide opportunities to engage seniors, and keep them active as they age and become increasing frail. The development of mixed generation communities should be guided by the assumption that these communities should not be prevented from occurring in either natural or planned settings (Lawler, 2001).

Calibrated support is the fourth and final component of successful aging-in-place programs. Here, calibrated support involves the development of both healthcare and housing infrastructures that assess for and deliver appropriate levels of coordinated care delivery. To ensure the avoidance of under-care or over-care delivery, ongoing assessment of healthcare and housing needs must occur. Additionally, a wide range of services must be provided to address the changing needs of those elders who are aging in place (Lawler, 2001).

Best Practices for Aging in Place

Best practices in the area of aging-in-place and care delivery have been identified for use by assisted living administrators. Factors that influence aging in place include state regulatory requirements that determine facility admission, retention, and discharge policies, and thus determine the feasibility of aging-in-place opportunities for elders. (National Center for Assisted Living, 2019). Also influencing the ability of elders to age in place is the availability of services within each state as well as state-regulated staffing and service requirements (National Center for Assisted Living, 2019).

In addition, there are a number of design influences that impact aging in place. Accessibility features, such as facility entrances that are at the ground level and do not require stairs, single-story facility construction, and the presence of ramps and elevators, are needed for elders who age in place as they become frail and experience an increase in mobility challenges. The presence of wider doorways, lever handles on doors, walk-in showers, grab bars around toilets, tubs, and showers, as well as the presence of handrails on walkways and ramps, also serve to reduce excess disability and reduce problems associated with gait and balance changes, along with grasp changes. Changes in facility design serve to increase independent functioning and enhance safety for assisted living community residents.

In a qualitative study conducted by Ball et al. (2004), the process of aging in place was investigated in five Georgia assisted living facilities during a 1-year time period. Through a process of purposive, maximum variation sampling, the five facilities were selected to reflect diversity in elderly residents, including race and socioeconomic status, size of the facilities, geographic location of the facilities, and resources available for the elderly residents. The researchers found that the ability of elders to age in place was primarily a function of "fit" between residents and facilities to manage resident decline. The managing of resident decline was a function of capacity to manage decline at the resident, facility, and community levels. Resident decline was approached through the process of decline prevention. This involved health education efforts as well as an adherence to treatment regimens. A second strategy involved responding to decline through a process of balancing resident needs with available resources. Finally, the researchers noted that resident and assisted living community fit was viewed as both an outcome as well as an influence on the decline process, with resident and facility risk both a consequence and intervening factor in resident decline. Their findings highlighted some of the complexities associated with aging in place and highlighted the need for residents to become well informed about assisted living communities (Ball et al., 2004).

Roles of Administrators, Staff, Residents, and Families in Aging in Place

Assisted living community administrators and staff play key roles in determining the capacity of individual facilities to successfully offer and support the services needed for aging in place. A number of factors determine whether aging in place can be offered in a facility, including both state and facility regulations, policies, and the physical environment of the facility, including whether or not changes can be made to make rooms and buildings accessible to residents growing frailer as they age in place. Staff members who work in facilities with aging in place must be able to provide the services that are needed by elders as they experience physical and mental decline. Staff must be qualified to provide additional nursing services, including medication administration and medication management, as well as services to deal with a number of physical problems such as incontinence, reduced mobility, and cognitive problems such as dementia.

Residents and family members play important roles in aging in place in assisted living communities. One key element of aging in place is the focus on needed services. Residents are encouraged to be in control of the services that are provided to them. Family members are also encouraged to become active participants in the care that their family members receive as they age in place.

ISSUES RELATED TO UNIVERSAL DESIGN

There are a number of issues associated with the use of universal design in assisted living communities. The economic benefits and benefits to residents, administrators, and staff will be briefly addressed. A number of the recognized challenges of relevance to administrators working with the concepts of universal design in assisted living communities will also be reviewed and discussed in the following section of this chapter.

Benefits Related to Universal Design

As noted earlier, the use of universal design provides a number of benefits. The economic benefits associated with universal design are well described for builders and contractors who use manufactured rather than custom-built materials, and for designers using standardized features, who will therefore require less time(Steinfeld, 1988). The benefits associated with the use of universal design for assisted living residents include increased accessibility and potential increases in mobility, functional status, and independence. The benefits to administrators include the creation of assisted living communities that increase the functioning and overall quality of life for residents. Staffing costs may be reduced in assisted living facilities if resident rooms and spaces are made more accessible with the use of universal design principles. Studies in hospitals indicate that changes that promote patient independence, reducing the use of nursing services, significantly reduce overall hospital costs (Mace et al., 1991). Staffing costs in assisted living communities could potentially be reduced if design changes to resident rooms and facility spaces also serve to improve accessibility and resident independence.

Challenges associated with the use of universal design are primarily associated with the costs of designing and building new facilities, or with alterations to existing facilities. Many argue, however, that the actual costs of assisted living community spaces are offset by the benefits accrued from increasing resident independence in accessible living spaces.

ISSUES RELATED TO AGING IN PLACE

There are a number of issues related to aging in place in assisted living facilities. Benefits of aging in place include resident and family benefits, alongside benefits in cost. Challenges associated with aging in place include resident challenges, facility challenges, and economic challenges. Some of the benefits and challenges associated with state regulations related to aging in place are of additional significance.

Benefits Related to Aging in Place

A number of benefits related to aging in place have been identified. As noted earlier, a major benefit associated with aging in place in assisted living facilities is the increased quality of life and enhanced well-being that residents experience when they participate in this care model. These settings should ensure that individuals, who are not fully able to care for themselves, can maintain the highest degree of independence, autonomy, human dignity, and personal fulfillment possible throughout the lifespan (Miller & Moore, 2006). Those individuals who are in assisted living communities practicing aging in place are placed at the center of caregiving activities and have their needs addressed, as opposed to being subjected to institutional or structural needs. This also serves to improve quality of life for assisted living community residents.

Aging-in-place programs offer a number of social benefits to residents in assisted living facilities. Aging in place increases resident self-sufficiency and offsets social isolation. In addition, aging in place prevents or defers relocation, which has been shown to involve the loss of friendships, social connections, and interactions with familiar staff and service personnel. Relocation can be associated with a decrease in quality of life, dignity, and personal control (Lawler, 2001). In addition, the negative effects of relocation and moving from one facility to another can be traumatic for residents who are experiencing loss of their functional independence. This may result in a number of negative consequences, including depression, dementia, and diminished abilities to perform a number of functional activities.

Lawler (2001) notes that healthcare delivery services to the elderly are more expensive when delivered in a production rather than in a customized model. Services that are provided in traditional assisted living facilities provide the same set of services and housing options to all residents, and care is provided to the median needs of the majority of residents rather than to the needs of each individual resident. The production model is more likely to deliver care that may be "too much" for some residents, while other individuals do not receive enough services. Overcare results in the delivery of services that are unnecessary, costly, and of lesser benefit to residents. The restrictions and loss of independence resulting from too much care can result in shorter and less productive lives for residents, who may also experience disorientation, increased likelihood of depression, and can diminished quality of life (Lawler, 2001). *Under-care* refers to services that are inadequate for residents in assisted living communities. A lack of necessary and appropriate services can put residents at risk for a number of problems, and is as debilitating for elders as is the provision of too much care.

Aging in place in assisted living communities not only provides physical, social, and emotional benefits to residents, but also provides a number of cost benefits. Chapin and Dobbs-Keppler (2001) noted that the care provided in assisted living facilities when targeted to the residents at the appropriate care level, can be more cost-effective than the care that is delivered in long-term care facilities. Aging-in-place programs, which keep residents in more cost-effective systems such as assisted living communities can create significant cost savings for individual residents as well as for a number of state programs. Residents who are less impaired and aging in place in assisted living communities will use fewer expensive institutional services, again creating savings in overall costs.

Challenges Related to Aging in Place

A number of challenges have been identified in assisted living aging-in-place programs. These challenges include aging inplace in rural versus urban contexts. As Lawler (2001) indicates, many individuals in rural areas note that elders who are unable to remain in their homes are forced to relocate to nursing facilities a distance away from their home settings. Administrators in rural communities indicated that they would be able to support assisted living facilities, but experienced difficulty in finding developers willing to build new facilities. Those individuals in urban settings reported that they also had a lack of housing options for aging in place and h concerns about a lack of support services (Lawlor, 2009).

Understanding the market for assisted living facilities, especially those with aging-in-place care plans, can be a challenge for individuals interested in these services, as well as the communities interested in sponsoring such facilities. Traditional market studies that assess indicators such as age, income, housing tenure, and other demographic data will not accurately predict whether communities can support either the expenses associated with the building of new assisted living facilities or the retrofitting of older facilities (Lawler, 2001).

State Regulations and Practices for Aging in Place in Assisted Living Communities

State agencies have adopted a number of regulations that allow for a broad level of service delivery to meet the needs of assisted living residents as they age in place. According to a study conducted of state-assisted living policies and practices by the National Academy for State Health Policy, 29 states and the District of Columbia supported regulations that promote the assisted living model of care, which is resident focused rather than facility focused (Mollica, 2005). The ability of elders to age in place is therefore reflected in each facility admission and discharge criteria, and also in the stated move-in and move-out policies and regulations (Mollica, 2005). A review of state regulations revealed considerable variability in the admission and retention criteria for residents wishing to age in place in a number of assisted living communities (National Center for Assisted Living, 2019). Assisted living community administrators will need to review the regulations for the state in which they work.

Future Directions for Aging in Place

The demand for aging-in-place programs in assisted living communities continues to grow as does the number of older adults who are either in assisted living facilities or considering entry into these settings. As the baby boomers age, the numbers of individuals who will need care services increases and will continue to increase. The benefits of aging in place with an emphasis on quality of life and well-being continue to be of great importance to those interested in aging-in-place services. The problems associated with long-term care institutions also are factors driving increased demand for aging-in-place programs. Although regulations vary widely from state to state, most states now have regulations in place that serve to facilitate aging-in-place programs in assisted living facilities.

Administrators can find resources and additional information about aging-in-place programs from a number of sources. Review of state regulations regarding aging in place is important so as to understand the parameters of many aging-in-place programs. There are a number of online resources that may offer administrators information about these regulations. The AARP Public Policy Institute and the National Institute on Aging are just two of these resources.

CASE STUDY

HG is a 78-year-old male who recently moved in to an assisted living community after living for 50 years in his suburban family home. The decision to move to the assisted living community was very difficult for HG, who did not want to move to many different facilities as he continued aging. Although the assisted living community that HG selected did not have a formal aging-in-place policy, HG was assured that he could anticipate spending many years in his new home.

Six months after moving into the assisted living community, HG fell and broke his right hip. Following surgery to stabilize his hip fracture, HG was informed that he also suffered from severe osteoporosis and would probably experience many future difficulties in walking independently and could expect to be spending a great deal of time in a wheelchair. HG became very depressed as he thought of having to move from the assisted living community and began to refuse to get out of bed, eat, or spend time with his friends and family.

The administrator and staff of the assisted living community met with HG to develop a plan that would allow HG to remain in the community. The doorway to his room and his bathroom facilitated wheelchair access, and the staff worked to make adjustments to ensure safety such as the removal of scatter rugs, changing the location of HG's bed and several small room tables, and making sure that HG was able to access the shower in his bathroom. The administrator also worked with specialists, including a physical therapist, occupational therapist, and registered nurse to address many of HG's physical and emotional needs.

The administrator and the staff of the assisted living community understood the importance of aging in place for elders such as HG. Their willingness to work with HG to make adjustments to his physical space as well as their work to assist HG emotionally were extremely helpful in HG's physical and emotional recovery from his hip fracture. HG's depression improved as he moved back into the assisted living community and informed his family and friends that he was living in the "best place on earth."

CONCLUSIONS

The areas of universal design and aging in place have the potential to improve the quality of living and well-being of elders in a number of settings, including assisted living communities. This chapter presents a basic understanding of both concepts as well as some benefits and challenges associated with universal design and aging in place. Services to residents can be enhanced through an awareness of the information provided herein.

REFERENCES

Ball, M. M., Perkins, M. M., Whittington, F. J., Connell, B. R., Hollingsworth, C., King, S. V., Elrod, C. L., & Combs, B. L. (2004). Managing decline in assisted living: The key to aging-in-place. *Journals of Gerontology Series B: Psychological Sciences and Social Sciences, 59*(4), S202–S212. https://doi.org/10.1093/geronb/59.4.S202

Center for Inclusive Design & Environmental Access. (2012). *The goals of universal design*. www.universal design.com/what-is-ud

The Center for Universal Design. North Carolina State University. (1997). *The principles of universal design*. https://projects.ncsu.edu/ncsu/design/cud/about_ud/udprinciplestext.htm

Centers for Disease Control and Prevention. (2013). *Healthy places terminology*. https://www.cdc.gov/healthyplaces/terminology.htm

Chapin, R., & Dobbs-Kepper, D. (2001). Aging-in-place in assisted living. Philosophy versus policy. *The Gerontologist, 41*, 43–50. https://doi.org/10.1093/geront/41.1.43

Guide to Retirement Living Sourcebook. (2018). *Research study, "aging in place in America."* https://www.retirementlivingsourcebook.com/articles/research-study"aging-in-place-in-america"-2270

Lawler, K. (2001). *Aging-in-place. Coordinating housing and health care provision for America's growing elderly population* [Report, Fellowship Program for Emerging Leaders in Community and Economic Development].

Mace, R. L., Hardie, G. J., & Place, J. P. (1991). Accessible environments: Toward universal design. In W. F. E. Pressler, J. Vischer, & E. T. White, (eds.), *Design interventions: Toward a more humane architecture*. Van Nostrand Reinhold.

Miller, E. A., & Moore, V. (2006). *Out of the shadows. Envisioning a brighter future for long-term care in America*. Brown University Center for Gerontology and Health Care Research.

Mollica, R. L. (2005). *Aging-in-place in assisted living: State regulations and practice*. American Seniors Housing Association.

National Center for Assisted Living. (2019). *Assisted living state regulatory review*. Author.

Peek, S. T. M., Eveline, J. M., van Hoof, J., Luijkx, K. G., Boeije, H. R., & Vrijhoef, H. J. M. (2014). Factors influencing acceptance of technology for aging in place; A systematic review. *International Journal of Medical Informatics, 83*(4), 235–248. https://doi.org/10.1016/j.ijmedinf.2014.01.004

Steinfeld, E. (1988). *Universal design: Housing for the lifespan of all people*. U.S. Department of Housing and Urban Development.

Touhy, T. A., & Jett, K. (2018). *Ebersole and Hess' gerontological nursing & healthy aging*. Elsevier.

Vespa, J. (2018). *The U.S joins other countries with large aging populations*. https://www.census.gov/library/stories/2018/03/graying-america.html

FURTHER READING

National Center for Assisted Living. (2006). HUD awards Assisted Living Conversion grants to six state projects. *Focus, 11*(12), 1–6.

HOME- AND COMMUNITY-BASED SERVICES AS AN ALTERNATIVE TO ASSISTED LIVING

WITH CONTRIBUTING AUTHOR PAULINE MOSHER SHATARA

LEARNING OBJECTIVES

Upon the completion of Chapter 15, the reader will be able to:

- Describe home- and community-based services (HCBS) in the context of the continuum of long-term care services, including assisted living.

- Discuss the historical evolution of HCBS.

- Explain the structure of three HCBS programs (State Plan, 1915c, and PACE [Program of All-inclusive Care for the Elderly]).

- Discuss the need for expansion of HCBS in light of the challenges that consumers face.

INTRODUCTION

The purpose of this chapter is to introduce the reader to HCBS as an alternative for consumers who want to avoid leaving their homes to reside in assisted living—that is, communities that provide a combination of care and housing in a group setting. To understand the benefits of HCBS, we first review the broad spectrum of long-term care services. Next, the historical evolution of HCBS is provided to help the reader understand the background and development of today's supportive services. Next, this chapter examines in more detail three existing HCBS programs. Closing the chapter is a discussion of the need for expansion of HCBS programs in light of the challenges experienced by consumers in accessing services.

The Long-Term Care Continuum

As people age, they need different levels of long-term care to meet their needs. The kind of services they need is not a function of age alone, however: A healthy and mobile 90-year-old may thrive in a relatively independent setting with minimal supportive services, whereas a 60-year-old who has survived two strokes may have relatively high needs for medical care and assistance with daily living.

Accordingly, long-term services and supports (LTSS) comprise a broad array of assistance provided to persons with a range of health states in a variety of settings. The settings can include the consumer's home, adult day healthcare centers, assisted living, or a skilled nursing facility (Reaves & Musumeci, 2015)

The portfolio of services that consumers may require are broadly classified as assistance with activities of daily living (ADL), such as eating, bathing, dressing, toileting, transferring, grooming, walking and continence care, and instrumental activities of daily living (IADL), such as meal preparation, house cleaning, medication management, and transportation. These services can be provided informally through family caregivers or formally through home care agencies, medical professionals, or paraprofessionals.

The highest level of care is provided in skilled nursing facilities. There are over 15,500 nursing homes nationally serving 1.3 million seniors and persons with disabilities. Medicaid is the primary source of payment for 60% of nursing home residents (Bocutti et al., 2015). For those who do not qualify under Medicaid, the average annual cost is $102,200 for a private room (Genworth, 2019).

The next highest level of care is typically found in residential care facilities for the elderly. There are 28,900 facilities with 996,100 beds (Harris-Kojetin et al., 2019). Although the combination of relative autonomy and access to services may make assisted living the preferred option for many consumers, costs are again often an insuperable obstacle. The monthly median cost for private-pay residents in a residential care facility for the elderly is $4,500 monthly (Genworth, 2019).

The lowest level of care is found in unlicensed care homes, where room and board and some levels of service are provided to two or more unrelated individuals. These facilities are sometimes operating legally or illegally without a license. Residents typically seek these types of facilities due to limited resources. Due to the particularly vulnerable populations these homes serve, such as individuals who are formerly homeless or mentally ill, there are concerns about quality and safety (Greene et al., 2015)

One thing all these settings have in common is that they require consumers to move from their homes. Ample evidence exists that leaving home is something many consumers and their families wish to avoid, and for good reason. A 2015 AARP study demonstrated the vast majority of people want to age in place, for reasons such as remaining in the community as long as possible to be close to family, friends, neighbors, churches, and other community services (Barrett, 2014). When aging individuals cannot access the support and services needed to safely stay in their home, they stand to lose much more than the physical home and possessions they have acquired over a lifetime. The transition out of the community into a facility can represent a loss of independence and choice oflifestyle and daily routine (Lecovich, 2014). Indeed, in most long-term care facilities little emphasis is placed on the importance of autonomy and choice to maintain quality of life (Sherwin & Winsby, 2010).

The HCBS Alternative

HCBS provided through state Medicaid programs offer humane alternatives to consumers seeking long-term care services without leaving their homes and giving up significant autonomy. Enabling seniors to receive affordable services in their homes allows them to stay engaged with their communities, remain an integral part of their families, as well as reducing the financial burden on the seniors, their families, and the state and federal governments which cover a large portion of the cost of services. Essentially, HCBS programs are a viable alternative to skilled nursing facilities for low-income individuals because they are paid for by Medicaid. Medicaid is jointly funded by the state and federal governments and is the largest source of coverage for LTSS, totaling $167 billion in 2016, 57% of which was spent on HCBS (Government Accountability Office, 2018a).

THE HISTORICAL EVOLUTION OF HCBS

The 1935 implementation of the Old Age Assistance program essentially launched federally influenced institutional bias in the United States. The new program provided income benefits to indigent individuals aged 65 or older, while explicitly prohibiting payments to residents in public institutions (otherwise known as poor houses). These restrictions created a need for a new type of institution, and thus began the emergence of the nursing home industry. Moreover, the 1950 amendment of the Social Security Act (SSA) enabled direct payments to licensed skilled nursing facilities further facilitating the tremendous growth of the industry (Institute of Medicine Committee on Nursing Home Regulation, 1986).

In 1971, the first PACE program began as the result of a community initiative, which came to be known as *On Lok Senior Health Services (On Lok)*. On Lok was created by a committee of San Francisco community leaders aiming to address a growing concern for the well-being of older adults in select neighborhoods of the city. The community-based system of care was developed to help older adults age in place and incorporated the use of community health centers offering hot meals, social services, health services, and daily social engagement activities. The program later added in-home support services to further improve care and health outcomes. On Lok was the first of its kind to launch a Medicare-funded consolidated model of long-term care pioneering future programs to do the same (National PACE Association, n.d.)

In 1974 the federal government began encouraging states to prevent or reduce inappropriate institutional care by making amendments to Title XX of the SSA (1974). The amendments authorized the appropriation of federal funds to states for social services, including homemaker services, protective services, transportation, adult day care, training for employment, nutrition assistance, and health support (Henry J. Kaiser Family Foundation, 2015). These amendments finally acknowledged the institutional bias towards unnecessary institutionalization, propelling the movement toward home and community-based services.

The year 1981 ushered in the development of new home- and community-based waivers under section 1915 (c) of the SSA. Despite the implementation of new programs and federal incentives to reduce unnecessary institutionalization, skilled nursing facilities for persons with disabilities and the elderly remained overwhelmingly dominant, resulting in the lawsuit *Olmstead v. LC* (The SCAN Foundation, 2011). The lawsuit alleged that the two plaintiffs had been discriminated against under Title II of the Adults with Disabilities Act (ADA) by being placed in institutional care rather than being provided community-based alternatives by the state. Title II of the ADA includes two major provisions: (a) state and local governments are to operate in the most integrated settings appropriate for the needs of the disabled individual and (b) state and local governments must make "reasonable modifications" to prevent disability-based discrimination. In 1999, the Supreme Court ruled that the unnecessary institutionalization of people with disabilities is in violation of the ADA. Following the ruling, the federal Centers for Medicare & Medicaid Services (CMS) confirmed that the principles in the decision applied to all qualified individuals with disabilities protected under ADA, including seniors.

The 1997 passing of the Balance and Budget Act allowed for PACE programs to become permanently funded, integrating a Medicare managed care plan and allowing providers to receive a capitated payment to deliver a wide range of services. As of 2020 there are 263 PACE centers in 31 states serving 51,000 participants (National PACE Association, n.d.).

In 2010, rebalancing became the focus of the Affordable Care Act (ACA). A significant savings component of the act was to enroll seniors and persons with disabilities into Medi-Cal managed care, thus changing Medi-Cal coverage from the traditional pay-as-you-go model (also known as "Fee for Service") to premium-based payment from the state to third-party healthcare providers.

In 2014, the Coordinated Care Initiative (CCI) was implemented as part of the ACA to promote better health outcomes and cost savings through rebalancing the delivery of LTSS services toward home- and community-based care. Also in 2014, the CMS released guidance to the states on the Home and Community Based Services final regulation of HCBS. The regulations improved the quality of HCBS and provide additional protections to participants receiving services through three of the major Medicaid authorities 1915(c), 1915(k), and 1915(i). The regulation requires all HCBS settings meet certain qualifications regarding integration in the community, individual rights, optimizing autonomy, and person-directed care. It also includes additional requirements for provider-owned or controlled HCBS settings, giving participants a legally enforceable agreement or lease, the right to privacy, right to control their own schedule, and the right to have visitors, and requires the setting to be physically accessible. The regulation also definesd permissible settings, excluding nursing facilities, institutions for mental disease, intermediate care facilities for individuals with intellectual disabilities, and hospitals. The regulation also provides states with added operational flexibilities (Department of Health and Human Services, 2014).

In 2019, a federal bill was introduced affecting married couples accessing HCBS programs. The ACA expanded the definition of *institutionalized spouse* to include a married individual enrolled in an HCBS program. The expanded definition provided the spouse at home, otherwise known as the *community spouse*, with additional financial protections to prevent impoverishment when qualifying for Medicaid. The ACA extended these provisions to HCBS participants but with a sunset date ending five years after the initial expansion. The federal bill proposed H.R 1343 to the 116th Congress, which seeks to make the expansion of the HCBS spousal impoverishment provisions permanent.

STATE PLAN AND WAIVER PROGRAMS

HCBS services through Medicaid are provided under one of two main authorities: the state plan or a waiver. Each authority has different rules it must abide by, affecting the services provided and who may be eligible. Table 15.1 breaks down the list of available state plan benefits and waivers available to each state.

State Plan

A state plan is a formal, written agreement between the state and the federal government, submitted by a single state agency (42 CFR 431.10) and approved by the CMS, describing how that state administers its Medicaid (Medicaid and CHIP [Children's Heallth Insurance Program] Payment Access Commission, n.d.). The federal government requires the Medicaid program to cover certain services such as long-term care in a skilled nursing facility and home healthcare. HCBS programs under the state plan are optional, leaving the states flexibility to decide what they will include in the benefit packages. Programs offered under the state can remain part of the state plan indefinitely, allowing for consistency in the delivery of services. (Newcomer et al., 2011). If a benefit package is offered under the state plan it must meet the requirements listed in Table 15.2.

Personal Care Services

Personal care services are provided as an optional benefit under the state plan. In 2005, 37 states offered a personal care services program. These services offer assistance with ADL, such as bathing, dressing, eating, toileting, and transferring, and other assistance related to IADL, such as home-making services, transportation, and money management. More than half the states allow

TABLE 15.1 STATE-PLAN BENEFITS AND HOME- AND COMMUNITY-BASED SERVICE WAIVERS

STATE-PLAN BENEFITS		
Home health services	• Part-time or intermittent nursing services; home health aide services; and medical supplies, equipment, and appliances suitable for use in the home • At state option—physical therapy, occupational therapy, and speech pathology and audiology services	Required
Personal care services	• Assistance with self-care (e.g., bathing, dressing) and household activities (e.g., preparing meals)	Optional
Community-first choice	• Attendant services and supports for beneficiaries who would otherwise require institutional care • Income up to 150% FPL or eligible for benefit package that includes nursing home services; state option to expand financial eligibility to those eligible for HCBS waiver	Optional
Section 1915 (I)	• Case management, homemaker/home health aide/personal care services, adult day health, habilitation, respite, day treatment/partial hospitalization, psychosocial rehabilitation, chronic mental health clinic services • Beneficiaries must be at risk of institutional care • Population targeting permitted	Optional
HOME- AND COMMUNITY-BASED SERVICE WAIVERS		
Section 191 5 (c)	• Same services as available under Section 1915 (I) • Beneficiaries must otherwise require institutional care • Secretary can waive regular program income and asset limits • Cost neutrality required (average per-enrollee cost of HCBS cannot exceed average per-enrollee cost of institutional care} • Enrollment caps permitted • Geographic limits permitted • Population targeting permitted	Optional
Section 1115	• Secretary can waive certain Medicaid requirements and allow states to use Medicaid funds in ways that are not otherwise allowable under federal rules for experimental, pilot, or demonstration projects that are likely to assist in promoting program objectives • Federal budget neutrality required • HCBS enrollment caps permitted	Optional

FPL, Federal Poverty Level.

Source: From O'Malley Watts, M., Musumeci, M., & Chidambaram, P., (2020). *Medicaid home- and community-based services enrollment and spending.* Henry J. Kaiser Family Foundation. https://www.kff.org/report-section/medicaid-home-and-community-based-services-enrollment-and-spending-issue-brief

participants to self-direct services, giving them the authority to hire, fire, and schedule the hours for their caregivers. A few states allow participants to hire relatives as care providers and even fewer states allow legally responsible relatives such as a spouse or parent (Musumeci et al., 2020).

TABLE 15.2 STATE PLAN SERVICE REQUIREMENTS

• Offered unilaterally: Services must be available to all beneficiaries throughout the state. • Comparibility of services: The same benefits must be offered to all eligible beneficiaries. • Freedom of choice: The beneficiary has the right to select the participating provider of choice.

HCBS Participant Characteristics

In 2012, over 5.9 million people accessed LTSS through HCBS programs. According to the Medicaid and CHIP Payment Access Commission factsheet, general HCBS participant demographics are:

- 63.9% eligible for Medicaid-covered HCBS due to disability
- 29.8% eligible due to age (aged 65 or older)
- 42.5% are male
- 49.9% were White (non-Hispanic)

To be eligible for most HCBS programs, an applicant must demonstrate a level of care consistent with care provided in a skilled nursing facility. The criteria for nursing facility level of care (NF/LOC) varies across states and programs. For example, NF/LOC could mean that an applicant requires assistance with three ADL, such as bathing, dressing, and toileting. Conversely, NF/LOC could also be determined because a person is cognitively impaired and requires 24-hour supervision. Each program conducts a distinct assessment process to determine whether the applicant meets the required criteria. Figure 15.1 lists the five most commonly reported HCBS medical conditions and highest cost HCBS users. Although these are the most common conditions reported,

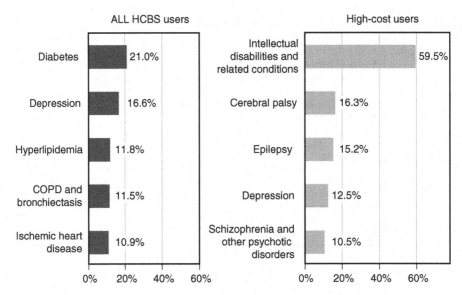

FIGURE 15.1 Five most commonly reported medical conditions and highest cost HCSB users.

COPD, chronic obstructive pulmonary disease; FFS, fee for service; HCSB, home- and community-based services.

Notes: The analyses include all states that had FFS HCBS expenditures, including states that provided HCBS through other program types and authorities, such as Section 1115 waivers, or provided FFS HCBS to specific populations not enrolled in managed long-term services and support programs, such as beneficiaries with intellectual or developmental disabilities. In 2012, 44 states were analyzed; Arizona, Colorado, Idaho, Kansas, Maine, Rhode Island, and Vermont were excluded. *High cost users* are defined as HCBS users with expenditures in the top 3% of the analytic sample by state. The top five most commonly reported conditions were identified from the top 20 conditions in each state across 201 D-2012. Conditions that did not occur in at least two states in at least 2 years were removed.

Source: From Medicaid and CHIP Payment Access Commission. (2018). *Medicaid home and community-based services: Characteristics and spending of high-cost users.* https://www.macpac.gov/wp-content/uploads/2018/06/Medicaid-HCBS-Characteristics-and-Spending.pdf

this is not an exhaustive list; many participants may experience multiple conditions, exacerbating their need for care. In addition to meeting the clinical criteria, an applicant must meet the Medicaid requirements. Each state has varying financial criteria and there can be multiple eligibility categories within a state.

CASE STUDY

CALIFORNIA PERSONAL CARE SERVICES

The Personal Care Services program in California is called *In-Home Supportive Services (IHSS)*. In 2015, it was estimated that the program served 467,000 Medi-Cal beneficiaries (Beck, 2015). The services are provided by a caregiver of one's choosing to assist with ADL and IADL such as bathing, dressing, meal preparation, shopping, laundry, and transportation to doctor's appointments. Service hours, which are approved by a task-based assessment given by a county social worker, are limited to a maximum of 283 hours a month and often do not fully satisfy the care needs. The average authorized number of hours provided to an IHSS recipient is 105 hours a month (Legislative Analyst Office, 2017).

IHSS participants use independent providers that they can hire, supervise, and fire at their discretion. The California Legislative Analyst Office (LAO) estimates a 33% turnover rate for IHSS workers, attributed to low home-care wages and poor working conditions (Thomason & Bernhardt, 2017). High turnover resulting in unfulfilled care hours for the consumer causes adverse health effects and ultimately nursing facility placement if the recipient is unable to replace the provider (Thomason & Bernhardt, 2017).

Almost two thirds of recipients receive care from a provider who is related to them (Thomason & Bernhardt, 2017). In addition, 46% of IHSS recipients receive care from either a parent, spouse, or adult child, and in about half of the cases, the provider-relative lives in the same home (Legislative Analyst's Office, 2017). Full-time family member's caregivers often rely on these low wages as their only source of income, impoverishing the entire household as a consequence (Thomason & Bernhardt, 2017). IHSS provider rates are closely tied to minimum wage, which varies by county, ranging from $13 an hour in rural counties to $16.50 an hour in San Francisco as of 2020 (Department of Social Services [DSS], 2020).

COMMUNITY FIRST CHOICE OPTION

Eight states (CA, CT, MD, MT, NY, OR, TX, and WA) offer the Community First Choice Option (CFCO) 1915 (k) (Government Accountability Office, 2018b). States offering the state plan option receive 6% enhanced federal matching. Services offered in the basic benefit package include assistance with ADL, IADL, health-related tasks, backup systems, and emergency response systems. Four states (CT, MD, OR, and WA) offer additional benefits, including institution to community transition costs (Musumeci et al., 2020). The future of this program is uncertain. If the proposed American Health Care Act is passed to replace the Affordable Care Act, a provision in the bill would repeal CFCO.

CASE STUDY

CALIFORNIA CFCO

California became the first state to implement the CFCO program in 2013, under a 1915 (k) waiver. The incentives to adopt the program included $573 million in additional funds for the first 2 years of implementation and a 6% increase in federal matching funds. Today about 40% of all IHSS participants are enrolled in the program (Legislative Analyst's Office, 2017). CFCO is one of the four IHSS programs offering additional services for individuals needing a skilled nursing level of care. The program provides cash for meal allowances, financial management services, development of individualized backup plans for emergency preparedness, and identifying back-up caregivers.

HCBS Waiver Programs

Waivers allow the states flexibility to provide alternatives to the basic services; however, in exchange for the flexibility, they must agree to strict budgetary criteria. Most waiver programs are required to be cost neutral (equal or less than the cost of providing institutional care). The 1115 waivers are required to demonstrate that actual costs will be reduced by implementation of the waiver. Renewals for the waivers must be submitted every two to five years, potentially causing drastic changes in services. Programs use the flexibility to waive federal requirements to then be able to meet the cost neutrality requirements. Table 15.3 lists the types of federal requirements waived.

Although the required medical criteria are more stringent for waiver programs, the state has the option to allow higher income limits up to 300% of the Federal Poverty Level (FPL). Forty-six states apply the 300% limit; California, however, does not exercise the option (Harrington et al., 2009). In California, financial eligibility for the 1915(c) waivers vary; the Assisted Living Waiver (ALW) in particular has a more stringent income threshold for single individuals. However, all California 1915(c) programs provide extra financial protections for married couples under the spousal impoverishment provisions.

Assisted Living and Home- and Community-Based Service Waivers

Assisted living is a key component of the Medicaid HCBS program in 48 states serving over 300,000 beneficiaries (Government Accountability Office, 2018a). It provides nonmedical care and supervision for individuals who can no longer safely stay in the home but do not yet need 24-hour skilled nursing care. Medicaid covers HCBS in an assisted living setting through the state plan, under waiver authority 1915(c) or 1115. Although the majority of states provide coverage for HCBS in assisted living, there is significant variation, including available enrollment slots and the participant's medical and financial eligibility (Molica, 2009).

TABLE 15.3 WAIVERS OF STATE PLAN PROVISIONS

- Offered statewide: Geographic limits permitted.
- Comparibility of services: Population targeting permitted, enrollment caps permitted, special income and resource standards permitted.
- Freedom of choice: State permitted to waive the requirement giving participants the right to choose any provider who accepts Medicaid (i.e., managed care).

CASE STUDY

THE CALIFORNIA ASSISTED LIVING WAIVER

The ALW was first initiated in 2006 in three counties and grew to 15 counties with full enroll-ment capped at 7,409 participants in 2020. The goal of the ALW is to facilitate nursing facility transition back into a homelike community setting, or prevent skilled nursing admissions for beneficiaries with an imminent need for nursing facility placement (Molica, 2009). The ALW offers participants the choice of residing in an assisted living setting or public subsidized housing (with augmented home health services) as an alternative to long-term placement in a nursing facility. Assisted living services, ranging by levels of care from tier one to five, are delivered by either Residential Care for the Elderly (RCFE) staff or licensed health agency staff based on the participant's choice of residential setting.

This program strives to achieve budget neutrality by waiving the following require-ments: state wideness and compatibility of services. Due to these waivers, the program is the least accessible of all the waivers targeting older persons in California. The program is offered in 15 counties with 377 participating facilities; the combined facilities have an overall capacity of 16,802 beds (Chen et al., 2019). Each participating facility can refuse to accept enrollment at any time and can limit the number of beds they make available to the program. The geographic distribution of facilities in the 15 counties is variable. Enrollment caps subject prospective applicants to the longest waitlist for all California HCBS pro-grams. As of February 2019, the ALW waitlist had 4,419 prospective participants (Chen et al., 2019). Available slots are dependent on participant attrition from death, entry into a skilled nursing facility, or improved condition. The program further restricts the target population by applying the most stringent Medi-Cal financial eligibility criteria, for most single participants this would mean an income less than or equal to 138% of the Federal Poverty level ($1,436 a month in 2020).

The monthly median cost for a private pay resident in an RCFE facility is $4,500 (Genworth, 2019). As a comparison, the ALW care rate is between $65 for tier one and $200 per day for tier five. The resident pays separately for the monthly room and board. For example, participants with monthly SSI income of $1,173.37, pay a room and board rate of $1,039.37. The Medi-Cal rate for a skilled nursing facility resident is $68,000 a year; the ALW saves the state over $51,523 annually on average for each participant (Department of Health Care Services [DHCS], 2017a). Low reimbursement rates may discourage potential providers and ultimately reduce consumer access. In geographic areas with high real estate values, the programs are not financially sustainable and almost nonexistent. Table 15.4 indicates the 2019 per diem tier rates and level of enrollment for each tier.

TABLE 15.4 CALIFORNIA ASSISTED LIVING WAIVER TIER STRUCTURE

TIER #	PER DIEM RATE	PARTICIPANTS (%)
Tier 1	$65.00	33
Tier 2	$77.00	17
Tier 3	$88.00	28
Tier 4	$102.00	22
Tier 5	$200.00	<1

PACE PROGRAM

As of 2019, PACE organizations were available in over 31 states, and the program served 50,000 participants (National Pace Association, 2020). The program is for individuals who are 55 years of age or older, need a nursing home level of care, and, with the appropriate support and services, can remain safely in the community. Participants are assessed for need and monitored by a team of healthcare professionals called an *interdisciplinary team*. The coordinated services can be provided in the home or one of 263 PACE centers nationwide. The average PACE participant is 76 years old; 70% are women and 30% are men. Twenty-six percent of participants need assistance with one to two ADL, whereas 35% require assistance with five to six ADL (National Pace Association, 2020).

PACE is distinct from the Medicaid Home- and Community-Based Services programs because it is a Medicare health plan that states can adapt as a state Medicaid option. Financing for this program is capped, allowing healthcare providers to deliver all necessary services without the fee-for-service limitation of reimbursement from Medicare and Medicaid (CMS, n.d.). Unlike the majority of the Medicaid waiver programs that have cost-neutrality requirements, PACE receives a capitated rate. The unique capitation rate provides an incentive to focus on cost-reduction methods such as avoiding costly hospitalization (Meret-Hanke, 2011). The capitated rate also gives the interdisciplinary team flexibility to tailor the program to individual needs and focus on services such as preventative care, clinical monitoring, and actively maintaining the care plan (Mukamel et al., 2007).

CASE STUDY

CALIFORNIA PACE PROGRAM

The California PACE Program operates 16 programs; statewide enrollment is at 10,090 participants in 2020. The participant population is multicultural: 41% of the participants are Hispanic and speak Spanish; 20% are Asian, of whom 13% speak Mandarin or Cantonese; 20% are White; and 10% are Black. All of the participants are Medi-Cal eligible, 73% of the enrollees are dually eligible, and 27% are Medi-Cal eligible only (CalPACE, 2019). The average capitation rate is $70,000 per year. In 2012, the average Medi-Cal capitation for dual eligibles in PACE was $3,800, and the average Medicare capitation was approximately $2,000 per member per month (CalPACE, 2020).

In 1979, the 30th Street Senior Center in San Francisco was the first PACE center to open. The 30th Street Center location offers seven programs and serves over 5,000 seniors. The average participant is 76 years old; the ethnic majority, or 67% of participants, are Latinx, 19% are Caucasian, 10% are Asian, and 1% are African American. More than 55% have incomes less than $12,000 a year. The program offers adult day healthcare at a PACE center or home health, meals at the center or delivered to the home, laundry services, physical and occupational therapy, primary and specialty care, as well as preventative care such as audiology, podiatry, dentistry, optometry, case management, and money management. It also offers durable medical equipment, prescription drugs, transportation, socialization, and recreation. The purpose of the program is to keep seniors safely in their homes; however, if the individual needs skilled nursing, PACE will cover it (On Lok Lifeways, n.d.).

Why the Disparity Between Preference and Options?

Although the majority of consumers prefer to age in place (Barrett, 2014) there are not enough programs available to meet the needs of our growing aging population, as evidenced by nationwide HCBS waitlists. In 2018, there were an estimated 820,000 people on HCBS waiting lists nationally (Musumeci et al., 2020). The disparity between preferences and the availability of comprehensive home- and community-based services is the result of a number of complex factors. A few of the major issues contributing to the disparity are as follows (a) Federal bias towards nursing home care. Coverage for skilled nursing care is mandatory under federal law. Anyone who is financially and medically eligible will be covered (Grabowski, 2006). (b) HCBS are only an optional benefit. Optional benefits lead to variation across the states and fragmentation within the states. (c) The cost-neutrality requirements limit access to prospective consumers (Newcomer et al., 2011). (d) There are no longitudinal studies reporting the efficacy of the built-in cost controls, therefore it is difficult to measure the true value of diverting institutionalization. Without compelling cost-saving figures it is challenging to persuade policy makers to increase funding allocations to HCBS (Harrington et al., 2009). (e) Low HCBS provider rates to PACE centers and assisted living facilities makes participation unattractive. Low caregiver wages contribute to the workforce shortage and increases the reliance on free or underpaid care provided by family.

RECOMMENDATIONS TO EXPAND CONSUMER ACCESS TO HCBS IN CALIFORNIA

Expanding HCBS is an urgent need for seniors who are unnecessarily institutionalized or are seeking services to remain in the community. California needs an infrastructure to be able to care for its population of over four million seniors, which is projected to increase by 40% by 2030. Medi-Cal, the largest payer of long-term care and the state's low-income health insurance program, covers over 1,160,314 seniors (DHCS, 2017b).

Eliminate Federal and State Barriers

Federal changes to allow viability of expansion should be implemented, such as eliminating cost-neutrality requirements and offering more support for program costs to reduce the burden on the state. In addition, the effectiveness of federal policies, such as restrictions on Medicaid reimbursement for room and board for noninstitutional settings, should be explored (Molica, 2009). Although there is a clear need for federal reforms to eliminate institutional bias, there are many expansion opportunities available within the federal law. Changes to the waivers must be enacted through the state legislature, then waiver amendments are submitted to to the CMS.

Expand Financial Eligibility Criteria

California uses draconian income and asset rules, and although the thresholds increase by a small percentage each year with federal cost of living adjustments, maintenance-need levels remain stagnant. Individuals over the income threshold are subject to a severely oppressive maintenance need of $600, which has not increased since 1989. Federal law allows the state to use a special optional eligibility category for HCBS, allowing individuals with income up to 300% of the FPL to qualify with no share of the cost. Forty-four other states allow income thresholds up to 300% of the FPL (Musumeci & Young, 2017). This increase would allow seniors with income up to $2,313 per month (Musumeci et al., 2020) to qualify for free HCBS services, compared to the majority of seniors who are cut off from free full-scope Medi-Cal if their countable income exceeds 138% of the FPL, or $1,436 monthly. Individuals over the threshold are subjected to an impossible living standard of $600 per month to pay for all other expenses. Granting a higher income eligibility standard for waiver programs provides an equitable choice between institutionalization and long-term care (Molica, 2009).

Medi-Cal asset limits are the same for an individual in a nursing home as they are for a person maintaining a residence and supplying their meals in the community. The $2,000 asset limit for an individual provides no safety net for the additional needs a person with complex medical needs or functional limitations may require. Federal law allows states to expand the asset levels to $6,000. Increasing the asset level could serve as a lifeline to individuals maintaining a car or a home, or supplementing extra care in case of emergency. The federal government should require California to expand the asset level to the federally allowable limit for HCBS (Harrington et al., 2009).

Eliminate Enrollment Caps and Expand Geographic Availability

Nationally, in 2015, more than 640,000 people were on 1915(c) waiver waiting lists, and the average wait time was 2 years (Ng et al., 2017). In California, all 1915(c) waivers institute some waitlists. At 2 years, the ALW has the most extensive waitlist. Program policies prioritizing skilled nursing residents put prospective community applicants at a disadvantage. By eliminating or expanding enrollment caps the waitlist times could be reduced to a reasonable length avoiding violation of *Olmstead*.

Geographic restrictions continue to be a commonly used cost control, which explicitly hurt seniors in the most rural areas. The ALW is only available in 15 counties in California and is not available in most rural areas. Policy makers must explore rollout strategies to target communities with unmet long-term care needs. To evenly distribute services, financial incentives should be offered to attract providers in geographic areas with high cost of living.

Create a Single Point of Entry and Universal Assessment Tool

In California there is not a single point of entry for HCBS programs; participants typically are referred by community advocates such as legal services, hospital social workers, geriatric care managers, and other community resources. Information about eligibility and how to apply is confusing to navigate even for professionals. To apply, individuals must contact the appropriate agency for the program in their respective county. The fragmented system for HCBS applications and assessment is inefficient and confusing for prospective enrollees. Although an applicant may be applying for more than one program, each program uses unique assessment processes and criteria. In addition, the information collected among programs is not shared in a centralized database, and as a result, programs collect duplicative information at a cost to the state (Taylor, 2015).

In 2012, the California legislature authorized a pilot implementation of a Universal Assessment Tool (UAT) to streamline eligibility and program assessment determinations for three HCBS programs (Multipurpose Senior Service Program [MSSP], In-Home Supportive Services [IHSS], and Community Based Adult Services [CBAS]; Wilber et al., 2013). A Universal Assessment Tool uses the same criteria to evaluate applicant's eligibility across the HCBS programs. In January 2015, the Legislative Analyst's Office released a report reviewing the current process and its problems. Ultimately, the report made many recommendations, including enacting legislation to implement a state-wide Universal Assessment Tool using a person-centered approach (Taylor, 2015). In the 2017-2018 budget, Governor Brown announced the termination of the development of the UAT and its pilot for the three primary HCBS programs (The SCAN Foundation, 2017).

Research has identified a single point of entry as an efficient way to make programs accessible to consumers (Wilber et al., 2013). Efforts to simplify the application and assessment process will help save the state money and provide better access to consumers. The decision to terminate the development of this tool will only serve to delay improvements to the programs and access.

Increase Provider Rates

Encouraging the expansion of existing programs relies heavily on providers who are willing and able to provide the required services at the provided rate while making a profit and maintaining quality care. Low provider rates paid to family member caregivers are incredibly problematic, creating a trickle-down poverty effect on the entire household (Thomason & Bernhardt, 2017). The low rates make it challenging to attract nonrelative providers, because prospective caregivers can find easier work with comparable pay in any other industry, furthering the shortage crisis of home-care workers. The state will need to work toward raising the rates where possible to ensure the quality of care and to combat scarcity of available services due to lack of providers.

There are wide gaps between the Medi-Cal rate and private industry rate. Private industry rates are significantly higher; the low Medi-Cal rates leave programs struggling to hire the myriad of required qualified staff, such as nurses, social workers, physicians, physical therapists, etc. Programs, such as community-based adult services and the ALW, the program must also pay facility operating costs and provide meals under the low rate. The inequitable rate compensation will continue to limit the number of available providers for the programs, ultimately leaving the consumer with fewer options and unmet needs.

CONCLUSIONS

Although HCBS programs have quickly grown in the last 30 years, barriers, such as existing state and federal laws, short-sighted budgets, and program limitations, continue to hinder their access to consumers. Program limitations should not discourage applicants from seeking services or joining waitlists if the desired service is unavailable. Waitlist enrollment serves as an indicator for consumer preferences and unmet need. National and state advocates continue to work on expanding programs and funding for Medicaid beneficiaries. In addition, constituents should notify their legislators about the importance of expanding HCBS. To find out about eligibility for Medicaid or HCBS in your state, contact your local Medicaid office or Area Agency on Aging.

REFERENCES

Barrett, L. (2014). *Home and community preferences of the 45+ population 2014.* https://www.aarp.org/content/dam/aarp/research/surveys_statistics/il/2015/home-community-preferences.doi.10.26419%252Fres.00105.001.pdf

Beck, L. (2015, November). *California's In-Home Support Program.* Public Policy Institute of California. https://www.ppic.org/publication/californias-in-home-support-program

Boccuti, C., Casillas, G., & Neuman, T. (2015). *Reading the stars: Nursing home quality star ratings.* Henry J. Family Ford Foundation. http://files.kff.org/attachment/issue-brief-reading-the-stars-nursing-home-quality-star-ratings-nationally-and-by-state

CalPACE, Community Leaders for California's Seniors. (2019). *PACE Cost-effectiveness*. http://www.calpace.org/wp-content/uploads/2017/12/PACE-Cost-Effective-Fact-Sheet-updated-2-21-20.pdf

CalPACE, Community Leaders for California's Seniors. (2020). *General fact sheet*. Retrieved from http://www.calpace.org/wp-content/uploads/2017/12/CalPACE-General-Fact-Sheet-02-19-20.pdf

Centers for Medicare & Medicaid Services. (n.d.). *Program of All-inclusive Care for the Elderly*. https://www.medicaid.gov/medicaid/long-term-services-supports/program-all-inclusive-care-elderly/index.html

Chen, O., Jordan, S., Lim, M., Lou, Z., & Segal, K. (2019, May). *Evaluating California's Assisted Living Waiver program*. http://www.canhr.org/reports/2019/Evaluating_the_ALW.pdf?utm_source=CANHR+News+%26+Notes+E-Newsletter&utm_campaign=489003cafd-EMAIL_CAMPAIGN_2019_07_03_04_22&utm_medium=email&utm_term=0_9af69b452e-489003cafd-224314829

Department of Health Care Services. (2017a, November). *Medi-Cal at a glance*. http://www.dhcs.ca.gov/dataandstats/statistics/Documents/Medi-Cal_at_a_Glance_Nov2017_ADA.pdf

Department of Health Care Services. (2017b, November). *Medi-Cal estimate assisted living waiver expansion*. dhcs.ca.gov

Department of Health and Human Services, Centers for Medicare & Medicaid. (2014). *Fact sheet: Summary of key provisions of the Home and Community-Based Services (HCBS) settings final rule* (CMS 2249-F/2296-F). https://www.medicaid.gov/sites/default/files/2019-12/hcbs-setting-fact-sheet.pdf

Department of Social Services. (2020). *County individual provider rates wage rates*. http://www.cdss.ca.gov/inforesources/IHSS/County-IHSS-Wage-Rates

Genworth. (2019). *Aging and cost of care*. https://www.genworth.com/aging-and-you/finances/cost-of-care.html

Government Accountability Office. (2018a). *Medicaid assisted living services. Improved Federal Oversight of Beneficiary Health and Welfare is Needed*. GAO-18-179.

Government Accountability Office. (2018b). *Medicaid Home and Community-Based Services. Selected states' program structures and challenges providing services*. GAO-18-628.

Grabowski, D. C. (2006). The cost-effectiveness of non-institutional long-term care services: Review and synthesis of the most recent evidence. *Medical Care Research and Review, 63*(1), 3–28. https://pdfs.semanticscholar.org/e2c9/873a1fae819f695065c24361bc6abb044d4f.pdf

Greene, A., Lepore, M., Lux, L. Porter, K., Vreeland, E. (2015, September). *Understanding unlicensed care homes: Final report*. U.S. Department of Health and Human Services.

Harrington, C., Ng, T., Kaye, S. H., & Newcomer, R. (2009). *Home and Community-Based Services: Public policies to improve access, costs, and quality*. http://citeseerx.ist.psu.edu/viewdoc/download?doi=10.1.1.585.393&rep=rep1&type=pdf

Harris-Kojetin, L. D., Sengupta, M., Lendon, J. P., Rome, V., Valverde, R., & Caffrey, C. (2019). *Long-term care providers and services users in the United States, 2015–2016*. Retrieved from https://www.cdc.gov/nchs/data/series/sr_03/sr03_43-508.pdf

Henry J. Kaiser Family Foundation. (2015, August 31). *Long-term care in the United States: A timeline*. https://www.kff.org/medicaid/timeline/long-term-care-in-the-united-states-a-timeline

Institute of Medicine (U.S.) Committee on Nursing Home Regulation. (1986). *Improving the quality of care in nursing homes*. National Academies Press. https://www.ncbi.nlm.nih.gov/books/NBK217556

Lecovich, E. (2014). Aging in place: From theory to practice. *Anthropological Notebooks, 1*, 21–33.

Legislative Analyst's Office. (2017, February 28). *The 2017–18 budget analysis of the human services budget*. http://www.lao.ca.gov/Publications/Report/3576/2

Medicaid and CHIP Payment Access Commission. (2018). *Medicaid Home- and Community-Based Services: Characteristics and spending of high-cost users factsheet*. https://www.macpac.gov/wp-content/uploads/2018/06/Medicaid-HCBS-Characteristics-and-Spending.pdf

Medicaid and CHIP Payment Access Commission. (n.d.). *Program administration, State Plan*. https://www.macpac.gov/subtopic/state-plan

Meret-Hanke, L. A. (2011). Effects of the Program of All-inclusive Care for the Elderly on hospital use. *The Gerontologist, 51*(6), 774–785. https://doi.org/10.1093/geront/gnr040

Molica, R. L. (2009). *State Medicaid Reimbursement Policies and Practices in Assisted Living*. https://www.ahcancal.org/ncal/advocacy/Documents/MedicaidAssistedLivingReport.pdf

Mukamel, D., Peterson, D., Temkin-Greener, H., Delevan, R., Gross, D., Kunitz, S., & Williams, T. (2007, August). Program characteristics and enrollees' outcomes in the Program of All-inclusive Care for the Elderly (PACE). *Milbank Quarterly, 85*, 499–531. https://doi.org/10.1111/j.1468-0009.2007.00497.x

Musumeci, M., O'Malley Watts, M., & Chidambaram, P. (2020, February). *Key state policy choices about Medicaid home and community-based services*. Henry J. Kaiser Family Foundation.

Musumeci, M., & Young, K. (2017, May). *State variation in Medicaid per enrollee spending for seniors and people with disabilities*. Henry J. Kaiser Family Foundation. http://files.kff.org/attachment/Issue-Brief-State-Variation-in-Medicaid-Per-Enrollee-Spending-for-Seniors-and-People-with-Disabilities

National PACE Association. (n.d.). *The history of PACE*. https://www.npaonline.org/policy-advocacy/value-pace#history

Newcomer, R., Harrington, C., Stone, J., Bindman, A. B., & Helmar, M. (2011). *California's Medi-Cal Home & Community-Based Services waivers, benefits & eligibility policies*, 2005–2008. University of California, San Francisco & California Department of Health Care Services. http://www.thescanfoundation.org/sites/default/files/camri_waiver_report_0_3.pdf

Ng, T., Musumeci, M., & Ubri, P. (2016, October). *Medicaid Home- and Community-Based Services programs: 2013 data update*. Henry J. Kaiser Family Foundation. https://www.kff.org/medicaid/report/medicaid-home-and-community-based-services-programs-2013-data-update/

O'Malley Watts, M., Musumeci, M., & Chidambaram, P., (2020). *Medicaid Home- and Community-Based Services enrollment and spending*. Henry J. Kaiser Family Foundation. https://www.kff.org/report-section/medicaid-home-and-community-based-services-enrollment-and-spending-issue-brief

On Lok Lifeways. (n.d.). *On Lok PACE program*. https://www.onloklifeways.org

Reaves, E. L., & Musumeci, M. (2015). *Medicaid and long-term services and supports: A primer*. The Henry J. Kaiser Family Foundation. https://www.kff.org/medicaid/report/medicaid-and-long-term-services-and-supports-a-primer

The Scan Foundation. (2011, January). *Implementing* Olmstead *in California* (Technical brief series No.5). https://www.thescanfoundation.org/sites/default/files/ltc_fundamental_5_0.pdf

Sherwin, S., & Winsby, M. (2010). A relational perspective on autonomy for older adults. *Health Expectations, 14*(2), 182–190. https://doi.org/10.1111/j.1369-7625.2010.00638.x

Taylor, M. (2015). *The universal assessment tool: Improving care for recipients of Home- and Community-Based Services*. Legislative Analyst Office. http://www.lao.ca.gov/reports/2015/hhs/uat/uat-012215.pdf

Thomason, S., & Bernhardt, A. (2017). *California's homecare crisis: Raising wages is key to the solution*. UC Berkeley Center for Labor Research and Education. http://laborcenter.berkeley.edu/californias-homecare-crisis

Wilber, K., Saliba, D., Fulbright, K., Lhasa, R., & Newcomer, R. (2013). *Memorandum on the current assessment approaches and domains used by three HCBS programs in California*. https://www.thescanfoundation.org/media/2019/07/usc-ucla-ucsf-current_assessment_approaches_domains_three_ca_hcbs_programs-9-25-13.pdf

FURTHER READING

Assistant Secretary for Planning and Evaluation Office of Disability, Aging and Long-Term Care Policy. (2015). *Understanding unlicensed care homes: Final report*. https://aspe.hhs.gov/system/files/pdf/200961/Unlicensed.pdf

Department of Health and Human Services, Centers for Medicare & Medicaid. (2019). *Assisted living waiver approval letter*. https://www.dhcs.ca.gov/services/ltc/Documents/ALW-Renewal-2019-2024-Approval-Letter.pdf

Health for California. (n.d.). *Covered California income limits*. https://www.healthforcalifornia.com/covered-california/income-limits

U.S. Government Accountability Office. (2018). *Medicaid Home- and Community-Based Services selected states' program structures and challenges*. https://www.gao.gov/assets/700/694174.pdf

INFORMATION AND COMMUNICATION TECHNOLOGY IN ASSISTED LIVING

WITH CONTRIBUTING AUTHOR BENJAMIN BONGERS

LEARNING OBJECTIVES

On the completion of Chapter 16, the reader will be able to:

- Understand what information and communication technology (ICT) is and how it can be of use in an assisted living community (ALC).
- Define general terminology when speaking about ICT.
- Know the history and evolution of ICT, and how it affects our everyday lives.
- Understand how the use of ICTs can aid both residents and caregivers in assisted living communities.
- Look to ICT as a tool for improving and safeguarding a resident's ability to age in place.
- Understand some of the surprises and challenges that occur when using ICT.
- Consider the quality of life enhancement that ICT may offer an assisted living community.

INTRODUCTION

The world population is living longer, and the birth rate is in steep decline. With 10,000 baby boomers retiring each day, the majority (87%) of adults aged 65 and over wish to continue living in their current homes or communities as long as possible (Harrell et al., 2014). However, there will not be enough people of working age (20 to 64 years old) to care for those in the "elderly" category by the year 2050 (United Nations, 2017). With worldwide longevity on the rise and birth rates in decline, the global "Silver tsunami" may in all actuality be forced to age in place, be it at home independent, or in assisted living with or without on-site human assistance.

In the United States, a little over 75% of older adults owned cell phones in 2014, with over 50% using tablets or smartphones (Smith, 2014). As technology has advanced, so has the acceptance of these communication devices by the older population. ICT is an emerging system that presents possible applications to assist the care of older adults, either directly or in a support capacity, and may provide needed assistance at a reduced cost.

OVERVIEW

Definition

ICT is defined as information technology and other equipment systems, technologies, or processes for which the principal function is the creation, manipulation, storage, display, receipt, or transmission of electrical data and information, as well as any associated content. Examples of ICT include but are not limited to computers and peripheral equipment, information kiosks and transaction machines, telecommunications equipment, customer premises equipment, multifunction office machines, software, applications, websites, videos and electronic documents (ICT Standards and Guides, 2015).

A Brief History of ICT

ICT has been around since the early 1960s with the advent of the Defense Advanced Research Project Agency (DARPA), which led to the creation of the internet in 1962. The internet allowed computers to communicate directly in research and military projects. In 1989, Tim Berners-Lee created the World Wide Web and wrote the first web browser in 1990.

The first handheld uses of functional ICT were the personal digital assistant (PDA), and the self-contained power source mobile telephone. The first PDA for the public (named *The Organizer*) was developed by Psion in 1984 and could only transfer input information onto a memory card, which would then have to be downloaded to a computer for processing (Castelluccio, 2004). Soon, Motorola[M], IBM, Nokia, Blackberry, and Apple would develop their own versions of the PDA that included touch screens and web connection. Incidentally, the term *personal digital assistant* was later coined by Apple's chief executive officer, John Sculley, in 1992.

Martin Cooper of Motorola created the first handheld, self-sustaining mobile phone in 1974. It was roughly 9 inches long, 5.185 inches deep, 1.75 inches wide, and it weighed approximately 2.5 pounds. Its battery life was only 30 minutes and took 10 hours for a full charge (Maisto, 2014). Soon came the Motorola DynaTAC 8000X, the Nokia 2100 Series, and in 2003, the Blackberry 6210.

The Blackberry 6210 was the first fully integrated PDA/mobile phone, and was the preferred tool of most businesspersons in the early 2000s. In 2007, the Apple iPhone hit the market and was the first touchscreen-controlled smartphone to gain popularity with the general public and soon spun off into tablet technology. Many of the businesspersons who used this ICT in the early 2000s are in retirement, now looking for assistance with aging in place through the use of today's ICT.

ICTs AND THEIR USE IN AIDING OLDER ADULTS

Use of Ambient Technology to Assist With Activities of Daily Living and Instrumental Activities of Daily Living

Ambient technology has been present in science fiction and cartoons for many years, but its practical uses are a recent development. With ICT, smartphones, and digital technology, comes the ability to track, monitor, and surveil people in their own environment. All this can now be done with little or no visible apparatuses or detection, thus keeping the feeling of "being watched" to a minimum. This section covers three areas of ambient technology: ambient assisted living, wearable technology, and smart homes.

Ambient Assisted Living

Ambient assisted living (AAL) is implemented by means of sensors that are embedded into the walls, ceiling, floor, and/or furniture of the person's home. These sensors monitor the action, activity, behavior, and motion of the resident in sequence (e.g., first pick up a glass, then turn on the tap for cold water, then hold glass under faucet, then turn off tap, finally drink water and set down glass). Through a hierarchy of algorithms, the sensors can detect early forms of frailty, dementia, and other chronic ailments such as Parkinson's or gait and balance issues. The array is scanning for low-level to high-level determinants of activity, capturing things like eye tracking, gait speed and distance, and repetition of movement or stalling of motion. The sensors also extract data on length of time to begin, manage, and complete a task, continually observing if all processes of the activity are completed (Thi-Hoa-Cuc et al., 2016). The data is then synthesized and compared to previous outcomes, helping to give early detection of changing conditions or new behaviors.

The AAL system has proven to be particularly useful in self-care for those older adults who have mild cognitive impairment (MCI) or ongoing dementia, and with the passage of time, the effected elders either did not realize they were being monitored or did not care. Many times the caregivers feel they are in better control of care and have a higher rate of relaxed interaction and increased personal time away from their older adult because the system is monitoring for any aberrational behavior.

Other benefits of AAL are care cost savings, reduced health risk through vitals monitoring, prompts and reminders for medication consumption, brain stimulation games, and video communication with family or medical personnel through an established web portal; all of these aid in enhancing mental dexterity and socialization skills necessary to age in place (Mitseva et al., 2012).

Wearable Technology

Due to compact size and longer-lasting battery power, AAL is now able to work in tandem with wearable technology. These "wearables" consist of anything worn or grasped by the person using or being monitored by the technology. Many of these have become everyday consumer products or applications with new innovations coming to market every day. Products like FitBit track not only steps, but also offer Global Positioning System (GPS) tracking and heart rate. More specialized applications are downloaded to a smartphone to sense balance or gait; two such products are the "Smartphone Balance Trainer" and the "Class CoreMotion" by Apple. Other ICT applications for smartphone health monitoring track blood pressure, heart rate and electrical impulses (EKG), electrical activity in the brain (EEG), glucose levels, fall risk, oxygen levels, and temperature, to name a few. The information can be downloaded to another device for easy tracking or monitored in real time by the wearer, a caregiver, or a physician if they have been approved to observe it.

Smart Homes

The term *smart home* makes one think of a science-fiction future come to life, and in many cases, it feels that way. A *smart home* by definition is a residence that uses internet-connected devices to enable the remote monitoring and management of appliances and systems (Rouse, 2017). An older adult could either move into a pre-existing smart home or have their present domicile retrofitted with the necessary equipment. By tracking activity and recognizing what an elder may be doing, the system creates a scalable solution to support optimizing the personalization of care (Fiorini et al., 2017). The results are then built into a model and fine-tuned in cooperation with a caregiver, creating a care plan over time. Through recognition of an elder's movement patterns, the computer model can recognize modal behavior clusters that have been proven to accurately track all activities of daily living (ADLs) with a 96.85% of accuracy, and can warn of possible change in condition (Nef et al., 2015).

Medical Assistance and Safety Measures Using ICT

Today, there are many new and different forms of assistive technology and practical aides based on smartphone or tablet technology. Through use of applications, ICT assists elders in rehabilitation, reminders, and positive feedback. The use of retail technology to track and report vital statistics to caretakers, caregivers, and stakeholders in older adults' well-being is fairly new and still being explored.

eHealth, teleMed, and mHealth

Electronic health (eHealth) started as usable ICT when visual and vocal screen technology became available. Mobile Health (mHealth) is a sub-category denoting specifically mobile devices such as smartphones or tablets. With the arrival of smartphones, tablets, and other robotics, the process has taken on a new life. In the United States, videoconferencing through use of home computers, smartphones, and tablets for medical purposes is becoming a trend. It has been conservatively estimated that at least one million doctor consultations were made by eHealth, teleMed, and mHealth in 2016 alone. And, because of low overhead and the expense of fewer in-office visits and lesser travel, some insurance companies are now offering these services free of charge (Harvard Health Letter, 2016).

Hospitals no longer "chart" on paper forms, and many surgeries are now done robotically. Now, through integration of electronic health records with ICT appendices and externals (smart watches, tablets, smartphones, computers, etc.), elders' vitals can be tracked and charted in real time and may eliminate time-consuming and expensive office visits. This is monumental for those who live in rural areas, for whom the closest medical facilities may be many hours away.

As with any program, there are drawbacks. All of the equipment used needs to be purchased and a fairly wide broadband-width network needs to be established prior to going online. But with the growth and expansion of technologies, this will be the wave of the future, especially for rural areas. Technologically connecting urban, suburban, and rural areas through ICT will allow elder adults to keep medical appointments, reduce travel time, and foster more proactive health awareness.

Tele-Monitoring

Because older adults have a higher risk of health concerns, they require more visits to medical facilities and caregivers may need to be present. These visits are time-consuming, expensive, and sometimes disturbing to older persons. One way of minimizing travel time, personnel costs, forgetfulness, and frustration is by tele-monitoring. Tele-monitoring tracks medication use, vital signs, falls, wandering, and elopement monitoring, as well as smoking cessation.

MEDICATIONS

Self-management of medications becomes a very real concern for older persons, not taking the correct dose at the right time accounts for 31.8% of medication errors (Field et al., 2007). Memory is one of the biggest concerns with self-administration of medication. There are now many ICT products on the market related to medication—timers, dispensers, and reminders of all varieties and prices. The keys to use of an elder's medication aid are ease of use, ease of training, reliability, and acceptability. One of the largest issues with self-medicating is memory.

DEFINED TRACKING

Today, it is a normal part of conversation to find out how many steps someone has taken that day. The idea of tracking distance is not new, but becomes invaluable when looking at the movement, calories burned, altitude ascended or descended, and position on a map of an older adult, particularly if they are showing signs of confusion or are in need of more exercise.

Through use of accelerometers, gyroscope sensors, GPS, and other new technology, specific criterion can be tracked and data reported through an appendage monitor (smart watches, smart bracelets, etc.), as well as smartphones and computers. This information can now be shared with caretakers, children, or doctors. Energy expenditure, caloric intake, blood glucose levels, and all forms of heart monitoring can easily be tracked.

FALLS

With age comes frailty and preventing falls becomes critical for older adults. Every year 2.8 million older adults are treated in emergency rooms for fall injuries due to clutter in walking paths, uneven surfaces, and tears in carpet or worn areas, and over 800,000 are hospitalized due to accidents (Centers for Disease Control and Prevention [CDC], 2017).

By using a smart bracelet or smartphone (which has an accelerometer built into it) falls can now by detected using an application. The secret to cessation of falls is still strength training and balance. The largest risks come from lower body weakness, difficulty with walking and balance, vision problems, foot pain or poor footwear, and tripping hazards. Through ICT, a tablet can be used in strengthening the core of the body, thus improving balance and the gait of an older adult. Through the application and monitoring by a physical therapist, an elder is tested physically to find the weak points in the physical action of walking.

WANDERING AND ELOPEMENT

With many MCI-based diseases and in those with Alzheimer's, wandering away from a home situation can be traumatic and/or dangerous. Depending on the condition and how it is manifested, the older person may be in good physical condition, yet become disoriented and lose reference to where "home" is. The person with these progressive conditions will, over time, need more and more care, thus increasing monitoring and expense.

Through use of GPS, ICT can not only can track those with MCI, but aid the person in finding their own way back to home. Through use of haptic-feedback (think of the vibrations in a smart watch or smartphone) and internal GPS systems, the elder can be guided back to their home (Me et al., 2017).

Tele-Rehabilitation

Maintaining physical strength through exercise is important for older adults' health. Exercise not only of the body's core, but of the arms and legs, has been proven effective in allowing an elder to age in place. Through use of any one of the many core-strengthening applications on a smart device, an older person can gain strength, increase balance, and become more flexible.

Another important use of tele-rehabilitation is chronic pain management in elders, particularly those living in rural areas where coming to a rehabilitation center several times a week may be impractical or impossible. In cooperation with a physician, physical therapist, and caregiver, a care plan can be created and implemented. Many subjects are able to reduce pain and regain movement after surgery and immobilization. After a prescribed time, a follow-up session in person can be created to check on the elder's form.

Robotic Assistance

Japan was the first country to explore human interactive robotics in the 1980s; since then, other countries have joined this research community. The thought is that robots can provide support for older adults in the instrumental activities of daily living by physically moving objects, aiding in mobility, giving reminders, ordering services, administering necessary items, and generally aiding in caregiving.

INTERACTIVE ROBOTS

In cooperation with smart-home technology, robotics is being used not just for go-and-fetch systems, but also communications, vital-sign assessment, and reminders. By use of sensors worn by the elder, a robot can interact with the person as if it was an intuited being. The robot comes on command, knows in which room of the domicile the human is located, and what direction they are facing. The robot can also detect, by verbal command and visual stimulation of hand activity, where the older adult would like them to go or what they would like them to retrieve, thus allowing the human greater autonomy and privacy.

In some cases, robots are now beginning developed as possible caregivers. In supportive apartment living (SAL), robots take on the role of physical, mental, and emotional support surrogates, many times at a lower cost and higher satisfaction rate than humans. Through home safety monitoring, efficient and accessible communication devices, and tele-health monitoring systems, robots in SALs are proving effective. The robot assistants can deliver items gotten outside the home (groceries, takeout food, etc.) and they are able to lift and move objects too heavy or cumbersome for the older adult to handle. They also engage in minor forms of conversation and question answering, thus giving the appearance of being sentient (Sefcik et al., 2018).

ALL-TERRAIN WHEELCHAIRS

All-terrain wheelchairs have been on the market for several years now and have proven very effective. In most cases, they have a multiplicity of wheels and joints allowing the user to go up and down staircases and that extend upward to different heights—simulating standing.

Another development in wheelchair dynamics is assisted by the self-driving automobile industry. The same technology of danger detection is now being tested in wheelchair trials and showing great promise. The effectiveness is proving a benefit to the autonomy and safety of elders in populated spaces or areas with terrain that may be uneven (Tuck-Voon et al., 2013).

Safety and Health Promotion/Prevention ICT

Safety in the home has been extended to an older person's appliances. There are several products on the market specifically developed for elders living at home with MCI or Alzheimer's disease that have safeguards built into them. Stovetops with a built-in timer that can be set either manually or remotely, allowing the unit to function for a set amount of time or during certain hours of operation. Other units have been developed to be functional if the operator is physically present. If they leave the unit's proximity for a predetermined length of time, the appliance will turn off (Nygård, 2009).

Physical safety does not come exclusively from safeguarding exterior elements. Physical and mental fitness are also primary safeguards. The easiest way of remaining vital is by adding activity and creating a physical fitness regimen. There are apps aimed toward behavioral changes and disease management that encompass topics from physical movement to depression treatment and psychological support groups. The older adult *must* be trained in the use of the technology for it to be effective. Many times, the best way of encouraging ICT use is through the elders' peer group (Helbostad et al., 2017).

Home Communication Tools for Socialization

Many times, elders may shy away from using ICT because they feel out of touch and/or unable to learn the new technology. The older the cohort, the less likely members are to use ICT. The primary reason given is that they do not see a need to use the technology. The thinking is that if people wanted to communicate with the older person, they would call, write, or come to visit. Another reason given is the complexity of the new communication. In the older person's mind, the "new technology" is unforgiving and must be used in a linear way; there are no obvious work arounds. The younger the cohort, the more able users are (Feist et al., 2010).

Because of this reluctance, elders rarely ask for one-on-one sessions to learn about the use of the technology. There are benefits in learning to use ICT in a group situation. A model that seems to be beneficial to both learning and socialization is having a teacher assist 10 to 12 students in a loosely structured situation. With few points to be learned, a class session's time can be extended for socialization—with finger food and drinks added. The greatest benefit to using this model occurs when an elder student masters understanding of a concept and aids the teacher in instructing their peers (Helbostad et al., 2017). Then, in a relaxed atmosphere, work in smaller groups or one-on-one instruction can happen organically.

Videoconferencing

Even in assisted living communities, isolation has been shown to lesson an older adult's willingness to socialize, keep up with personal care, and live longer (Shankar et al., 2015). As older adults become stationary, many begin to detach from socialization and become reclusive, which causes disassociation, loneliness, and eventual depression. Through use of simple ICT (particularly, texting, email, and videoconferencing through apps such as Skype, FaceTime, and Instant Message), or using more advanced platforms (Google's Home Hub, Amazon's Alexa Echo Show, and FaceBook's Portal), an older adult has the ability to keep in contact with family, friends, and associates easily.

Email, Messaging, and the Internet

In many cases, older adults have diminished hearing or eyesight. Emailing and messaging either by text or by other means allows clear communication. Font size can be increased, and differing colors of screen and type can be used for those with sight issues. The use of emailing and texting is also valuable for memory prompts. By saving the electronic communication, dates, times, and other information can be stored for future reference.

Another point of comfort through written ICT communication is not having to look or listen for cues from the person with whom they are conversing. The person can carry on a conversation with ease and request more information if necessary. They can also pick up or leave the communication at their leisure; there does not have to be a set time.

Transportation Driving Surrogacy

The freedom and autonomy of driving or continuing with an alternative transportation arrangement is very important for an elder. There are many reasons for elders to hang up their keys: maladies of sight and hearing, possible medication reactions, or slowing of reflexes. The ability to be mobile and travel is crucial for older adults to maintain their everyday lives. There are social events, doctor's visits, and shopping to do. So, if unable to drive themselves, the choices should be simple: they must hire transportation.

Today, depending on how urban or rural the area, elders have several choices. In in an urban area, taxi services or application transport vompanies (ATCs; Lyft, Uber, etc.) are the easiest to arrange. However, there is a built-in "fear factor." The elder does not know the driver and may or may not know the route they will be taking. There is also fear using mass transit in that many major cities no longer accept currency, only electronic transit passes, which older persons may not be familiar with.

The services that offered fall into three categories: curb-to-curb, door-to-door, and door-through-door. Curb-to-curb is a basic taxi service. Door-to-door drivers will assist in helping a mobile person to their destination and return to the point of origination; however, they will not generally help with assistive technology (e.g., wheelchairs, walkers, etc.). Door-through-door services will assist in getting a person with needs to and from the destination, then help the elder in and out of a wheelchair or assist with walkers and carry any necessary packages to and from the vehicle.

Rural elders have a harder time with unified transportation systems. Currently, there is no unified elder-transport agency in any state. And in most cases, if there is a rural elder transport, it is strictly for medical visits.

Online Outlets

Online shopping is a major pastime of the baby boomer generation. The main reason given is simplicity; many are unable to physically get to a shopping area for reasons of health or proximity. Online, an older person can compare prices, sizes, and all other criterion before purchasing. As most elders are on a fixed budget, comparing prices before purchase is a major benefit. Through use of online ordering, an older adult can shop for food, clothing, entertainment, and personal hygiene items that will be delivered. Remember, the ability to shop, dress, and either prepare or order food is a basic need that is considered part of the ADL and instrumental activities of daily living (IADL) criteria for aging in place.

Online Banking and Financial Monitoring

The IADL criterion requires older persons do their own banking and financial transactions proficiently. Inter- and intrabankfund transfers are now done worldwide exclusively through ICT. However, the majority of older adults are afraid they will be taken advantage of if they use electronic banking and run a higher risk than any other cohort of identity theft (AARP, 2011; Department of Homeland Security, 2018; Fox, 2013). The older population feels they have been marked as trusting and unsuspecting. Internet scams against the elderly are listed as number six on the National Council on Aging's "Top 10 financial scams" list, only behind Medicare/health insurance scams, counterfeit drugs, funeral/cemetery scams, fraudulent anti-aging scams, and telemarketing/phone scams (National Council on Aging, 2018).

The U.S. Department of Homeland Security (2018) has two fact sheets on how to avoid cyber-crime, with one specifically created for older adults (Cybersecurity & Infrastructure Security Agency, 2020). The two fact sheets may seem very basic to a digital native, but for someone from the baby boomer generation or older, many of the tactics and/or protection processes offer real value. Things like when and when not to give out personal information, how to check for security on banking sites, and the need to always look at your checking account and charge statements when you have made an online purchase are helpful reminders.

The older adult information sheet (Cybersecurity & Infrastructure Security Agency, 2020) does not consider a deeper level of security; for that information the elder needs to look at the Basic Tips and Advice page (Department of Homeland Security, 2018). This page talks about the need for enhanced password protection, current security software, and offers the motto, "when in doubt, throw it out" for suspicious email (Department of Homeland Security, 2018). Both sheets tell the reader to look for the "**s**" in the web addresses (e.g., https:// versus http://). The addition of the "**s**" gives the site a security locking system, thus keeping all data safe from external leaks.

Online finance (basic banking, stock and bond purchases, annuities, etc.) is here to stay. With education from the financial institutions and personal security safeguards in place, an older adult can continue their own money management. If the elder feels they may not be able to keep up with the online changes, they may be able to hire an online service through their financial institution or allow a trusted proxy to monitor their accounts.

ICT Surprises, Drawbacks, and Security Issues

Due to the relative newness of assistive ICT in long-term care, there are several unexplored, unthought-of, or—worse yet—hindrances to its use for elders and caretakers. This section explores the burgeoning field's progress, failures, and frustrations to expose mistakes and ensure the ability to learn from them. With ICT devices increasing in power and decreasing in size, wearable technology is no longer something from science fiction or Dick Tracey comic books. Wrist monitors, smartphones, and other noninvasive technologies are now sold around the world in the same outlets where you buy breakfast cereal and coffee makers. But how is this technology being used? Who is reviewing it?

Unrestricted Secondary Informational Use and Privacy Apprehension

Considered a "surprise" in this category would be the insurance industries' interest in tracking by use of ICT (e.g., wearable sensors, extremity monitors, etc.) for the companies' benefit. Insurance companies are now exploring the

> Adoption of wearable devices in senior citizens by describing various researches for moni-toring physical activity indicators, such as energy expenditure, posture transitions, activity classification, fall detection and prediction, gait and balance analysis, also by adopting con-sumer-grade fitness trackers with the associated limitations regarding acceptability. . . [and] the impact of wearable devices on life and health insurance companies, with a description of the potential benefits for the industry and the wearables market [analyzing the] example of the potential emerging market drivers for such technology in the future. (Tedesco et al., 2017, p. 1)

The insurance industry claims its concern is to aid the health and well-being of its customers by use of vital-sign tracking. In 2014, 3% of insurers were already using the data given by twearable technology, and 22% of insurers are now developing a strategy to use vital sign tracking as a part of their industry (Tedesco et al., 2017). This shows that activity tracking not only works but soon may become mandatory for many insurance companies. By agreeing to the updates already on these devices, the consumer may someday be agreeing to allow the insurance industry to track their vital signs, thus allowing the price of their insurance to rise or fall with the data analysis.

1. Not Enough Proof in Testing and Ethical Concerns

With many products, there is a real concern for lack of critical analysis before they are put on the market. As a case in point, testing showed that the Android-based fall detection system had no real framework or data to validate its claims (Casilari et al., 2015). The study found that there was simply not enough memory, computing power, or battery life in the unit to do all the calculations the detection system claimed a smartphone could deliver.

There is also an inability to gage the measure of users' (e.g., caregivers, older adults, family members, etc.) real-life experience with ICT to aid an oelder person(Connelly et al., 2014; Roberts et al., 2015). For example, there is no real model to show what good caregiving is versus computer-generated supposition. Was it the observation of a skilled caregiver or the computer's analysis that first found signs of MCI in the older adult? There is no way to confirm or deny either at this point. With the newness and rapid development of this technology, not only in the aging category, but concerning all testing and marketing, many safeguards and data are not taken into consideration, or worse yet, not done at all (Connelly et al., 2014).

The lack of social contact is another major concern in ITC use, particularly for elders living rurally who are geographically limited compared to those elders living in an urban setting with transportation options and available assisting personnel. Using effective eHealth, tele-medicine, and mHealth, most older adults' chronic conditions can be managed and monitored with accuracy and ease; however, a part of "good medical care" is also social interaction with the patient. There is quite a marked difference in outcomes for urban studies of care versus those on the outskirts of urban areas or in rural areas (Roberts et al., 2015). The reason given was the older adult and caregiver both enjoyed the personal contact more than they did the outcome of the condition, thus proving that many forms of ICT should not be used exclusively, but in tandem with personal caregiving.

To aid the ethical creation of applications for ICT, in January 2018, the American Medical Association, American Heart Association, DHX (Digital Health eXcellence) Group, and Healthcare Information and Management Systems Society created and implemented a cooperative guideline for consumers and developers alike. This early guideline assesses the security, privacy, operability, and content of health applications. This development is a first step to adding ethics to ICT's wild frontier (The Xcertia mhealth app Guidelines, 2018).

Desire and Divide

As mentioned previously, there is a very real digital divide between those who have been raised in the electronic age and elders who did not begin using ICT until they were past 60 years of age. Fears of looking incompetent, thinking they may "break something expensive," and not feeling a real "need" for the use of ICT are naturally feelings in the elder community.

The most successful form of elder instruction seems to be done in cooperation with the social event itself. The elders learn through small successes that they share with others in their cohort. After 10 classes the older adult's self-efficacy level rises and anxiety over ICT drops precipitously (Tsai et al., 2015).

Further reinforcement is also beneficial to both the care companion and the elder. "[I]t is necessary to communicate concrete benefits to the older adult and, at the same time, reduce technology-related concerns specific for that individual." and "[w]hen an older adult does not see the need for a technology, it is highly unlikely that he or she will be inclined to start using it" (Peek et al., 2014, p. 246).

2.   What We Don't Know Is a Lot

Who is developing most of the ICT that we are seeing on the market today for elder use? The top seven companies responsible for innovation and most of the research and development (R&D) of ICT show a lack of effort to incorporate older adults' perspectives and/or input into the design process (Allen, 2016). There is little to no elder advice or tutelage in helping to determine elders' needs.

Unfortunately, the creation of ICT for older adults today is a "young-man's game." Many companies are doing R&D, testing, and marketing of "elder care technology" without ever having had an elder see the product in development. Over the last few years, a few companies began basing their R&D in cooperation with older adults. Companies like World Wide Web Consortium (W3C), Aging 2.0, and Google are beginning to use ointo lder adults as R&D resources.

All Systems

The new voice-activated assistant (VAA) holds great promise. Google Home, for example, is a VAA, Amazon's Alexa, Apple's HomePod, or FaceBook's Portal can be given a voice command and the system will follow through with a simple action. Things like turning on lights, reading the news, and ordering dinner or a car service are as simple as speaking the commands. VAAs will make lists, play music, and call family members or doctors—either by phone or audio/visual means. VAAs can turn on certain televisions, play movies on command, and change the lighting in the room to set a mood or environment. They can tell users about scheduled appointments, remind them of medications to take, and call for help in case of emergencies. Other external items connected to and managed by VAAs are light bulbs, electric plugs, cleaning robots, and cameras with home security systems—with more and varied items coming to the market every day.

As with all new technological systems, some things need to be worked out. Requests must be singular and asked clearly, in a logical, sequential, and timely manner with no pauses. This narrows the user base considerably and would exclude those with MCI or speech impediments due to muscular or cognitive issues.

So, will elders live like *The Jetsons* or be "beamed up" onto the bridge of the *Enterprise*? Will older adults have the opportunity to age in place for the duration of their life? The answer is yes and no. We are beginning to use robotics the way Rosie was portrayed in *The Jetsons*, and the original "clam shell" mobile phones and iPads™ were created to mimic the "communicators" and "info tablets" of *Star Trek* fame. In fact, there are now universal real-time translators, holodeck projection rooms, phasers, and hypo-sprays for medication absorption through the skin—all fantasy just a few years ago,and now a reality in the years to come. . .

EXAMPLES OF PRACTICAL USE

According to a Pew Research survey, four in 10 older adults now use the internet and own smarphones—up 50% from 2014 to 2018 (Anderson & Perrin, 2017). Jewish Senior Life, a continuing-care retirement community in Rochester, New York, has a strong understanding of how technology can help enrich the lives of their residents. Through resident training by their staff, the population uses ICT to enhance connections with family and friends. By using voice-activated assistants, webcams, email, and texts, the residents stay engaged, informed, in touch, and in control—even those who have never used computers before (King, 2018).

Minds are stimulated and technology-enhanced rehabilitation programs are used to improve hand–eye coordination through use games and puzzles. By using ICT, the resident's quality of life is augmented by a wide range of cognitive and physical ability technologies, adapted just for them.

By using Google Home throughout the facility, voice-activated smart speakers gives instant access to news, entertainment, and communication, as well as providing reminders for appointments and medications. The system is also used in paying bills, ordering products, and summoning transportation.

Another system incorporated in the Jewish Senior Life center is It's Never 2 Late (iN2L). The iN2L system is a touch-based system that uses pictures as prompts, aiding those with cognitive issues. The system is personalized for each resident's immediate needs.

Aiding those with Sundowners syndrome is Music & Memory Hearing familiar music from the elder's past is calming and decreases episodes of agitation. The music is loaded onto iPods and a playlist is created specifically for each resident with the syndrome.

The use of ICT in communities is very new and continues to be a cutting-edge improvement for the lives of residents. As new products come to market, communities not utilizing these products will be at a distinct disadvantage.

CONCLUSIONS

Although in early development, ICT is viable to aid older adults in everyday life. Practical ICT is now used in elder medical tracking of vital signs, medical visits, physical therapy, communication, shopping, banking, and safety alerts. Through ambient technology, those with MCI and neurological issues are being afforded more personal autonomy and freedom to travel in their own "neighborhoods." Through use of eHealth, teleMed, and mHealth, older adults in rural and urban areas alike can have an easier connection with their medical and rehabilitation teams and an elder's social life, be it with family or friends, can be full and engaging.

However, there are a few areas of concern that still need review and more practical study. Elders are seldom used as a part of the process from product inception to completion, and there is a need for practical education for elders and caregivers to be able to use ICT effectively. And what about infrastructure in most care centers? Will their Wi-Fi be able to handle an influx of double, triple, or quadruple forms of ICT?

There are also ethical and security issues for elders using ICT who are more susceptible to fraud and hacking. Another concern is price. Typically, elders have fixed incomes, and ICT is not inexpensive. Moving forward, there will need to be research and lobbying for many of the ICT systems and products to be purchased through Medicaid/Medicare. Although VAA systems, while relatively inexpensive and already on the market, have proven to assist elder autonomy, they still need to be purchased, set up, and maintained.

With training on ICT use the older population will continue living as they have in the past technological modifications. Their sight will go and they will not be able to drive a motorcycle anymore, but they can always call out, "Alexa, call me a car" and be on their way. Hearing will dim, but through a better cochlear implant, one will hear all the frequencies heard years before. Memory will slip, but through nanobots in the bloodstream, I'll be able to do higher calculus in seconds.

Sounds like science fiction? Probably. But so did the submarine to Jules Verne, HAL to Stanley Kubrick and Arthur C. Clark, and the communicator to Gene Roddenberry. With time, research, and cooperation, older adults will be able to age in place longer with ICT than without. Live long and prosper.

REFERENCES

AARP. (2011). *Aging in place: A state survey of livability policies and practices*. https://assets.aarp.org/rgcenter/ppi/liv-com/aging-in-place-2011-full.pdf

Allen, R. (2016) Average age of tech company's employees. *Smart Insights*. https://www.smartinsights.com/manage-digital-transformation/average-age-tech-companys-employees-chartoftheday

Anderson, M., & Perrin, A. (2017, May) Tech adoption climbs among older adults. *Pew Research Center*. https://www.pewresearch.org/internet/2017/05/17/tech-adoption-climbs-among-older-adults

Casilari, E., Luque, R., & Moron, M. (2015). Analysis of android device-based solutions for fall detection. *Sensors, 15*(8), 17827–17894. https://doi.org/10.3390/s150817827

Castelluccio, M. (2004). Writing on the screen. *Strategic Finance, 85*(11), 59–60.

Centers for Disease Control and Prevention. (2017, February 10). *Important facts about falls*. https://www.cdc.gov/homeandrecreationalsafety/falls/adultfalls.html

Connelly, K., ur Rehman Laghari, K., Mokhtari, M., & Falk, T. (2014). Approaches to understanding the impact of technologies for aging in place: A mini-review. *Gerontology, 60*(3), 282–288. https://doi.org/10.1159/000355644

Cybersecurity & Infrastructure Security Agency. (2020, January). *Stop. Think. Connect. Older American resources*. https://www.cisa.gov/sites/default/files/publications/Cybersecurity%20and%20Older%20Americans.pdf

Department of Homeland Security. (2018). *Basic Tips & Advice. Stop. Think. Connect*. https://stopthinkconnect.org/resources/preview/tip-sheet-basic-tips-and-advice

Feist, H., Parker, K., Howard, N., & Hugo, G. (2010). New technologies: Their potential role in linking rural older people to community. *International Journal of Emerging Technologies & Society, 8*(2), 68–84. https://www.researchgate.net/publication/257536625_New_Technologies_Their_Potential_Role_in_Linking_Rural_Older_People_to_Community

Field, T. S., Mazor, K. M., Briesacher, B., DeBellis, K. R., & Gurwitz, J. H. (2007). Adverse drug events resulting from patient errors in older adults. *Journal of the American Geriatrics Society, 55*(2), 271–276. https://doi.org/10.1111/j.1532-5415.2007.01047.x

Fiorini, L., Cavallo, F., Dario, P., Eavis, A., & Caleb-Solly, P. (2017). Unsupervised machine learning for developing personalized behavior models using activity data. *Sensors, 17*(5), 1–17. https://doi.org/10.3390/s17051034

Fox, S. (2013). 51% of adults bank online. *Pew Research Center*. Retrieved from http://www.pewinternet.org/2013/08/07/51-of-u-s-adults-bank-online/

Harrell, R., Lynott, J., Guzman, S., & Lampkin, C. (2014). What is livable? Community preferences of older adults. *AARP Public Policy Institute, 4*(1), 8–9. https://www.aarp.org/content/dam/aarp/research/public_policy_institute/liv_com/2014/what-is-livable-report-AARP-ppi-liv-com.pdf

Harvard Health Letter. (2016). Virtual doctors visits: A new kind of house call. *Harvard Health Letter, 41*(12), 4. https://www.health.harvard.edu/staying-healthy/virtual-doctor-visits-a-new-kind-of-house-call

Helbostad, J. L., Verejken, B., Becker, C., Todd, C., Taraldsen, K., Pijnappels, M., Aminian, K., & Mellone, S. (2017). Mobile health applications to promote activity and healthy aging. *Sensors, 17*(3), 1–13. https://doi.org/10.3390/s17030622

Information and Communication Technology Standards and Guidelines. (2015). *Advance notice of proposed rulemaking*. https://www.access-board.gov/attachments/article/1702/ict-proposed-rule.pd

King, M. (2018, September). *Smart technology takes hold in retirement communities*. NextAvenue.org. https://www.nextavenue.org/smart-technology-retirement-communities

Maisto, M. (2014, January). Mobile phone's history in 10 industry-changing devices. *Eweek*. Retrieved from http://www.eweek.com/mobile/mobile-phone-s-history-in-10-industry-changing-devices

Me, R. C., Andreoni, G., Biamonti, A., & Mohd Saad, M. R. (2017). Wearable haptic-feedback navigational assistance for people with dementia: Preliminary assessment. *Technology & Disability, 29*(1/2), 35–46. https://doi.org/10.3233/TAD-150116

Mitseva, A., Peterson, C. B., Karamberi, C., Oikonomou, L. C., Ballis, A. V., Giannakakos, C., & Dafoulas, G., E. (2012). Gerontechnology: Providing a helping hand when caring for cognitively impaired older adults—Intermediate results from a controlled study on the satisfaction and acceptance of informal caregivers. *Current Gerontology & Geriatrics Research, 2012*, 1–19. https://doi.org/10.1155/2012/401705

National Council on Aging. (2018). *Top 10 financial scams targeting seniors*. https://www.ncoa.org/economic-security/money-management/scams-security/top-10-scams-targeting-seniors

Nef, T., Urwyler, P., Büchler, M., Tarnanas, I., Stucki, R., Cazzoli, D., Müri, R., & Mosimann, U. (2015). Evaluation of three state-of-the-art classifiers for recognition of activities of daily living from smart home ambient data. *Sensors, 15*(5), 11725–11740. https://doi.org/10.3390/s150511725

Nygård, L. (2009). The stove timer as a device for older adults with cognitive impairment or dementia: Different professionals' reasoning and actions. *Technology & Disability, 21*(3), 53–66. https://doi.org/10.3233/TAD-2009-0273

Peek, S. T., Wouters, E. J., vanHoof, J., Luijkx, K. G., Boeije, H. R., & Vrijhoef, H. J. (2014). Factors influencing acceptance of technology for aging in place: A systematic review. *International Journal of Medical Informatics, 83*(4), 235-248. doi: 10.1016/j.ijmedinf.2014.01.004

Roberts, A., Philip, L., Currie, M., & Mort, A. (2015). Striking a balance between in-person care and the use of ehealth to support the older rural population with chronic pain. *International Journal of Qualitative Studies on Health & Well-Being. 10*, 1–11. https://doi.org/10.3402/qhw.v10.27536

Rouse, M. (2017, October) Definition: Smart home. *Techtarget internet of things agenda*. http://internetofthingsagenda.techtarget.com/definition/smart-home-or-building

Sefcik, J., Johnson, J., Yim, M., Lau, M., Vivio, T., Mucchiani, N., & Cacchione, C. (2018). Stakeholders' perceptions sought to inform the development of a low-cost mobile robot for older adults: A qualitative descriptive study. *Clinical Nursing Research, 27*(1), 61–80. https://doi.org/10.1177/1054773817730517

Shankar, A., Rafnsson, S. B., & Steptoe, A. (2015). Longitudinal association between social connections and subjective well-being in the English Longitudinal Study of Aging. *Psychology & Health, 30*(6), 686–698. doi:10.1080/08870446.2014.979823

Smith, A. (2014). *Older adults and technology use*. Pew Research Center. http://www.pewinternet.org/2014/04/03/older-adults-and-technology-use

Tedesco, S., Barton, J., & O'Flynn, B. (2017). A review of activity trackers for senior citizens: Research perspectives, commercial landscape and the role of the insurance industry. *Sensors, 17*(6), 1–39. https://doi.org/10.3390/s17061277

Thi-Hoa-Cuc, N., Nebel, J., & Florez-Revuelta, F. (2016). Recognition of activities of daily living with egocentric vision: A review. *Sensors, 16*(1). 1–24. https://doi.org/10.3390/s16010072

Tsai, H. S., Shillair, R., Cotton, S. R., Winstead, V., & Yost, E. (2015). Getting grandma on line: Are tablets the answer for increasing digital inclusion for older adults in the US? *Educational Gerontology, 41*(10), 695–709. https://doi.org/10.1080/03601277.2015.1048165

Tuck-Voon, H., Wang, R. H., & Mihailidis, A. (2013). Evaluation of an intelligent wheelchair system for older adults with cognitive impairments. *Journal of Neuroengineering & Rehabilitation (JNER), 10*(1), 1–16. https://doi.org/10.1186/1743-0003-10-90

United Nations. (2017). *World Population Aging*. http://www.un.org/en/development/desa/population/publications/pdf/ageing/WPA2017_Report.pdf

The Xcertia. (2018). *mHealth app guidelines*. http://www.xcertia.org

V

RESIDENT CARE MANAGEMENT

DIVERSITY ISSUES

Upon the completion of Chapter 17, the reader will be able to:

- Define the concepts of culture ethnicity and heritage consistency.
- Describe the concept of diversity and cultural groups within the United States.
- Identify elements of selected cultural groups.
- Discuss health disparities within selected diverse elder groups.
- Understand selected diversity issues for selected groups.

INTRODUCTION

Assisted living administrators represent and work with residents and staff from diverse cultural and social groups. Understanding the differences among theses groups is beneficial for both administrators and for seniors. Information about the concepts of culture and ethnicity is provided to aid in this process. In addition, diversity is explored through discussion of selected cultural groups, including African Americans, Hispanic Americans, Asian Americans, and Native Americans. Issues and challenges related to caring for diverse elders in several cultural groups are presented as are select best practices in service provision to diverse elders, including African Americans, Asian Americans, and Native Americans.

CONCEPTS OF CULTURE, ETHNICITY, AND HEALTH DISPARITIES

Touhy and Jett (2018) report a marked increase in ethnically diverse elders within the United States and project that this trend will continue into the near future, underscoring the importance of understanding concepts of culture, ethnicity, health disparities, and health inequities. Culture can be viewed as the total of characteristics that are inherited by humans in varied groups and transmitted from one generation to the next generation. It includes the sum of beliefs, habits, norms, customs, rituals, likes, dislikes, and practices that are handed down through generations (Spector, 2012). The essential components of culture are frequently modified or altered by social, political, and economic forces and by the society in which individuals reside (Spector, 2012). Cultural diversity refers to recognition that there are different groups with differing values and viewpoints.

Ethnicity refers to social groups within social or cultural systems accorded status on the basis of variable and complex traits (Spector, 2012). Ethnicity can also be viewed as characteristics common to and shared by members of a specific group. These characteristics include the following: race; common geographic origin; language and dialect; shared traditions; religious faith; shared values; common literature, music, and folklore; food preferences; migration status; political special interests; institutions that provide specific group services; the internal sense of distinctiveness; the external perception of distinctiveness; and the presence of ties that transcend family and community boundaries (Spector, 2012). Cultural background is also noted to be an important component of the concept of ethnicity. A number of ethnoracial groups are found in the United States, including African Americans, Asian Americans, Hispanic Americans, Native Americans, and multiracial groups.

Health disparities can be defined as differences in diseases, violence, or injury and differences in opportunities to achieve optimal health outcomes, such as to an increase in illnesses in one or more groups compared to other group occupants (Centers for Disease Control and Prevention, 2014; Touhy & Jett, 2018). Significant health disparities are the result of age, gender, race, and ethnicity and are also factored into differences in how elders receive health promotion and disease prevention services (Mauk, 2018). Health inequities refer to differences occurring as a result of wealth distribution between identified groups and are often are the result of current or historical injustices (Touhy & Jett, 2018). Understanding how the concepts of culture and ethnicity are interrelated and interconnected in elders who are often marginalized due to aging can provide administrators with information needed to provide services that are both sensitive and relevant for elders residing in assisted living facilities.

Diversity and Cultural Groups

Multiple cultural groups reside in the United States. Demographics in the United States reveal that White Americans are the racial majority. African Americans are the largest racial minority and comprise 12.7% of the population, whereas Hispanic and Latinx Americans represent the largest ethnic minority at 17.8% of the American population (U.S. Census Bureau, 2016). In addition, the numbers of African Americans, Hispanic Americans, Asian Americans, and Middle Eastern Americans are expected to increase throughout the United States (Touhy & Jett, 2018).

Assisted living administrators may have interactions with both elders and staff reflecting one or more of many cultural or social entities. Information about elders residing in selected groups, including African Americans, Hispanic Americans, Asian Americans, Native Americans, and members of the LGBTQ communities, can enhance understanding necessary for the provision of adequate or enhanced senior services to these individuals. Data regarding aspects of each of these cultural groups, including ethnicity, family, and health, will be briefly discussed.

African Americans

As noted, African Americans constitute about 12.6% of the total U.S. population (Agency for Healthcare Research and Quality [AHRQ], 2016). Increases in overall diversity during the late 20th century have resulted in a population increase in African Americans, and this group remains larger than other non-White groups in selected regional areas, with 55% of the African American population residing primarily in southern states. It is important to note that many African Americans identify themselves as Black in combination with one or more races, indicating a significant interracial and diverse population (AHRQ, 2016).

For many African Americans, slavery formed the basis of their culture within an essentially White, European American society. Effects of slavery evident in this culture include discrimination and psychological barriers. Continuing elements of racism continue in the United States in the present day, contributing to many of the problems experienced by African Americans, including race-related stress as a result of racial discrimination (Adomoko, 2019).

The values held by African Americans are widely varied and may reflect cultural practices from a number of African societies, from adapted American cultural norms, or from personal experiences. A history of slavery served to influence the cultural beliefs for many of these individuals, creating a heterogeneous cultural group. Many older African Americans place great value in connections with their churches. The Black church serves an important function in African American culture and communities, providing social and economic connections for elders as well as other members of this group.

There are variations in African American family structures representing both married-couple families, single-parent families,—many headed by females—and intergenerational families. As noted, many older African Americans serve as grandparent caregivers for their families or for unrelated children. Education, social structure, cultural identity, and personal experiences are also determinants of African American families, and changes in families also reflect changing views on racism and discrimination in the United States. It is also important to note that many of the traditions evolving from African American experiences in the southern United States elevate the status of elders in both families and society. Elders are thought to possess wisdom and knowledge as the result of prior experiences and are given elevated status in their homes, churches, and communities.

Health disparities experienced by African Americans are reflected in an increased incidence of chronic conditions within this population, including hypertension, heart disease, diabetes, cancer, and arthritis (Mauk, 2018).

Hispanic Americans

The United States classifies Hispanic Americans as members of a specific ethnic group, and not as a specific race. *Hispanic* is the term used to refer to individuals of Spanish heritage who originate from Spain or Spanish countries in the Americas, and who speak the Spanish language. This is in contrast to Latinx Americans, who originate from Mexico, Central America, or South America, and may also speak the Spanish language. Currently, these terms are used interchangeably to identify individuals representing groups from all geographic areas.

Hispanic Americans represent the largest minority group in the United States. The Hispanic American older population is the fastest-growing segment of the U.S. population and by 2050 is projected to comprise 19.8% of all older Americans (Administration on Aging, 2010).

There is significant variability in the origins of this ethnic group in the United States. Individuals from Puerto Rico are more likely to live in the northeastern United States and are more likely to have been born in the United States than other ethnic groups. Individuals from Mexico are more likely to live in the western United States and are more likely to hold lower socioeconomic status. Individuals from Cuba live primarily in the southern United States and are more likely to hold higher levels of education and socioeconomic status than other Hispanic Americans (Alegria et al., 2008).

Historically, many Mexicans immigrated to the United States to build railroads in the southwestern areas of the country. During the time period from 1940 to 1960, experienced agricultural laborers immigrated to the United States to work in agricultural industries. Currently, many farmworkers are undocumented, and while representative of younger age groups, these individuals will increase the numbers of aging Mexican Americans residing in the United States (Miller, 2009).

Many Cubans immigrated to the United States during the 19th century to work in the tobacco industry, and a large number of Cubans came to the United States between 1959 and 1979 for political reasons. These Cubans came primarily from middle and upper-middle-class families, and represent a significant population of aging individuals, primarily residing in the southern United States. Puerto Ricans, granted citizenship status in the United States in 1917, moved for primarily economic, social, and family reasons, and have mainly stayed in the northern parts of the United States (Miller, 2009).

Many Hispanic Americans work in lower-paying agricultural or service jobs. Socioeconomic disadvantages create a number of problems for Hispanic Americans in many of the different ethnic groups.

Many Hispanic Americans hold strong family ties and family values. The emphasis on family connections and collaborative efforts to protect and provide for all family members are characteristics held by this ethnic group. The needs of individual family members are placed above the needs of individuals within these ethnic groups. Many older Hispanic Americans are more likely to live with family members or with family support than to live in institutional settings. Much of the family caregiving responsibility resides with Hispanic American women.

Health disparities experienced by Hispanic elders include an increased incidence of chronic diseases, including heart disease, diabetes, cancer, and strokes (Mauk, 2018). Many note that Hispanic Americans are less likely to receive preventive healthcare services, including flu vaccines and mammograms, compared to White elders. Health inequities can be connected to socioeconomic disadvantages, including higher poverty levels, lower educational levels, higher unemployment rates, and work in lower paying jobs (Mauk, 2018). Many Hispanic Americans encounter a number of socioeconomic barriers and are considered to be overrepresented in low-paying jobs, and underrepresented in professional and higher paying employment.

Asian Americans

The term *Asian Americans* refers to many diverse subgroups of individuals living in the United States. The term *Asian* refers to those individuals from the Far East, Southeast Asia, as well as the Indian subcontinent, which includes China and India.

Immigration from mainland China and Taiwan resumed during the late 1960s and 1970s, with many Chinese students, families, and professionals entering the United States (NKI Center of Excellence in Culturally Competent Mental Health, 2008b). Early immigrants lived together in communities called Chinatowns, many of which still exist in a number of urban settings. Currently, many of these well-educated professionals live in urban areas in California, Hawaii, New York, Texas, and Illinois.

Japanese immigrants came to the United States in the mid-19th century. In 1942, all Japanese Americans were relocated into internment camps. Immigration increased in the mid-1960s when many immigration restrictions were relaxed (Miller, 2009). Filipinos and Koreans immigrated to the United States initially to assume positions as laborers in agricultural settings. Current immigrants are much more likely to be students, college educated, or professionals. Vietnamese and Cambodian immigrants have entered the United States fairly recently as political refugees, many coming from war zones or refugee camps (Miller, 2009).

The concept of family is of critical importance to most Asian Americans. The family is considered to be the backbone of Chinese society and the family functions as a collective unit where family members assume interdependent roles. The Confucian concept of filial piety, or *Xiao,* is central to the Chinese family, Children expected to provide their elders with respect, loyalty, material goods, obedience, and physical care (Heying et al., 2006). In general, Asian American older adults are less likely to live alone than elders in the general United States population. Language barriers are variable, with many Asian Americans born in the United States exhibiting bilingual capabilities and many elders and immigrants able to speak only their native language.

Health disparities for Asian Americans are reflected in increased rates of heart disease, diabetes, stroke, and cancer (Mauk, 2018).

Native Americans

The terms *Native American* and *American Indian* are used to refer to individuals who are direct descendants of indigenous peoples residing in North America prior to the arrival of European settlers. A number of these indigenous groups, identified as tribes or nations, hold cultural practices that are influenced by geographic, regional, and socioeconomic factors and vary from group to group (Reynolds et al., 2006). In 2016, the American Indian and Alaska Native population was about 259,000 and is projected to increase to 648,000 by 2060, reflecting a total of 0.7% of the total older population (Administration for Community Living, 2017c). It is important to note that about 60% of Native Americans currently live in urban settings rather than rural or tribal land settings (Yurkovich & Lattergrass, 2008). Many Native Americans reside in the western United States, but there are Native Americans currently living in Texas, Michigan, New York, Florida, and Alaska (Miller, 2009).

Demographically speaking, many Native Americans are poor, living either with their family members or alone. Younger Native Americans are likely to speak English; older Native Americans speak either English or one of a number of indigenous languages. Many Native Americans have low educational levels with a high school education or less (Miller, 2009).

In general, Native Americans hold cultural beliefs that are holistic in design, and view humans as connected physically, mentally, spiritually, and emotionally. The mind–body split that is common in Western thought is viewed as adverse to many Native Americans (Yurkovich & Lattergrass, 2008). Group membership, connections to nature, respect for the environment, respect for elders, and honor are all viewed by many Native Americans as essential for sustaining their culture. Spirituality and trustworthiness are important to Native Americans.

Family structures and roles are varied among Native American tribes. The concept of extended family is very strong within Native American culture, providing a network of relationships beyond individual families and tribal groups. Extended families and communities take precedence over the demands of individuals, and frequently include a connection to ancestors through tribal history. Additionally, families are usually multi-generational, including caregiving for both children and for elders.

The roles of many Native American women are significant in many tribes and societies. Women serve important roles in the preservation and transmission of culture and values. Women are regarded as life givers, teachers, healers, doctors, and seers, with many viewing women and women's roles as essential for the health of communities (Walters et al., 2006).

The overall life expectancy for American Indians has increased from 52 years in 1940 to 74 years in 2018 (Bylander, 2018). Health disparities for Native Americans are significant (Mauk, 2018). Leading causes of death in this population are heart disease, diabetes, stroke, and cancer (Mauk, 2018). It is important to note that Native Americans have the highest rates of diabetes in the United States and experience higher rates of obesity, mental health problems, and substance abuse (Mauk, 2018). Health inequities for Native Americans are reflected in higher rates of poverty and in many areas limited access to services, including health services and preventive services.

DIVERSITY ISSUES

Although assisted living administrators do not provide direct-care services to elders, they can improve elder-care services and also enhance staff care delivery through an understanding of diversity and diversity issues. Selected diversity issues faced by older African Americans, Hispanic Americans, Asian Americans, and Native Americans will be identified and discussed further.

African Americans

Diversity issues faced by many aging African Americans occur in the areas of family values, as well racial disparity, poverty, and prior history of discrimination. For many African Americans, family members are expected to provide caregiving services to elders and the use of assisted living facilities or other institutional settings remains limited or unused in many communities. In addition, many African American elders are the primary caregivers for children or grandchildren, making it difficult for them to receive care as needed.

Although there are services and assisted living facilities dedicated to service provision specifically for African Americans, issues related to the number and location of these facilities have been identified. As Howard et al. (2002) noted, African Americans tend to seek services in facilities used by African Americans, whereas White Americans reside in facilities primarily used White elders. Facilities for African Americans were located in primarily rural African American communities. These facilities also tended to have lower cleanliness and maintenance ratings (Howard et al., 2002).

Despite these limitations, African Americans may actually benefit from care received in assisted living communities with predominately African American residents and staff. The major reasons for potential benefits include: (a) African Americans require services that address many of their unique physical and social cincerns; and (b) African American care providers have a better understanding of the cultural and social context of many of the illnesses within this community (Howard et al., 2002).

Issues related to poor health status as a result of poverty, inadequate access to healthcare services, and underutilization of healthcare services have been identified in African American communities. African Americans have higher rates of morbidity, disability, and mortality than do Whites in similar age groups. Poverty for many African Americans does not occur with aging but rather is the result of lifelong patterns of discrimination and many disadvantages unique for African Americans

Best practices for care delivery to African American elders need to be developed. These practices should focus on care that take into consideration the social, cultural, and economic issues faced by this population. As previously noted, facilities have been designed for this population, but they remain geographically limited. Many facilities do not meet current or minimal care standards, making care for this cultural group a future priority.

Hispanic Americans

There are a number of diversity issues experienced by Hispanic American elders. These issues include communication problems, inadequate family structures, poverty, and the presence of a number of chronic illnesses.

Many of these elders experience significant communication problems related to an inability to speak English and the inability of care providers to communicate in Spanish. These language barriers create problems in the delivery of safe and effective care, and increase frustration and difficulties for Hispanic American seniors.

For many Hispanic Americans, cultural values are associated with strong family connections. Family members are expected to provide care when needed to their elders. Problems and issues develop when families are unable to help family members and must use other options. There are a limited number of assisted living facilities providing culturally relevant services for Hispanic American seniors, creating problems not only for seniors and their families, but also for staff members and facility administrators.

The poverty experienced by many Hispanic American elders is an issue. Many individuals experience chronic illnesses connected to inadequate healthcare and poor nutrition. Many of these illnesses result in increased morbidity and mortality for Hispanic American elders. Rates of obesity, diabetes, metabolic syndrome, heart disease, and hypertension are increased in this ethnic group as opposed to members of other ethnic and cultural groups. Additional issues of decreased care access are identified in Hispanic American elders.

Asian Americans

Diversity issues affecting many aging Asian Americans include language barriers and poverty. Many Asian American elders have communication problems because they do not speak English and frequently must rely on care services from non-Chinese-speaking providers or translators. These language difficulties exacerbate existing problems and create new problems for elders both in the community as well as in assisted living and other long-term care facilities. Assisted living administrators must take language barriers into consideration as they plan services for many Asian American residents.

The family values held by many Asian Americans give elderly family members great respect and status within family units. Many elders expect to receive caregiving services from family members and do not plan for aging in institutional settings. This creates potential problems when family members are not available to provide care services or when family members have to work both inside the home as well as hold outside jobs. Because many of these cultural groups stress social responsibilities to the family over individual rights, care for aging family members can create increased family stresses, especially when elders are placed in assisted living facilities or other institutional settings.

Poverty is another issue that contributes to many of the problems experienced by Asian American elders. Poverty creates an environment in which elders are at increased risk for health issues related to inadequate nutrition, inadequate healthcare delivery, and poorer healthcare outcomes. Elders working in substandard working conditions during their lifetimes are also at increased risk for a number of chronic illnesses that increase morbidity and mortality.

Administrators and staff in a number of assisted living communities and organizations can benefit from the identification of best practices for service delivery to Asian American elders. One such best practice is seen in assisted living facilities designed specifically to address the diversity of this population. Aegis Gardens in Fremont, California, offers services for Asian American elders in a for-profit facility. Facility staff speak Chinese, the facilities have been designed with Chinese decorations and gardens, and Chinese food is served to residents who access services specific to their culture.

Another example of a best practice in caring for Asian American elders is seen in Self–Help for the Elderly, which operates facilities for Chinese elders in San Francisco, Santa Clara, and San Jose, California. These facilities provide residents with staff who are multilingual and able to communicate in several Chinese dialects. Residents are also able to access culturally specific services, including games such as Mahjong, arts and crafts, festivals, and the availability of Chinese food (Self-Help for the Elderly, 2009).

Native Americans

Diversity issues identified in this population include access to culturally relevant assisted living facilities, challenges associated with cultural differences, prevalence of chronic illnesses, and past history of discrimination.

There are very few assisted living communities available in the United States providing culturally relevant and appropriate services for Native Americans who represent a heterogeneous group of individuals. The United States Indian Health Service is designated as the primary healthcare service provider for Native Americans. Most of these services are in the form of clinics providing acute or crisis-focused services, and most clinic facilities are located on reservations. Access to these services is limited for many Native Americans who live in urban areas rather than on reservations.

Beliefs in holism and the connection of physical, emotional, spiritual, and cognitive aspects of humans are central to Native American culture. These beliefs are frequently in conflict with the mind–body approach associated with Western medicine. Many assisted living communities use a medical model of care that is in direct conflict with Native American beliefs and values. Also, many Native Americans rely on spiritual and traditional healing methods that are incongruent with traditional medical interventions. These cultural conflicts must be addressed by assisted living administrators and staff as they work to provide care to Native American residents.

Native Americans as a group are at risk for a number of significant chronic illnesses. Rates of diabetes, obesity, heart disease, hypertension, and metabolic syndrome are increased in this population, becoming more severe as Native Americans age (Mauk, 2018). Major psychiatric problems for Native Americans include alcoholism, substance abuse, pathological gambling, depression, stress, and anxiety. Some researchers note a lifetime diagnosis of alcoholism in this population (Mauk, 2018). Assisted living administrators and those caring for Native Americans must have an awareness of the risks associated with these problems, and must also be prepared to provide services needed to combat these severe and chronic illnesses.

A final diversity issue facing those caring for Native American elders is the history of past discrimination faced by Native Americans. For many Native Americans, prior U.S. laws and governmental practices have created a climate of mistrust for any services provided by agencies or institutions, either private private or government sponsored. This mistrust creates barriers for those caring for Native American elders and presents challenges for administrators and staff members who must work with these individuals.

Although administrators and staff working in assisted living communities and organizations need to provide culturally relevant services to support Native American elders, few facilities providing these services currently exist.

CASE STUDY

DG is the administrator of a small assisted living community located in a small western community who has been asked to mediate a dispute between the assisted living community staff and several residents. The staff are concerned about requests from two residents, one of whom is African American and one of whom is Asian American, for what staff describe as "ethnic foods and activities." One staff member was reportedly unhappy about

(continued)

CASE STUDY

"foreigners" asking for favors. The Asian American elder asked for ginseng served with her meals, whereas the African American elder wanted to have family members attend a Kwanza candle lighting in the facility living room. Although the facility has a policy regarding diversity, the majority of the residents and the staff are described as Caucasian.

DG recognizes that there are many issues related to elder care of diverse groups, and is committed to the provision of culturally competent care that is acceptable and useful to elders' cultural backgrounds and expectations. She also notes that culturally competent care involves an awareness of provider personal biases, knowledge of population-specific cultural values, and provider skills in working with diverse populations. DG arranges for members of the local Asian and African American communities to speak to the facility staff regarding issues important to these diverse residents. Additional sessions are also arranged for the staff to discuss their feelings about care of ethnically diverse elders and to review and modify the facility policies to support and include cultural activities as well as diets modified to include a wider variety of foods. Following these changes, DG notes that many of the facility staff has a better understanding of how to care and respect diverse elders. Several of the residents asked to have ginseng served with meals and staff members have expressed interest in participating in an upcoming Kwanza celebration.

CONCLUSIONS

Assisted living administrators can improve their work with elders through improved understanding of culture and cultural issues identified in a number of diverse groups. As noted in this chapter, awareness of selected cultural differences seen in aging African Americans, Hispanic Americans, Asian Americans, and Native Americans can provide assisted living community administrators and their staff members with valuable information. This knowledge can then be used to enhance important services to elderly residents.

REFERENCES

Adomoko, F. (2019). *African American older adults and race-related stress.* American Psychological Association Office on Aging.

Agency for Healthcare Research and Quality. (2016). *Chartbook on healthcare for blacks.* https://www.ahrq .gov/research/findings/nhqrdr/chartbooks/blackhealth/index.html

Alegria, M., Canino, G., Shrout, P. E., Woom M., Duan, N., Vila, D., Torres, M., Chen, C., & Meng, X. (2008). Prevalence of mental illness in immigrant and non-immigrant U.S. Latino groups. *American Journal of Psychiatry, 165*(3), 359–369. https://doi.org/10.1176/appi.ajp.2007.07040704

Bylander, J. (2018). *Meeting the needs of aging Native Americans health affairs blog.* https://www.healthaffairs .org/do/10.1377/hblog20180305.701858/full

Centers for Disease Control and Prevention. (2011). *Office of Minority Health and Disparities.* https://www .cdc.gov/minorityhealth

Centers for Disease Control and Prevention. (2014). *Minority health.* http://www.cdc.gov/minorityhealth

Heying, J. Z., Guangya, L., & Guan, X. (2006). Willingness and availability: Explaining new attitudes toward institutional elder care among Chinese elderly parents and their adult children. *Journal of Aging Studies, 20*(3), 279–290. https://doi.org/10.1016/j.jaging.2005.09.006

Howard, D. L., Sloane, P. D., Zimmerman, S., Eckert, J. K., Walsh, J. F., Bule, V. C., Taylor, P. J., & Koch, G. G. (2002). Distribution of African Americans in residential care/assisted living and nursing homes: More evidence of racial disparity? *American Journal of Public Health, 92*(8), 1272–1277. https://doi .org/10.2105/AJPH.92.8.1272

Mauk, K. L. (2018). *Gerontological nursing. Competencies for care.* (4th ed.). Jones & Bartlett.

Miller, C. A. (2009). *Nursing for wellness in older adults* (5th ed.). Lippincott, Williams, & Wilkins.

Office of Minority Health, U.S. Department of Health and Human Services. (n.d.). HHS.gov

Reynolds, W. R., Quevillion, R. P., Boyd, B., & Maackey, D. (2006). Initial development of a cultural values and beliefs scale among Akota/Nakota/lLakota people: A pilot study. *American Indian and Alaska Native Mental Health Resarch, The Journal of the National Center, 13*(3), 70–97.

Self-Help for the Elderly. (2009). *Kwok Yuen assisted living in San Jose.* http://www.selfhelpelderly.org/ services/assisted_living/san_jose/kwok_yuen/index.php

Spector, R. E. (2012). *Cultural diversity in health and illness* (8th ed.). Prentice Hall.

Touhy, T. A., & Jett, K. (2018). *Ebersole and Hess' Gerontological Nursing & Healthy Aging.* Elsevier.

U. S. Census Bureau. (2016). https:// www.census.gov/data.html

U. S. Census Bureau. (2020). census bureau.gov

Walters, K. L., Evans-Canpbell, T., Simoni, J., Ronquillo, T., & Bhuyan,R. (2006). My spirit in my heart. Identity experiences and challenges among American Indian tow-spirit women. *Journal of Lesbian Studies, 10*(1/2) 125–149.

Yurkovich, E. E., & Lattergrass, I. (2008). Defining health and unhealthiness: Perceptions held by native American Indians with persistent mental illness. *Mental Health, Religion and Culture, 11*(5), 437–459. https://doi.org/10.1080/13674670701473751

FURTHER READING

Administration on Aging, Department of Health and Human Services. (2010). *A profile of older Americans: 2010.* https://aoa.acl.gov/Aging_Statistics/Profile/2010/2.aspx

Aronson, D. (2002). *Civil Rights Journal.* http://findarticles.com/p/ articles/mimOHSP/is_1_6/ai_106647784

Ebersole, P., Hess, P., & Luggin, A. S. (2004). *Toward healthy aging: Human needs and nursing response* (6th ed.). Mosby.

LGBTQ ISSUES IN ASSISTED LIVING

WITH CONTRIBUTING AUTHOR BRIAN DE VRIES

LEARNING OBJECTIVES

Upon the completion of Chapter 18, the reader will be able to:

- Understand why LGBTQ older adults face substantial barriers as they age.
- Define key terms and concepts related to the LGBTQ population.
- Recognize LGBTQ issues and challenges for assisted living communities.
- Consider best practices and resources important for developing LGBTQ-welcoming communities.
- Learn about national and state initiatives supporting LGBTQ seniors.
- Learn about a model community for LGBTQ residents in need of long-term care.

INTRODUCTION

More than 70 years ago, psychologist Henry Murray and anthropologist Clyde Kluckhohn (1948) wrote (paraphrasing the gendered language that was used) that in many respects, a person is (a) like all other people, (b) like some other people, (c) like no other person. Murray and Kluckhohn were proposing the fundamentals of personality formation: the somewhat startling observation (at that time) that there are universal human characteristics (in a period of personality science when the focus of research was on what is unusual and distinguishing); that there are shared characteristics—described as "socio-cultural unit[s];" and that there are unique characteristics based on what they saw as the inescapable fact that each individual's particular modes of feeling, needing, and behaving are never duplicated by any other individual. This may be a useful and evocative framework for considering older adults and particularly older adults in assisted living communities.

There are probably universal characteristics of older assisted living (AL) residents (however "old" is defined) in terms of basic needs for nutrition or activities of daily living. Concomitantly, older adults, and all individuals, have unique histories, identities, and life circumstances that demand attention (and are the focus of person-centered care) and, as such, are unlike any of their peers—past, present, or future. In between are some of the familiar social organizations of life (the so-called sociocultural units, like gender, biological sex, and sexual orientation, for example, that render us comparable to some and different from others.

In many ways, LGBTQ AL residents adhere to the "universal" patterns of activities of daily living (ADL) and instrumental activities of daily living (IADL) care needs; diseases and chronic conditions do not seek traditional sexual orientation and gender identity affirmation. In many ways, LGBTQ AL residents are like no other persons (of any sexual orientation or gender identity) in their individual histories and circumstances—true individuals in the formal sense of the word. LGBTQ AL residents are also like some other persons through their shared social and life experiences of grappling with a sexual orientation and gender identity that differs from traditional norms and values, and in dealing with the associated stigma, discrimination, and consequences of a lifetime of such negotiations. Herein lies the level of analysis of this chapter.

What follows are definitions of the important terms and concepts included in this chapter and a detailed presentation of some of the central LGBTQ issues and their implications for assisted living.

DEFINTIONS

- *Cisgender* refers to having a gender identity that corresponds to the traditional expectations of the biological sex of birth; one's internal gender identity thus conforms to the cultural expectations of one's biological sex and gender presentation (American Psychological Association [APA], 2015).

- *Gender identity* refers to one's sense of self and identification as male, female, or transgender as influenced by biological, social, and cultural factors (APA, 2015). Gender identity is independent of sexual orientation; a transgender person may be gay, lesbian, bisexual, heterosexual, or something else.

- *Sexual orientation* refers to one's enduring sexual attraction to male partners, female partners, or both (APA, 2015). *Heterosexuality* refers to cross-sexuality attraction (e.g., male to female); *homosexuality* refers to same-sex attraction (e.g., male to male, or gay; female to female, or lesbian); bisexuality refers to attraction to both sexes (American Psychological Association, 2015). Recently, discussions of asexuality have appeared in the literature.

- *Transgender* is an overarching term that characterizes individuals whose gender identities are incongruent with those typically associated with the biological sex assigned at birth.

CONCEPTS

- *Minority stress* refers to the elevated and chronic levels of stress experienced by persons subjected to stigmatization as members of marginalized groups (Meyer, 1995).

- *Stigma* refers to the negative regard, inferior status, and relative powerlessness that is assigned by society to individuals and groups that are associated with a variety of attributes, conditions, and/or statuses (Institute of Medicine, 2011).

LGBTQ ISSUES IN ASSISTED LIVING

Shared by LGBTQ persons, and distinct from heterosexual, cisgender (i.e., most) others, is a sense of "otherness": the experience of nonconformance to the cultural norms of exclusive (some say compulsory) heterosexuality with the attendant traditional gender roles and expectations on multiple levels (Institute of Medicine, 2011). This "otherness" is associated with stigma, prejudice, and discrimination. The current cohort of older LGBTQ persons spent much of their (early) adult years in an environment wherein they were labeled "sick" by their medical system, "immoral" by their churches, "illegal" by their government, and "unfit" by their military (Kochman, 1997). Many of these labels have since been either withdrawn or attenuated (though certainly not all), but their effects often remain—both among those who were supported in hurtling such labels and especially those at whom they were hurtled. Attitudes and experiences persist even when formal labels may not and this has pervasive implications both for LGBTQ persons in assisted living, and those with whom they share such spaces. For example, notwithstanding California's progressive laws related to LGBTQ persons for facility staff and long-term care providers (e.g., Senate Bill [SB] 1729: senior care training requiring skilled nursing facilities to provide biannual training on working with LGBTQ people; SB 219: LGBT Senior Bill of Rights prohibiting long-term care facilities from taking discriminatory actions based on the actual or perceived sexual orientation, gender identity, gender expression, or HIV status of residents; California Advocates for Nursing Home Reform [CANHR], 2019), the attitudes and behaviors of other residents can only be broadly managed—and are sources of some significant anxiety for LGBTQ persons (de Vries et al., 2019).

The theory of minority stress (Meyer, 2003) has been productively applied to LGBTQ persons recently supporting the chronic stress that emanates from ongoing stigma and discrimination. This stigma may be objective, with behaviors ranging from disdainful looks to exclusion to physical violence; the stigma may also be subjective, depending on an individual's experience, and may range from concealment of one's identity or orientation (for fear of reprisal) to internalized homophobia or a type of self-directed stigma. Research based on this theory has demonstrated pervasive costs and consequences of such long-term exposure to stress—with extensive implications for those in assisted living.

It is important to note that owing to this stigma and discrimination, as well as changing norms and variations in definition and social conditions, estimates of the prevalence of LGBTQ persons vary widely (de Vries, 2006). Using identity labels, a recent Gallup poll (2018) found that 4.5% of Americans *identify* as lesbian, gay, or bisexual—more than 11 million adults in the United States. The poll further reveals that less than 2% of those born before 1945 identify as LGBTQ, 2.4% of baby boomers so identify, as do 3.5% of Generation Xers, and 8.2% of millennials. Not all persons who have sex with persons of their same gender, however, identify as LGBTQ; fewer older persons and persons of color use these labels (Adelman et al., 2006; Fredriksen-Goldsen et al., 2013). As such, these estimates likely undercount the percentages, especially of older persons.

Personal observations (Joy Silver, personal communication, August 9, 2019) suggest that LGBTQ older adults present themselves to assisted living providers often at later ages with more severe manifestations of disease and higher care needs. Substantial research notes the lack of LGBTQ awareness and acceptance on the part of aging services (Sussman et al., 2020), the associated fear and mistrust with which older LGBTQ adults approach healthcare institutions (National Senior Citizens Law Center, 2011), and the consequent delay in seeking formal care (MetLife, 2010). Several studies demonstrate that LGBTQ older adults delay seeking care—between 17% and 30% of LGBTQ respondents have reported doing so in a California health interview study (Movement Advancement Project, 2010). Reasons for such delay are primarily based on a reluctance to disclose one's sexual orientation and/or gender identity fearing reprisal, rejection, and discriminatory behaviors from health and other care providers. Recall that it was during the young-adult years of these LGBTQ older adults that the American Psychiatric Association removed homosexuality from the *Diagnostic and Statistical Manual of Mental Disorders* (2nd ed.; DSM II; American Psychiatric Association, 1968) as a mental illness—in 1973, when today's 75-year-old LGBTQ person was 29 years old, for example. Seeking care involves presenting oneself and being vulnerable to the same system that earlier in their lives had pronounced them as mentally ill.

Other reasons for such delays include the shame (i.e., internalized homophobia, biphobia, and transphobia) that LGBTQ older adults may experience (Cook-Daniels & Munson, 2010). Among transgender older adults in particular, sizable proportions report a delay in seeking care because they believe appropriate services (e.g., tailored to the needs of transgender persons) are not available or that staff are not cognizant of the particular needs of transgender persons (Pang et al., 2019); insufficient financial resources were also noted as a reason for delaying care (Cook-Daniels & Munson, 2010). Along such lines, Choi and Meyer (2016) note that financial vulnerability is a major concern among LGBTQ older adults owing to lifetime disparities in income (through restricted employment opportunities, denied advancement, and lower overall compensation) as well as discriminatory social support programs for older adults.

Directly related to delays in seeking care are the higher rates of disability noted among LGBTQ older adults. Fredriksen-Goldsen et al. (2011), in a national study of LGBTQ older adults, report that nearly half of their large sample reported a disability (a physical, mental, or emotional disorder and use of assistive device), including almost two thirds of transgender older adults (62%), 54% of bisexual men, 53% of lesbian women, 51% of bisexual women, and 41% of gay men. Several studies have found higher rates of cancer among older lesbians and gay men (Chin-Hong et al., 2004; Valanis et al., 2000) and much higher rates of HIV especially among gay men (Emlet et al., 2019). The U.S. Centers for Disease Control and Prevention (2018) noted that in 2016, almost half (49%) of new HIV diagnoses were among gay and bisexual men; about the same proportion (47%) of Americans with HIV were at least 50 years of age in 2015.

Concomitant with the preceding concerns are the much higher rates of mental health challenges, including depression (Mills et al., 2004), stress, anxiety, and suicide ideation (Fredriksen-Goldsen et al., 2011) among LGBTQ older adults. The theory of minority stress places many of these mental (and physical) health challenges as outcomes of the stresses of life as a member of a sexual and/or gender minority. Negotiating disclosure and identity presentation over many decades and across myriad situations has significant costs in both physical and mental health. That is, consider the cost to a person if that person has to survey the safety of the environment and decide how much, if any, information to disclose and what might be the consequences of such disclosure; each encounter takes a toll that results in a substantial cost over the course of a long life.

Research has often revealed that disclosure rates vary across groups and situations. With a community sample of LGBTQ adults ranging in age from 21 to over 90 years of age (and consistent with other research), Gardner et al. (2013) found that about one third of midlife and older lesbians and gay men maintained some fear and anxiety about disclosing their sexual orientation—this was particularly the case for lesbians, who also placed more conditions on disclosure (also noted in de Vries et al., 2019). Fredriksen-Goldsen et al. (2011) and a variety of other studies have examined the proportions of LGBTQ older adults who are "out" to their healthcare providers, and results typically reveal that between one quarter and one third of respondents do not disclose their sexual orientation. Given that trust is likely a basis of effective healthcare dynamics, this disclosure may have many and significant implications and health consequences, perhaps related to seeking the care available in assisting living environments.

Choosing not to disclose is not an option for many transgender persons. De Vries et al. (2019), in their qualitative study of LGBTQ older persons and end-of-life decision-making, reported several trans persons who noted that, "it is impossible not to 'come out' as a transsexual [in healthcare settings] because your medical file follows you everywhere." They further cite a transwoman who reported that her "greatest reason for having [gender reassignment] surgery was to ensure that her anatomy agreed with the gender she was living; she didn't want to be in a nursing home with breasts and a penis" (p. 369). Across all dimensions, transgender persons experience more and often more significant challenges.

Many distressing accounts of the insensitivity of healthcare providers have been noted in research studies. One masculine transwoman spoke of being left on a hospital gurney in a hallway for several hours with her breasts exposed; it was a custodial staff person who covered her. A transman, for example, reported that he visited 42 physicians before he could find one who would even accept him as a patient. Another transwoman commented on her feelings of vulnerability in assisted living settings:

> You [a facility] could say you're trans friendly, queer friendly, but does it happen in practice and how are these things enforced? And when you're in a home for [the] aged you're very vulnerable regardless, even if you're not trans or intersex or two-spirit or gender queer, but if you are, even more so, and if you haven't had full surgical transition and your body looks different . . . the people there could freak out. . .even if they may not do anything blatant, there's still that subtle 'othering' that goes on. If you have a nurse there or personal support worker, they're going to know at some point. So there's a vulnerability around that. . . (Pang et al., 2019)

Pang et al. (2019) also describe past negative experiences of being mis-gendered by medical professionals, some intentionally, and the particular impact and challenges that exist when cognitive impairment is also involved.

Relative to heterosexual, cisgender women and men of comparable ages, LGBTQ older adults are more likely to live alone (up to 3 times more likely) and are less likely to be partnered (up to one third less likely; Adelman et al., 2006; MetLife, 2010; Wallace et al., 2011). This often-surprising finding has been replicated in many community surveys and in the few representative studies conducted in this area. Men, especially transmen and gay men, are particularly likely to both live alone and to not have a partner (MetLife, 2010). This, of course, means that these men lack the support of a partner. Further, LGBTQ persons, and again particularly gay and transmen, are less likely to have children—about 5 times less likely (Statistics Canada, 2011). In a large study of San Francisco LGBTQ older adults, only 15% of the over 600 participants reported that they had children, and 60% of these parents noted that their children were not available to help them if needed (Fredriksen-Goldsen et al., 2013).

Many of these serious and life-limiting health conditions just described are exacerbated by these sociocultura (to use Murray and Kluckhohn's term) demographic characteristics. That is, research reveals a heteronormative pattern of support seeking (e.g., Cantor & Mayor, 1978) wherein care is both expected and first sought from immediate (i.e., biological) kin and then more distant kin, followed by "others" and formal services. For those without or alienated from biological kin, this pattern places them at a significant disadvantage. In such cases, their first turns are often to those individuals (i.e., friends) removed from the center of established (i.e., heteronormative) care. The positive news is that friends are both more prominent and influential in the lives of LGBTQ persons (de Vries & Megathlin, 2009; MetLife, 2010); there is a substantial literature describing the "chosen families" (Weston, 1997) or the "logical kin" (Maupin, 2007, a contrast to biological kin) of LGBTQ adults—those people with whom an LGBTQ person feels emotionally close and may consider to be "family" even in the absence of a biological or legal connection. The less positive news is that such friendship networks lack the structure and support of those kinship systems that are so strongly linked to care in later life (Barker, 2002). That is, friends may rise to the challenges of care in the absence models of how to do so and amidst questions about the appropriateness of their actions (Barker, 2002)—both potentially generating greater stress in the provision of care.

It is worth noting that this family-dominant pattern, combined with society's reticence about end of life and preparations for the same (de Vries et al., 2020), also suggests that LGBTQ people are also less likely to have the opportunities to engage in discussions about future care; after all, sources or courses of care are not typical (i.e., "polite") discussion topics at social gatherings. As rare as these discussions might be, they are, in general, family-centered (often initiated by a concerned child and raised in a "family conference" setting). This suggests that LGBTQ older adults may be both more hesitant about seeking care and less certain about on whom they might call for care; LGBTQ persons may be even less prepared for care and later life than comparably aged heterosexual, cisgender persons. This is mitigated somewhat by the findings that a greater likelihood of LGBTQ persons have completed wills and advance directives than comparably aged heterosexuals—though these people are still among a minority of midlife LGBTQ persons (MetLife, 2010).

The preponderance of the preceding discussion (and the professional literature) has focused, appropriately, on the many challenges experienced by LGBTQ persons as they age—and as they seek care. Often masked in such discussions and more recently addressed are some of the many strengths LGBTQ older persons may bring to their later years. Early evidence described a crisis competence along the lines of "that which challenges us ultimately makes us stronger" (de Vries, 2015, p. 63). That is, having successfully endured the many challenges of living, LGBTQ people develop skills and resources that can be applied to subsequent challenges. Others have described this in terms of positive marginality (Unger, 2000), in which through attempts to reduce stress and adversity, those who experience marginalization can also find meaning in their experience of stigma—and perhaps thrive as a consequence. Along such lines, a variety of studies have found (in addition to the stigma, discrimination, and related hardships) that older LGBTQ people describe an enhanced self-concept (which they attribute to their extensive coping experiences) and a commitment to social justice and community (Meyer et al., 2011), including significantly higher rates of caregiving (MetLife, 2010); LGBTQ older adults tend to be more highly educated, perhaps attributable to their search for information and meaning (Adelman et al., 2006). These more positive attributes do not justify the stigma and discrimination, but they do provide a more holistic characterization of LGBTQ older persons.

One further issue merits attention that returns us to Murray and Kluckhohn's (1948) characterization of personality: LGBTQ older people are more than their sex, sexual orientation, gender identity, and age; they are also individuals from different races, cultures, ethnicities, with varying socioeconomic status, HIV statu, and social groups—among myriad other factors and identities that influence the lives and well-being of LGBTQ persons. An intersectional perspective provides a focus on the multiple transecting dimensions of marginality and inequality and how they influence each other. This perspective encourages the examination of not only commonalities and differences between groups (between marginalized and dominant groups)—but also within groups (Gamson & Moon, 2004) of LGBTQ persons. A person-centered approach to care recognizes the unique intersections of these sociocultural groups among the universal experiences of aging.

BEST PRACTICES: KNOW YOUR RESOURCES

There is no perfect solution to best serving the LGBTQ population in assisted living communities. Issues of gender identification versus orientation exist. Furthermore, there are considerations that include cultural, religious, and ethnic identification. Similar to the straight elder community, there are generational divides that exist. For example, there are those who lived before marriage equality or the AIDS epidemic. Therefore, when addressing the needs of LGBTQ seniors in assisted living communities one must consider the lessons learned and best practices, but—most important—one must be committed to the development of a practical and flexible plan that prioritizes and empowers resident choice.

Fortunately, there has been a national movement to understanding how to provide inclusive service and care for LGBTQ people, including in long-term care communities. Key stakeholders have published relevant guides, trainings, and books that the assisted living administrator can draw from to create their plan of action. Although it is beyond the scope of this book to identify all best practices on the topic, some key resources and examples are identified

In their guide, Inclusive Services for LGBT Older Adults: A Practical Guide to Creating Welcoming Agencies (2012), the National Resource Center on LGBT Aging and SAGEUSA (Services and Advocacy for LGBT Elders; 2012) offer solutions for dealing with topics such as client intake policy, confidentiality, staff training, and inclusive marketing. For example, to avoid common misconceptions relative to LGBT adults, they suggest:

1. *Do* presume your agency has LGBT clients. Aging service providers should always work from the premise that they have LGBT clients, even if no one has openly identified as LGBT.

2. *Do not* assume you can identify LGBT individuals by appearances, experiences, or external characteristics. LGBT older adults do not all look the same way or adopt the same mannerisms or ways of dressing. They also may have past life experiences, such as being previously married or having children or grandchildren, that conflict with common assumptions about LGBT people.

3. *Do* remember that a client's sexual orientation and gender identity are only two aspects of a person's overall identity and life experience. In addition to sexual orientation and gender identity, each client brings with them their racial, ethnic, and cultural heritage, as well as their unique individual history. For example, LGBT older adults who are also racial and ethnic minorities will often face the highest levels of disparities, due to racism, among other factors.

4. *Do* ask your clients about their sexual orientations and gender identities in a safe and confidential manner. The more a service provider knows about their clients, the better they will be able to provide person-centered support and care. Remember that while it is important to ask about sexual orientation and gender identity along with all of the other key components of care, LGBT people have significant histories of discrimination and stigma, which makes them far less willing to disclose these parts of their identities. Ask the questions as you would any other factual question, but do not force anyone to answer. If a client looks uncomfortable, anxious, or refuses to answer, move on to the next question.

5. *Do not* assume that treating everyone the same, regardless of sexual orientation or gender identity, is effective or will make LGBT older adults feel safe or welcomed. More often than not, treating everyone the same translates to treating everyone as heterosexual and glossing over the particular challenges LGBT older adults may have faced, including discrimination, physical and emotional stress, and violence.

The National Resource Center on LGBT Aging and SAGEUSA offer many other references and resources that are worthy of consideration.

With his 2020 book, *Welcoming LGBT Residents: A Practical Guide for Senior Living Staff,* Tim R. Johnston published the first comprehensive book that provides a road map for working with LGBT older adults in senior- iving settings. The chapters in this exemplary book include:

1. Getting to know LGBT older adults

2. First impressions

3. Move-in day and collecting information

4. LGBT programming and services

5. Staff opinions, beliefs, and training

6. Addressing bullying and conflict between residents

7. Navigating family dynamics

8. Sexuality and sexual health

9. Bisexuality and aging

10. Gender identity and expression

11. Older adults with HIV/AIDS

12. Dementia, memory care, and LGBT people

13. Rights and protections

14. Strategic planning and diversifying the board

Lavender Seniors of the East Bay, an LGBTQ advocacy group based in Oakland, California, has a mission to support older LGBTQ residents to achieve and maintain a high quality of life through community building, education, and advocacy. Developing current and effective training programs helps them achieve their goals. They have produced a free, five-video online training series that covers the basics of creating an inclusive care environment. Topics include LGBTQ senior social and mental health concerns, as well as appropriate policies and procedures. Pre- and postcourse quizzes help you monitor your understanding of the issues. The training also features downloadable forms that your assisted living community can adapt and use, including an inclusivity checklist and a nondiscrimination statement (Creating a Healthcare Practice Welcoming to LGBT Seniors; https://lavenderseniors.org/training).

FEDERAL AND STATE INITIATIVES

Deciding where to live as you age and your care needs increase, is an important decision for any adult. LGBT older adults must also consider finding a welcoming community that can meet their needs. SAGEUSA (n.d.) has developed a National LGBT Elder Housing Initiative to address many of the challenges faced throughout the country. This initiative includes the following:

- Building LGBT-friendly housing in New York City,
- Advocating nationally against housing discrimination,
- Training eldercare providers to be LGBT culturally competent,
- Educating individuals about housing rights,
- Helping builders across the United States replicate LGBT-friendly housing.

Some, but not all, states have developed laws and regulations to protect LGBT seniors from discrimination, as well as protect their rights. One example of a comprehensive bill, known as the *LGBT Long-Term Care Facility Resident's Bill of Rights*, was recently passed in California (California Legislative Information, 2017). S.B. 219, written by Senator Scott Weiner and signed into law by Governor Jerry Brown, requires facilities to refer to residents by their preferred name or pronoun and prohibits facilities from denying admission, involuntarily discharging, evicting, or transferring a resident within a facility or to another facility based on anti-LGBT attitudes of other residents or a person's actual or perceived sexual orientation, gender, gender identity, gender expression, or HIV status. Facilities are now required to post a notice regarding LGBT discrimination where the current non-discrimination policy is posted.

A MODEL PRACTICE

According to Leading Age, the largest provider organization serving not-for-profit organizations representing the entire field of aging services, one New Jersey life-plan community is making itself very welcoming to LGBTQ elders (Simon, 2018). Green Hill was founded in Newark, New Jersey, in 1866 by 13 widowed and single aging women who were without familial support. Recognizing the need for more person-centered care, Green Hill added the first Green House homes in New Jersey in 2011. The person-directed care that characterizes the Green House approach required retraining of the team, and at that time it became clear to Green Hill that understanding and acknowledging an elder's sexual orientation and/or identity were important to its success in serving the growing senior LGBTQ community and their families. Green Hill, in 2016, became the first senior living community to complete SAGECare, cultural competency training for LGBTQ care. The Green Hill team looks for actionable steps for what to do next to create a welcoming community for LGBTQ elders. Their work continues as they identify additional best practices and aim for continual quality improvement.

CONCLUSIONS

This chapter illustrates the urgent need to acknowledge and learn about the unique fundamentals of LGBTQ older adults. A historical context and critical issues are discussed to build a foundation for learning. In the context of assisted living administration, ways to address the challenges and barriers faced by LGBTQ residents are considered and addressed by including useful information, applicable research, best practices, and resources. Enhancing programs within assisted living communities that are specific to LGBTQ residents is vital for all administrators today.

REFERENCES

Adelman, M., Gurevitch, J., de Vries, B., & Blando, J. (2006). Openhouse: Community building and research in the LGBT aging population. In D. Kimmel, T. Rose & S. David (Eds.) *Lesbian, gay, bisexual, and transgender aging: Research and clinical perspectives* (pp. 247–264). Columbia University Press.

American Psychiatric Association. (1968). *Diagnostic and statistical manual of mental disorders* (2nd ed). Author.

American Psychological Association. (2015). *APA dictionary of psychology* (2nd ed.). Author.

Barker, J. (2002). Neighbors, friends, and other nonkin caregivers of community living dependent elders. *Journal of Gerontology, 57*(3), 158–167. https://doi.org/10.1093/geronb/57.3.S158

California Advocates for Nursing Home Reform. (2019). *Legislation for LGBT rights.* http://www.canhr.org/lgbt/relevant-laws.html

California Legislative Information. (2017). *SB-219 Long-term care facilities: rights of residents.* http://leginfo.legislature.ca.gov/faces/billNavClient.xhtml?bill_id=201720180SB219

Cantor, M. H., & Mayer, M. (1978). Factors in differential utilization of services by urban elderly. *Journal of Gerontological Social Work, 1*(1), 47–61. https://doi.org/10.1300/J083V01N01_05

Centers for Disease Control and Prevention. (2018). *HIV/AIDS among persons 50 and older.* https://www.cdc.gov/hiv/group/age/olderamericans

Choi, S, K., & Meyer, I. H. (2016). *LGBT aging: A review of research findings, needs, and policy implications.* The Williams Institute.

Chin-Hong, P. V., Vittinghoff, V., Cranston, R. D., Buchbinder, S., Cohen, D., Colfax, G., Da Costa, M., Darragh, T., Hess, E., Judson, F., Koblin, B., Madison, M., & Palefsky, J. M. (2004). Age-specific prevalence of anal human papillomavirus infection in HIV-negative sexually active men who have sex with men: The EXPLORE study. *Journal of Infectious Diseases, 190*(12), 2070–2076. https://doi.org/10.1086/425906

Cook-Daniels, L., & Munson, M. (2010). Sexual violence, elder abuse, and sexuality of transgender adults, age 50+: Results of three surveys. *Journal of GLBT Family Studies, 6*(2), 142–177. https://doi .org/10.1080/15504281003705238

de Vries, B. (2006). Home at the end of the rainbow: Supportive housing for LGBT elders. *Generations, 29,* 64–69.

de Vries, B. (2015). Stigma and LGBT aging: Negative and positive marginality. In N. Orel & C. Fruhauf (Eds.), *Lesbian, gay, bisexual, and transgender older adults and their families: Current research and clinical applications* (pp. 55–71). American Psychological Association Press.

de Vries, B., Gutman, G., Humble, A., Gahagan, J., Chamberland, L., Aubert, P., Fast, J., & Mock, S. (2019). End-of-life preparations among LGBT older Canadians: The missing conversations. *International Journal of Aging and Human Development, 88*(4), 358–379. https://doi.org/10.1177/0091415019836738

de Vries, B., Gutman, G., Soheilipour, S., Gahagan, J., Humble, A., Mock, S., & Chamberland, L. (2020). Advance care planning among older LGBT Canadians: Heteronormative influences [Special Issue: LGBT End of Life]. *Sexualities.* https://doi.org/10.1177/1363460719896968

de Vries, B., & Megathlin, D. (2009). The meaning of friends for gay men and lesbians in the second half of life. *Journal of GLBT Family Studies, 5,* 82–98. https://doi.org/10.1080/15504280802595394

Emlet, C. A., O'Brien, K. K., & Fredriksen Goldsen, K. I. (2019). The global impact of HIV on sexual and gender minority older adults: Challenges, progress, and future directions. *International Journal of Aging and Human Development, 89*(1), 108–126. https://doi.org/10.1177/0091415019843456

Fredriksen-Goldsen, K., Kim, H.-J., Hoy-Ellis, C., Goldsen, J., Jensen, D., Adelman, M., Costa, M., & de Vries, B. (2013). *Addressing the needs of LGBT older adults in San Francisco: Recommendations for the future.* San Francisco Department of Public Health.

Fredriksen-Goldsen, K. I., Kim, H.-J., Emlet, C. A., Muraco, A., Erosheva, E. A., Hoy-Ellis, C. P., Goldsen, J., & Petry, H. (2011). *The aging and health report: Disparities and resilience among lesbian, gay, bisexual, and transgender older adults.* Institute for Multigenerational Health.

Gallup. (2018). *In U.S., estimate of LGBT population rises to 4.5%.* https://news.gallup.com/poll/234863/estimate-lgbt-population-rises.aspx

Gamson, J., & Moon, D. (2004). The sociology of sexuality: Queer and beyond. *Annual Review of Sociology, 30*(1), 47–64. https://doi.org/10.1146/annurev.soc.30.012703.110522

Gardner, A., de Vries, B., & Mockus, D. (2013). Aging out in the desert: Disclosure, acceptance, and service use among midlife and older lesbian and gay men in Riverside County. *Journal of Homosexuality, 61*(1), 129–144. https://doi.org/10.1080/00918369.2013.835240

Institute of Medicine. (2011). *The health of lesbian, gay, bisexual, and transgender people: Building a foundation for better understanding.* National Academies Press.

Johnston, T. (2020). *Welcoming LGBT residents: A practical guide for senior living staff.* Routledge.

Kochman, A. (1997). Gay and lesbian elderly: Historical overview and implications for social work practice. In J. Quam (Ed.), *Social services for senior gay men and lesbians* (pp. 1–25). Haworth Press.

Lavender Seniors of the East Bay. (n.d.). *Lavender Seniors training films.* https://lavenderseniors.org/training

Maupin, A. (2007). *Michael Tolliver lives.* HarperCollins.

MetLife Mature Market Institute. (2010). *Still out, still aging.* MetLife Mature Market Institute.

Meyer, I. H. (1995). Minority stress and mental health in gay men. *Journal of Health and Social Behavior, 36,* 38–56. https://doi.org/10.2307/2137286

Meyer, I. H. (2003). Prejudice, social stress, and mental health in lesbian, gay, and bisexual populations: Conceptual issues and research evidence. *Psychological Bulletin, 129,* 674–697. https://doi .org/10.1037/0033-2909.129.5.674

Meyer, I. H., Oullette, S., Haile, R., & MacFarlane, T. (2011). "We'd be free": Narratives of life without homophobia, racism, or sexism. *Sexuality Research and Social Policy, 8,* 204–214. https://doi.org/10.1007/s13178-011-0063-0

Mills, T. C., Paul, J., Stall, R., Pollack, L., Canchola, J., Chang, Y. J., Moskowitz, J. T., & Catania. J.A. (2004). Distress and depression in men who have sex with men: The Urban Men's Health Study. *American Journal of Psychiatry, 161*(2), 278–285. https://doi.org/10.1176/appi.ajp.161.2.278

Movement Advancement Project. (2010). *Improving the lives of LGBT older adults.* https://www.lgbtmap.org/file/improving-the-lives-of-lgbt-older-adults.pdf

Murray, H. A., & Kluckhohn, C. (Eds.). (1948). *Personality in nature, society, and culture.* Alfred A. Knopf.

National Resource Center on LGBT Aging and SAGE. (2012). *Inclusive services for LGBT older adults: A practical guide to creating welcoming agencies.* https://www.lgbtagingcenter.org/resources/resource.cfm?r=487

National Senior Citizens Law Center. (2011). *LGBT older adults in long-term care facilities: Stories from the field.* https://www.justiceinaging.org/lgbt-older-adults-in-long-term-care-facilities-stories-from-the-field

Pang, C., Gutman, G., & de Vries, B. (2019). Later life care planning and concerns of transgender older adults in Canada. *International Journal of Aging and Human Development, 89(1),* 1–19. https://doi.org/10.1177/0091415019843520

SAGEUSA. (n.d.). *National LGBT housing initiative.* https://www.sageusa.org/what-we-do/national-lgbthousing-initiative

Simon, A. (2018). *Building an inclusive culture for LGBT elders.* https://www.leadingage.org/magazine/july-august-2018/Building-an-Inclusive-Culture-for-LGBT-Elders-V8N4

Statistics Canada. (2011). *Gay pride by the numbers.* Author.

Sussman, T., Brotman, S., MacIntosh, H., Chamberland, L., MacDonnell, J., Daley, A., Dumas, J., & Churchill, M. (2018). Supporting lesbian, gay, bisexual & transgender (LGBT) inclusivity in long-term care (LTC) homes: A Canadian perspective. *Canadian Journal on Aging, 37(2),* 121–132. https://doi.org/10.1017/s0714980818000077

Unger, R. K. (2000). Outsiders inside: Positive marginality and social change. *Journal of Social Issues, 56,* 163–179. https://doi.org/10.1111/0022-4537.00158

Valanis, B. G., Bowen, D., J., Bassford, T., Whitlock, E., Charney, P., & Carter, R. A. (2000). Sexual orientation and health: Comparisons in the women's health initiative sample. *Archives of Family Medicine, 9(9),* 843–853. https://doi.org/10.1001/archfami.9.9.843

Wallace, S. P., Cochran, S. D., Durazo, E. M., & Ford, C. L. (2011). *The health of aging lesbian, gay and bisexual adults in California.* UCLA Center for Health Policy Research.

Weston, K. (1997). *Families we choose: Lesbians, gays, kinship.* Columbia University Press.

FURTHER READING

Centers for Disease Control and Prevention. (2010). Prevalence and awareness of HIV infection among men who have sex with men—21 cities, United States, 2008. *Morbidity and Mortality Weekly Report, 59(37),* 1201–1207.

Green Hill. (n.d.). *Green Hill.* https://www.green-hill.com

Kuyper, L., & Fokkema, T. (2010). Loneliness among older lesbian, gay, and bisexual adults: The role of minority stress. *Archives of Sexual Behavior, 39(5),* 1171–1180. https://doi.org/10.1007/s10508-009-9513-7

National Institute on Aging. (2010). *Fact sheet: Disability in older adults.* https://archives.nih.gov/asites/report/09-09-2019/report.nih.gov/nihfactsheets/ViewFactSheet31ba.html?csid=37&key=D#D

Statistics Canada. (2010). Health promoting factors and good health among Canadians in mid- to late life. *Health Reports.* Author.

PHYSICAL ASPECTS OF AGING

Upon the completion of Chapter 19, the reader will be able to:

- Describe selected normal physiologic changes associated with aging.
- Discuss nutritional assessment in aging individuals.
- Describe strategies to maintain healthy nutrition in aging individuals.
- Identify elements of mobility assessment.
- Discuss strategies to promote mobility in aging individuals.
- Identify risk factors and assessment strategies for fall prevention.
- Discuss strategies for sleep assessment in aging individuals.
- Discuss strategies to improve sleep conditions in aging individuals.
- Describe assessment of chronic pain in aging individuals.
- Discuss selected treatments for chronic pain in aging individuals.
- Discuss selected best practices in mobility, fall prevention, and pain management.

INTRODUCTION

Although assisted living administrators do not usually provide direct clinical services to older persons, an understanding of how the normal aging process impacts a number of important body systems can provide useful information used in the decision-making needed to effectively provide resident services. Age-related changes to selected systems, including the cardiovascular, pulmonary, muscular, orthopedic, gastroenterological, genitourinary, neurologic, and skin and lymphatic systems, are identified, as are issues related to physiological aspects of aging. In addition, nutrition, mobility, falls, sleep, and chronic pain issues are briefly discussed. Strategies and best practices identified in improving and dealing with selected physical aspects of aging are presented throughout this chapter.

OVERVIEW OF NORMAL PHYSIOLOGIC CHANGES ASSOCIATED WITH AGING

Age-Related Changes to the Cardiovascular System

The cardiovascular system consists of the heart and the vascular system, a series of arteries and veins that carry oxygen and nutrients from the heart to all body systems, and remove carbon dioxide and waste back to the lungs. Structural changes to the heart muscle occur with aging as the heart muscle increases in size, and the heart chambers and heart cells increase in size and thicken. These changes, especially in the left ventricle or major pumping chamber of the heart, cause reductions in muscle flexibility and make the heart a less effective pump. The ability of the heart to contract or exert force to pump blood throughout the body does not appear, however, to change with normal aging (Mauk, 2018).

As arteries age, the walls of these blood vessels become stiff and twisted due to increased collagen levels and decreased elastin levels. This creates an increased resistance to blood flow requiring increased pressure to pump blood from the heart to arteries throughout the body. Increases in pressure then lead to additional changes and damage to these important blood vessels. Veins, the blood vessels designed to return deoxygenated blood from the periphery of the body, also undergo aging changes. With aging, veins become thicker, more dilated, and less elastic. The valves in veins also become less efficient in returning blood back to the heart (Mauk, 2018). These changes make blood return to the heart less efficient, and also cause blood to remain in the extremities. This can result in dependent edema in the lower extremities, especially after sitting for long periods of time.

Age-related changes to cardiovascular physiology are thought to be minimal, and healthy elders have heart muscles that are able to adapt to a number of physiologic changes and stressors. Functional changes associated with aging include decreased adaptive responses to exercise, decreased blood flow to the brain, and increased risk for the development of chronic cardiovascular illnesses (Mauk, 2018). Normal cardiovascular changes seen with aging include a moderate increase in blood pressure or hypertension, and an overall increased stiffness of both the heart muscle, and arteries and veins.

Age-Related Changes to the Respiratory System

The respiratory system is composed of organs that assist with breathing, including the airways (mouth, nose, and trachea), the diaphragm and chest muscles, and lungs. Aging changes to the airways can cause decreases in the ability to clear mucus and other secretions, especially from the trachea. Age changes to the chest wall include an increase in stiffness, due to a loss of elasticity, and increases in calcium in the cartilage connecting the ribs to the chest wall. This stiffness causes a decline in muscle strength. Decreases in the ability of the chest to expand and contract during breathing mean that elders use the diaphragm or the major respiratory muscle located at the bottom of the chest for chest expansion and contraction. The diaphragm may also weaken with age, making breathing more difficult (Mauk, 2018).

Age-related changes in the lung tissue also occur. The alveoli are spongy air sacks located in the lung tissue. The alveoli serve as the site for gas exchange with oxygen exchanged for carbon dioxide within these structures. With aging, the alveoli become more flat and shallow, decreasing the surface area available for oxygen exchange and reducing the amount of oxygen available for consumption. The lung tissue itself is designed to be elastic, expanding and contracting during inhalation and exhalation. Aging causes decreased lung elasticity. This in turn causes the lungs to close prematurely, trapping air and decreasing the efficiency of oxygen delivery (Mauk, 2018).

Some negative functional consequences of aging include decreased cough and gag reflexes, making choking a greater possibility in elders. Additionally, there is an increase in the energy required for breathing, an increased use of accessory muscles, including the diaphragm and other major respiratory muscles, and decreased efficiency of oxygen exchange in the lungs. These aging changes increase elder's susceptibility for a number of respiratory infections (Miller, 2009). In effect, the mechanics of breathing usually change with aging.

Age-Related Changes to the Muscular System

The body is composed of three types of muscles, including skeletal muscles, smooth muscles, and cardiac muscles. Skeletal muscles make up the majority of the body's muscle mass and are also most impacted by age-related changes. Reduction in muscle mass known as sarcopenia occurs with normal aging. This loss of muscle mass is thought to be individualized, due in part to genetics and lifestyle (Mauk, 2018). Loss of skeletal muscle mass involves a decline in the number and size of muscle fibers, a loss of motor units or skeletal muscle fibers and the motor nerves that innervate the muscle fibers. This condition is influenced by hormonal changes, altered protein synthesis, nutritional factors, and a lack of physical exercise (Mauk, 2018). These age-related changes may make walking and other functional activities of daily living more difficult for elders.

Loss of overall muscle strength or a muscle's ability to generate force is thought to be influenced by age-related changes in muscle mass. These changes related to age are thought to occur in both men and women, and increase as part of the aging process (Mauk, 2018). Age is also connected with changes in muscle quality or the strength generated per unit of muscle mass and this is variable among men and women. Many research studies have demonstrated increases in skeletal muscle mass and muscle strength in aging muscles through the use of resistance exercises and training (Mauk, 2018). The benefits of resistance exercises in the improvement and maintenance of skeletal muscle function should be viewed positively, and administrators should consider the addition of resistance training programs for residents in assisted living facilities.

Age-Related Changes to the Orthopedic System

The skeleton consists of a system of 206 bones and joints connecting the bones together, and serves to shape, support, and protect the body. Movement occurs because tendons attach muscles to the skeleton. Bones that comprise the skeletal system serve the function of mineral storage and the maintenance of a balance of mineral homeostasis, where bone is constantly reabsorbed and reformed. Aging alters the balance between the formation and re-absorption of bones throughout the body, resulting in bone mineral density loss. Changes in mineral density of bone are thought to occur starting at around age 30, and increases with age in both men and women. Research has demonstrated that reduction in estrogen levels play a key role in bone demineralization with increases in bone porosity occurring in postmenopausal women. Men also undergo age-related changes in bone density. Current research indicates that this loss is due to declining estrogen rather than testosterone levels (Mauk, 2018).

Bone strength is thought to decline as a result of normal aging processes. With aging, bones become more porous and thus more brittle. These changes result in an overall loss of bone strength. Younger bones are more flexible, able to withstand force with resilience. Aging bones are more brittle, less flexible, and therefore less able to withstand force (Mauk, 2018). These changes put elders at increased risk for bone fractures.

Joints are the connections or junctions between two or more bones. There are three types of joints in the body. Immovable joints use collagen fibers to bind bones tightly together and prevent bone movement. Skull bones are examples of immovable joints. With aging, the collagen fibers that bind bones together actually become coated with bone and the bones fuse or join together. This results in a strengthening of the joints, an example of joint changes that are actually improved with the aging process. Cartilaginous joints allow for slight movement through the use of cartilage which separates two connected bones. Ligaments may also serve to connect the bones together (Mauk, 2018). With aging, both the cartilage and the ligaments become stiff and lose elasticity. This results in a reduction of movement and an increase in overall stiffness.

Synovial joints are the third type of body joints. Bones are connected together by a layer of connective tissue at the bone ends, and the joint capsule is lined with a membrane that secretes a thick and slippery fluid that serves in part to absorb the shock of bone movement. These joints serve to provide a great degree of movement and are located in the arms, legs, shoulders, and hips. Functional decline in synovial joints occurs with normal aging. The cartilage lining these joints becomes stiffer, thinner, and less resilient. This results in reductions in range of motion and joint function, putting elders at risk for joint injuries, balance changes, and falls. Additionally, aging causes changes in the synovial fluid surrounding the joints. This fluid becomes less viscous and thinner, which in turn causes disease and discomfort with joint movement (Mauk, 2018). The number of joint injuries and decreases in overall activity are also seen as components of the joint aging process.

Age-Related Changes to the Gastroenterological System

The gastroenterological system includes body structures from the mouth to the anus. Age-related changes to a number of these structures are briefly discussed. The mouth serves to moisten food with saliva in order to enhance the passage of food to the pharynx and esophagus. Age-related changes to the teeth and related atrophy of jaw and mouth muscles can make chewing more difficult. Age-related changes to the esophagus include stiffening of the walls of the esophagus, as well as decreased sensations of discomfort and pain. These changes can make swallowing more difficult, which can potentially lead to serious consequences for elders. Although researchers do not find significant age-related changes in either stomach or small intestine functioning, age-related changes in the large intestine or colon include decreases in colonic motility. These changes result in a lengthening of total colonic transit time, or the amount of time required for both fluid and excrement to travel the length of the colon. This increase in transit time puts elders at increased risk for constipation. This may be worsened by poor nutrition, lack of exercise, and the use of many different medications. The rectum is located at the end of the colon before the anus. Age-related changes to this structure include an increase in fibrous tissue and a decreased ability to stretch as feces are excreted from the body (Mauk, 2018). Age-related changes to the rectum make excretion of feces more difficult, and in the setting of poor nutrition, lack of exercise, poor hydration, and decreases in colonic transit time may predispose elders to fecal impactions.

The liver serves to secrete bile into the small intestine as well as to filter blood from both the stomach and small intestine for toxins and excessive nutrients. Researchers note that as the body ages, overall liver size and the amount of blood flowing through the liver decreases by at least 30% to 40% (Mauk, 2018). One consequence of these changes is a decrease in the body's ability to remove drugs from the system, creating potential problems for elders taking both prescription and over-the-counter medications. The liver's ability to filter and remove alcohol from the blood stream is also decreased as a result of age-related liver function changes. As noted earlier, this can have a significant impact on elders who consume large quantities of alcohol.

Age-Related Changes to the Genitourinary System

The genitourinary system includes the kidneys, bladder, ureters, and urethra. This system is designed to: (a) remove a number of wastes and toxins from the blood; (b) regulate osmotic pressure in the blood; (c) regulate levels of calcium, potassium, sodium, magnesium, and phosphorus in the blood; (d) regulate blood pressure; (e) control acid-base balance; (f) regulate vitamin D;

and (g) stimulate the production of erythropoietin, a hormone responsible for red blood cell production in the bone marrow (Mauk, 2018). Age-related changes in the kidneys include both a decline in organ length and weight, decreased blood flow to the kidneys, as well as diminished glomerular filtration rates (Mauk, 2018). These changes result in age-related decline in kidney functioning, especially in the ability to remove toxins, other wastes, and medications from the blood. This potentially puts elders at risk for problems associated with an accumulation of harmful substances.

Age-related changes to the bladder include an overall decrease in size as well as the development of fibrous changes in the bladder musculature, as well as decreased stretching capabilities. The filling capacity of the bladder declines with age, as it does not have the ability to hold urine and withstand voiding. These age-related changes increase the potential for urinary incontinence, a significant problem for elders in assisted living communities. Changes in the genitourinary system that occur with aging cause additional alterations in genital structures, changes in hormone levels, changes in voiding behaviors, and decreases in the removal of toxins and medications from the body (Mauk, 2018). These changes can impact the physical, social, emotional, and psychological functioning of elders, especially when changes result in urinary incontinence. Understanding changes associated with aging is important when considering the receipt of services delivered to elders in assisted living facilities.

Age-Related Changes to the Neurologic System

The nervous system consists in part of the brain and peripheral nerves. Age-related alterations within the brain include, (a) a decreased number of neurons and an increased accumulation of changes in brain tissue, (b) an overall decrease in brain size and weight, (c) decreased blood flow to the brain, (d) increases in sleep disorders and insomnia, and (e) decreases in short-term memory (Tabloski, 2006). Changes in brain function impact a number of cognitive functions, including memory, and any of these alterations can be of significance in the elderly. Changes in brain function can lead to changes in senses, including vision, hearing, taste, and touch, and profoundly impact the functional status of elders.

The peripheral nervous system consists of billions of nerve cells and nerve fibers that connect the central nervous system to the rest of the body (Mauk, 2018). The speed of nerve conduction slows with aging, causing changes in overall motor speed, reaction times to a variety of stimuli, and sensory abilities such as vision and taste. Changes in these nerve pathways cause movements to become slower, less coordinated, and less accurate. In addition, elders become slower in their recognition of a number of stimuli making their actions and reactions to these stimuli slower and more difficult (Mauk, 2018). Impaired reaction times, impaired coordination, and decreased sensation to light touch, pain, and joint positioning are also seen in the aging peripheral nervous system (Tabloski, 2006). Again, understanding age-related changes to the peripheral nervous system provides understanding and insight into problems that many elders may experience, or may be at risk for experiencing.

Age-Related Changes to the Skin and Lymphatic System

The skin is the largest body system, as it covers the entire body, and provides protection from trauma, microorganisms, and sun exposure. I addition, the skin performs the following functions: (a) regulatesf body temperature, (b) aid in touch and proprioception, (c) works in the synthesis of vitamin D, and (d) prevents loss of bodily fluids (Tabloski, 2006). There are a number of age-related changes to the skin that represent changes in both function and appearance. Aging is associated with thinning and graying of the hair. Baldness may occur in both men and women. Skin color changes are common in the aging skin with areas of hyperpigmentation and increased pigmentation occurring on the face as well as throughout the body. Decreased elasticity, loss of subcutaneous tissue, and thinning of the dermis or the second layer of the skin are associated with aging. Decrease in elastin results in an increase in wrinkling, while an increase in skin dryness is seen as the result of decreased secretions from sebaceous glands. Aging also produces an increase in the number of vascular lesions such as petechia and telangiectasia, which are benign and seen throughout the body. Additionally, the aging process decreases the skin's ability to provide photoprotection from harmful ultraviolet radiation (Tabloski, 2006).

Elders are at risk for pressure ulcers and skin breakdown as a result of decreases in blood flow to the skin and overall skin thinning which occurs as part of the aging process. In addition, decreased blood supply to the skin with aging can result in decreased responses to injury and reduced thermoregulation capabilities. Age-related decreases to the touch receptors in the skin result frequently in the slowing of reflexes and diminished pain sensation throughout the body. Finally, decreases in skin regeneration may create potential delays in both wound healing and vitamin D production (Tabloski, 2006).

Understanding of the many skin changes that are associated with normal aging is essential for providing comprehensive services to elders in assisted living facilities. Of special importance is awareness that thinning and drying create skin that is fragile and a less effective barrier. This can put elders at risk for potentially lethal skin breakdowns and ulcerations.

A number of factors that are associated with aging can impact functioning of the immune system, a highly complex biological defense mechanism designed to protect the body from foreign bodies, chemicals, microorganisms, and parasites. Stress, co-existing diseases, changes in nutrition, and exercise all have the potential to alter immune functioning. Aging has also been shown to alter immune functioning through: (a) overall decreases in immune responses; (b) decreases in immunity through decreases in B cells, and increases in autoimmune responses to self; and (c) decreases in cellular immunity with impairment of immune system regulation. The aforementioned alterations in immune system functions place elders at risk for a number of acute and chronic illnesses in which the immune system plays a significant role (Tabloski, 2006). Administrators can benefit from an understanding that changes in immune system functioning can increase risks for infection and illness in an elderly population, especially within institutional settings like assisted living facilities.

Best Practices in Improving Physical Problems Associated With Aging

Administrators, staff, and residents in assisted living facilities can use new technologies as best practices to promote wellness and improve physical problems. Web-based support groups can provide improved outcomes for elders with a number of physical, social, and emotional problems (Mauk, 2018). The Wellness Community is an example of one approach using the internet to support services for elders dealing with cancer (Mauk, 2018). New technologies are in development in an emerging field of gerotechnology for use with elders. Smartphone tracking of cardiac rhythms, GPS positioning systems for tracking of dementia patients, blood glucose sensors, and emerging health applications for use in smartphones, watches, and tablets are examples of how new technologies can improve the monitoring of physical problems in an aging population (Mauk, 2018).

CASE STUDY

The administrator of a large urban assisted living community has an understanding of many of the normal physiologic changes that occur with aging but is concerned that facility staff are not adequately assessing residents' abilities to routinely perform many daily activities. This concern was highlighted by an interaction with Ms. S, an 85-year-old female who has been a facility resident for 3 years. As the administrator talked with Ms. S, she noted the very strong smell of urine and also noted that Ms. S's clothes were food stained and that the laces of her shoes were untied. Ms. S seemed unaware of these problems.

A best practice in this situation is the use of the Katz Index of Independence in Activities of Daily Living (ADL) as described in Touhy and Jett (2018). The index includes a list of six activities, including bathing, dressing, continence, feeding, toileting, and transferring. An older persons ability to perform these tasks is scored either as 1 (independence) or 0 (dependence) with a total score of 6 indicating independence in all ADL and a total score of 0 indicating significant dependence in all ADL. Use of the Katz Index of Independence in ADL can provide staff with valuable information about determining the functional status of elders and can be also used to monitor the functional status of elders over time.

When the administrator had staff use the Katz Index of Independence in ADL, Ms. S received a score of 3, scoring in the dependent range in the areas of bathing, toileting, and feeding. Further evaluation revealed that Ms. S had experienced a recent and unidentified stroke. The administrator and staff were then able to work with Ms. S to provide her with assistance in bathing, toileting, and feeding herself, thus improving her appearance and overall health.

ISSUES RELATED TO SELECTED PHYSICAL ASPECTS OF AGING

Assisted living administrators will need to have an awareness and comprehension of issues related to selected physiologic changes associated with aging that are relevant for many elders residing within assisted living facilities. The development of programs and services within these facilities can be enhanced through an understanding of physiologic issues. Five such issues, including nutrition, mobility, fall prevention, sleep, and pain management, are briefly explored and discussed.

Nutrition Issues

The importance of nutrition in elders residing in assisted living facilities cannot be understated. Good nutrition is essential for well-being and for the prevention and treatment of a number of diseases. Healthy People 2020 identifies the 2020 goals of health promotion and chronic disease reduction through the consumption of healthy diets and maintenance of healthy body weights (Healthy People 2020, 2019). Although there is agreement that adequate nutrition is essential for elders, many factors exist which influence the presence or absence of good nutrition, and therefore the nutritional status of elders. These include lifestyle, medication use, the presence of chronic illnesses, changes in body function and composition, lifetime eating habits, heredity, socioeconomic status, and social interactions (Linton & Lach, 2007). Many elders are at risk for malnutrition or undernutrition with implications for quality of life, health, and independence. Malnutrition is a serious concern as a lack of appropriate nutrients serves to compromise health and contributes to a number of acute and chronic illnesses. This is sometimes referred to as the *anorexia of aging*. For other elders, obesity or overnutrition becomes problematic, again creating a number of health risks and increasing complications for many chronic diseases, including diabetes, hypertension, and cardiovascular disease.

A number of nutrition-related changes have been associated with aging. Some of these changes include decreases in metabolic rates, decreased bone mineral density, and loss of lean body mass (Clegg & Williams, 2018). Social factors are also associated with nutritional changes in aging. Some commonly occurring social factors, including social isolation, loss, grief, reactions to life changes such as retirement, and changes in financial status, can result in altered nutrition. Awareness of age-related nutritional alterations helps administrators in assisted living facilities as they work to ensure that residents maintain adequate diets.

Nutritional Assessment

Administrators can utilize the services of dieticians, nurses, or nutritionists in the creation of nutritional assessments for elders in assisted living facilities. Assessments should include a diet or nutritional history. Dietary recall involves asking elders to recall their total food and beverage intake for a 24-hour time period. Elders are asked a series of open-ended questions to determine the specific foods eaten, the types of food, the amount of the food ingested, and the times that food was eaten during the given time period. Additional questions regarding the use of beverages, including alcohol, are also included in this dietary recall. Additional questions about food preparation, food preferences, and food shopping can provide additional information about nutritional status. Limitations of this assessment strategy include difficulties in recalling total food intake for a complete 24-hour time period. This may influence the accuracy of the data collected. Strengths of this assessment strategy include ease of administration for both elders and clinicians.

Nutritional assessments can also be obtained by asking elders to keep food records. This assessment strategy requires elders to list all food and beverage intake for a specific time period, usually a three to five-day time period. Once the food record is completed, clinicians can review the records to determine the nutritional adequacy of total food intake. The data from these assessments then serves as the basis for recommendations to improve nutritional status for individuals. Elders must be able to recall food intake for an extended time period. Gaps and difficulties in remembering food intake are limitations of this assessment approach. Strengths of this assessment include the ability of elders to provide information about diet and nutrition that reflect cultural and social preferences.

There are a number of screening tools available for nutritional assessment. Assessment should consider the following: (a) an inability to feed oneself; (b) chewing problems; (c) swallowing problems; (d) mouth pain; (e) weight loss; (f) altered taste; (g) hunger complaints; and (h) nutritional approaches such as therapeutic diets, supplement use, and the use of weight gain programs (Tabloski, 2006). This nutritional assessment may be of value in the assessment and ongoing screening of elders in assisted living facilities.

Nutritional assessments should also take into consideration a number of factors that impact eating. Physical changes related to dentition, with tooth loss, dentures that may fit poorly, or changes in the ability to adequately chew and swallow food. Sensory alterations should also be assessed. Elders who experience decreased taste and smell will frequently experience eating problems and are at risk for malnutrition.

Strategies to maintain healthy nutrition of elders living in assisted living facilities include the use of diets to promote health. Administrators are required by state regulations to provide food that meets minimal nutrition standards. Understanding a number of diets designed to promote health in aging populations can be used in conjunction with standard diets. A number of diets that can be of benefit to elders will be briefly discussed. Low-caloric diets are of use with elders who are overweight or obese. The goal of these diets is to reduce the total number of calories consumed by elders on a daily basis and thus reduce weight. Reductions in calories of 500 to 1,000 calories per day can result in weight loss of 1 to 2 pounds per week. More extensive weight loss is generally not recommended in elders. Low-fat diets are designed to reduce the amount of saturated fat in daily food intake. For elders who have cardiovascular disease, hypertension, or diabetes, diets that reduce fat intake can be of benefit in promotion of improved health.

There are a number of dietary recommendations for elders with diabetes. Nutritional guidelines for patients with diabetes include diets that are low in fat with saturated fat limited to 10% of total daily calories, and diets low in sugar with limits on simple carbohydrates and limits on alcohol. The lowering of sodium consumption is also recommended, limiting sodium to 2 g or less per day. Diets that are high in fiber are recommended for many elders. These diets are thought to be of benefit to elders with diabetes and cardiovascular disease. Because aging causes decreases in colonic transit time with resulting constipation, diets that increase fiber can improve or prevent the painful complications of constipation.

Malnutrition or under-nutrition remains a significant problem for many elders. Poor appetite, muscle wasting, weight loss, and insufficient diet define inadequate nutrition, and malnutrition results in poor health. This decreased quality of life encompasses multiple social and physical factors. Assessment of malnutrition is needed to determine optimal treatment options for elders with this problem includng specific treatment options based on the problems causing the malnutrition. Diets that provide adequate amounts of protein and calories should be offered to elders with malnutrition. Underlying social and physical problems should be assessed, and strategies to resolve the problems proposed (Clegg & Williams, 2018).

Nutritional supplements are recommended for elders who have specific problems and dietary deficiencies. Vitamin D supplementation is recommended for elders because they have less exposure to sunlight, have skin changes that decrease vitamin D absorption, and frequently have diets deficient in this vitamin. Calcium supplementation is recommended for elders again because many diets are deficient in calcium, and also because elders are at risk for age-related bone loss resulting in brittle bones. Older adults should consider the addition of 1,500 mg of calcium supplementation per day to moderate bone loss (Linton & Lach, 2007).

Administrators can obtain information regarding healthy nutrition from a number of resources. Experts in the field of nutrition, including dieticians and nutritionists, are available for consultation. Physicians and nurses can also play a role in nutritional assessment and recommendations for healthy diets in elderly individuals. Online resources include the websites associated with a number of organizations, including the American Heart Association, the American Diabetes Association, the American Association of Retired People, and the National Institutes of Health. Information from online resources may be current, relevant, and research-based and is also easy for busy administrators to access and review.

Mobility Issues

Mobility is the second issue related to the physical aspects of aging. Mobility, or the ability to move and function, is fundamental to quality health and quality of life (Webber et al., 2010). Mobility is influenced in older adults by age-related changes in muscles, bones, joints, and nervous system functioning. Although mobility promotes healthy aging, mobility declines with advancing age and changes are first noted in complex and demanding tasks (Rantanen, 2013). Factors that influence mobility include age-related decreases in muscle mass, degenerative joint changes, thinning or demineralization of bones, and sensory deficits, including decreased vision and hearing (Rantanen, 2013). Age-related changes create functional problems, including an inability to conduct ADL, including walking and balancing, and increasing the risk for serious falls. The presence of decreased mobility with associated loss of independence creates a number of social and psychological problems for elders. Loss of independence results frequently in a lessening in the quality of life for elders with even minimal mobility loss. Depression is a problem associated with decreased mobility.

Mobility assessments will provide information related to both physicality and functioning, and should include a health history that can be obtained by physicians, nurses, geriatric specialists, physical therapists, or other clinicians working in assisted living communities. The health history should include questions about the muscles, especially if muscle pain, weakness, or cramping is present. Questions about bones should be focused on the presence or absence of pain, deformities, and a history of prior fractures or bone problems. Information about joints should focus on the presence or absence of pain, decreased mobility, stiffness, and swelling. Questions should also be focused on an elder's ability to perform ADL, including bathing, dressing, feeding, moving, shopping, preparing meals, performing housework, and independently completing physical activities (Linton & Lach, 2007). Data obtained from a mobility assessment can be used to address both current and potential mobility problems in elders.

Exercise is considered to be an essential component of mobility, and the goal of exercise is to maintain or improve musculoskeletal functioning. Aerobic exercises should be encouraged for at least 20 to 30 minutes per day. Aerobic activities can include walking, swimming, biking, or dancing, and must be individualized for each individual participant. Passive exercises to maintain joint mobility are recommended for elders who are unable to exercise independently or unassisted. Resistive exercises or strength training exercises are now recommended to improve both musculoskeletal and cardiovascular functioning. Research indicates that regular participation in strength training programs increases both muscle strength and muscle mass. Isometric exercises involve muscle contractions without the use of joints, and can be effective in muscle strength training. Balance exercises are used to provide an additional form of strength training for elders. Tai Chi is one example of a balance exercise that is successfully used by many elders in both independent and group settings.

There are a number of assistive devices available for elders with changes or impairments in mobility. Understanding how devices, including canes, walkers, and wheelchairs, can assist walking, and thus improve mobility, is important for administrators working in assisted living facilities.

Canes are mechanical assistive devices that increase balance by broadening the base of support and absorbing body weight when partial weight bearing is required (Perry & Potter, 2010). There are a number of canes available for use, including a standard or straight-leg cane, a tripod cane with three feet, and the quad cane with four feet (Berman et al., 2009). The canes with three or four feet provide additional stability for elders with balance problems and also serve to improve security with use of these assistive devices. Walkers are assistive devices that improve mobility by providing additional support, especially for elders who need help with partial weight bearing. Standard walkers are lightweight, made of polished aluminum, and have four legs. Walkers with rollers or wheels do not need to be picked up to be moved forward, but are less stable than standard walkers. Elders who use walkers must have at least partial strength in hands, wrists, and elbows, as well as strong shoulder muscle depressors (Berman et al., 2009).

There are two types of wheelchairs in use to improve mobility. Manual and electric wheelchairs are commonly in use, and come with adjustable foot and leg rests. The wheels and tires on the front of the wheelchair should be selected according to use. Larger wheels move easily over bumps or obstructions but are harder to turn and also take more room to turn (Berman et al., 2009). Ease of turning wheelchairs and the ability to turn wheelchairs in assisted living environments with space limitations should be considered when selecting wheelchairs. Additionally, the seat used in a wheelchair should also be considered. Rigid wheelchair backing and solid seating with foam or air cushioning should be considered for those elders using wheelchairs on a long-term basis (Berman et al., 2009).

Administrators working with elders using assistive devices to enhance mobility must make sure that facility physical spaces are designed for the safe use of devices. Flooring must be designed to prevent skids or slips when elders use canes or walkers. Corridors and rooms must be free of furniture and equipment that would create problems or impede the use of walkers and wheelchairs. As noted, elders in wheelchairs must be able to freely move and turn the chairs in rooms and hallways. Administrators can refer to state regulations regarding the development of physical space in assisted living facilities for assistance in developing environments that ease elder mobility, with or without the use of assistive devices.

Fall-Prevention Issues

Fall prevention is a third issue related to the physical aspects of aging. Assisted living administrators should have an understanding of this important issue to prevent potential problems for all facility residents. The importance of fall prevention is underscored by statistics indicating that falls are a major cause of morbidity and mortality in elders. Older adults who fall account for about 60% of all injury-related emergency room visits and over 50% of injury-related deaths annually in the United States (Haddad et al., 2018). Approximately half of the elders living in institutions will experience falls annually (Mauk, 2018). The economic costs of treating elders who fall and require either hospitalization or treatment are significant for all segments of the population. In 2015, direct medical costs totaled $31.3 billion for nonfatal injuries (Burns et al., 2016). The social costs of treating elders who fall are also significant with changes in mobility creating both physical and functional impairments that can impact the quality of life for elders. Falls can be prevented through modifications of visual impairments, monitoring of medication adverse effects, and assessing for postural hypotension and vestibular problems (Haddad et al., 2018). Fall-prevention programs can effectively reduce the economic, physical, and social burdens associated with falls. The development of fall-prevention programs can reduce fall rates and the significant costs associated with falls.

There are a number of risk factors associated with falls experienced by elders. Commonly occurring risks include the following: (a) poor vision; (b) cognitive impairments, including memory changes, poor judgment, confusion, and dementia; (c) impaired mobility, including changes in gait, balance, and problems with lower extremities); (d) difficulties in movement, especially in getting out of a chair or bed; (e) weakness from illnesses or therapies; and (f) the use of a number of medications that can cause changes in orientation or mobility (Berman et al., 2009). Understanding the risks related to falls is important in falls assessment and the implementation of fall-prevention programs.

Although administrators in assisted living facilities will not conduct assessments for falls, understanding fall-assessment risk is an initial step in the creation of strategies to prevent falls, and the physical, social, and economic problems associated with falls. There are a number of falls assessment instruments that are available for use by clinicians, assessment instruments that focus on physical factors, history of prior falls, medication utilization, and environmental factors. Each area will be briefly presented and discussed.

Assessment of physical factors associated with increased risk of falls includes evaluation of motor and sensory problems, balance problems, along with memory and cognitive problems. Elders with existing medical problems that create fatigue, musculoskeletal weakness, incontinence, changes in cognition or mental functioning, or changes in vision or hearing are at increased risk for falls, and should have these problems assessed. Assessment of prior falls should include questions to assess the presence of any symptoms at the time of the fall, location of prior falls, time at which prior falls occurred, activities that were taking place at the time of the prior falls, and the presence or absence of trauma at the time of the falls. Special attention should be paid to the medications used by elders. There are a number of medications that increase falls risks in older adults. Antidepressants, sedatives, sleeping medications, antihistamines, steroids, antihypertensives, diuretics, muscle relaxants, cardiac medications, and hypoglycemics are some of the medications that may be problematic for elders. Elders should also be assessed for use of over-the-counter medication, as well as the use of vitamins and herbal supplements that may contribute to the risk of falling.

Environmental factors should be evaluated in falls risk assessment. Factors that contribute to falls include the physical environment, and are affected by lighting, flooring surfaces, physical plant design, clutter in rooms and hallways, and safe use of mobility assistive devices. Stairs with uneven step height, absence of railings, furniture with unsteady bases, and bathrooms without grab bars, with slippery floors, and with inappropriate toilet heights should also be assessed as potential risks for falls. Additionally, the clothing and footwear worn by residents in assisted living facilities are of high importance, and the use of nonskid footwear should be considered.

Fall-prevention programs should be implemented following careful falls risk assessment. Effective fall-prevention programs include the following elements: (a) medication reviews and medication modification as needed; (b) modification of environmental factors that increase falls risk; (c) use of assistive devices as needed; (d) exercise and strength training to enhance mobility; and (e) education of older adults to reduce falls risk.

Best Practices in Falls Prevention

The Centers for Disease Control and Prevention have developed an initiative that serves as a best practice in fall assessment and prevention. The Stopping Elderly Accidents, Deaths, and Injuries (STEADI) initiative serves as: (a) a guide for healthcare providers to screen and identify patients at risk for falls; (b) an assessment tool in the identification of modifiable risk factors; and (c) an intervention using effective clinical and community strategies (Haddad et al., 2018).

Best practices, including a series of community-based programs to prevent falls, have been cited by the National Council on Aging (2017). Programs include: (a) A Matter of Balance, an eight-session workshop to increase activity and reduce the fear of falling; (b) Otago Exercise Program of muscle strengthening and balance, including exercises for frail elders; (c) Stepping On, a 7-week program for elders to increase self-confidence through fall-prevention strategies; and (d) Tai Chi to increase balance through gait training and controlled movements (National Council on Aging, 2017).

Sleep Issues

Sleep issues occur frequently and exist as a fourth area related to the physical aspects of aging. Sleep is essential for healthy physical functioning. During sleep, a number of physiologic processes occur, including increased production of growth hormone, acceleration of protein synthesis and tissue repair, deceleration of metabolic processes, as well as the filtering and organization of cognitive and emotional information. Researchers have noted a number of age-related changes in sleep patterns. There is objective evidence that aging causes changes in sleep architecture, with increased fragmentation and an increase in the number of arousals and awakenings as well reductions in sleep efficiency and total sleep time (Cooke & Ancoli-Israel, 2011).

It is important to note that sleep problems are not solely considered to be the result of normal aging processes (Rodriguez et al., 2015). Many sleep disturbances are noted in older adults. These problems include insomnia, with difficulties in falling asleep or staying asleep, snoring, which may be an indicator of sleep apnea, breathing pauses which may also indicate sleep apnea, and tingling or discomfort in the legs which may indicate restless leg syndrome (Mauk, 2018). Insomnia is also connected with both comorbidities and medication side effects (Suzuki et al., 2017). Frequent nighttime awakenings, early morning awakenings, and difficulties falling asleep may also be seen in aging adults as age-related sleep changes, or as the result of co-existing medical problems. Additional age-related changes to sleep patterns involve decreased time in deep sleep stages, decreased time spent dreaming, and increased time spent in light sleep stages. Elders may experience a number of functional changes resulting from age-related sleep alterations. An overall increase in the time needed to fall asleep, frequent arousals during the night, increased difficulty in returning to sleep once aroused or awakened, an increase in the amount of time spent in bed with a decreased amount of overall sleep time, and poorer sleep quality also occur in older adults (Miller, 2009).

It is important to note that although assisted living administrators will not be conducting sleep assessments, the information obtained from such assessments can be valuable in understanding problems that elders may experience in regards to the design of interventions to assist in the promotion of healthy sleep patterns.

Sleep assessment should involve the assessment of commonly occurring risk factors affecting sleep and sleep patterns, including physiologic factors, psychosocial factors, medications, environmental factors, and pathologic problems such as sleep apnea. There are a number of physiologic factors that can alter sleep patterns such as chronic illnesses like cardiovascular disease and respiratory problems, physical discomfort or pain from chronic illnesses such as arthritis, neuromuscular disorders such as foot or leg cramping, and urinary problems that cause increased nighttime urination such as prostatic enlargement (Miller, 2009).

Psychosocial factors serve as risk factors for sleep disturbances. Problems, such as stress, anxiety, depression, and dementia, are frequently associated with a number of sleep issues. Elders with depression take longer to fall asleep, experience more light sleep, awake more during the night as well as the early morning, and feel much less rested upon awakening. Elders who feel alone or who have few work responsibilities, social demands, or environmental stimuli, or who experience increased stress, may also be at risk for a number of sleep problems (Miller, 2009). Questions to determine the presence or absence of these psychological risks should be included as part of the psychological sleep assessment.

Medication assessment is an important part of sleep assessment. There are a very large number of medications that have the potential to alter sleep patterns, including over-the-counter medications and herbal supplements (Cooke & Ancoli-Israel, 2011). Caffeine is a central nervous system stimulant that can lengthen sleep latency as well as increase awakening during the night. Nicotine interferes with sleep because of stimulant and respiratory effects. Alcohol increases the number of nighttime awakenings as well as suppressing REM sleep (Miller, 2009). In older adults, small quantities of caffeine, nicotine, and alcohol can create significant sleep problems.

Sleep assessments should include questions about environmental factors that may create sleep problems. Increased noise, changes in sleep routines, and alterations in temperature (rooms that are too warm or cold) may increase the risk for sleep problems. Increased lighting can create sleep problems as well. A lack of bright light during daylight hours can create problems by interfering with circadian rhythms and the production of melatonin, a hormone that regulates sleep, body temperature, and circadian rhythms (Miller, 2009).

Sleep apnea is another problem that should be assessed in elders at risk for sleep disturbances. Obstructive sleep apnea is defined as an involuntary cessation of airflow for a minimum of 10 seconds or longer, and the presence of five to eight of these episodes per hour is an indication of serious problems (Miller, 2009). Assessment data indicating the presence of sleep apnea requires that the elder with this problem be referred to a physician or sleep specialist. Administrators should also note that there are a number of sleep assessment tools available to obtain additional sleep assessment data. Consultation with sleep experts can assist in the use of specific sleep assessment tools.

Once sleep assessment data are obtained, administrators can work with clinicians to develop strategies to improve sleep conditions for elders. Educational programs can provide older adults with information about sleep changes associated with aging. There are a number of strategies that can enhance good sleep hygiene. Older adults should work to structure conditions that are conducive to good sleep. Going to bed the same time every evening, use of relaxation strategies—such as warm milk, warm baths, relaxing music, or relaxing reading—can improve sleep conditions. Environmental changes, including soft lighting, cool temperatures, and quiet, noise-free conditions, are also recommended, as are aromatherapy and massage. Use of daytime exercise, relaxation exercises, and stress management strategies can also improve sleep problems for older adults.

There are a number of medications available to treat sleep problems in elders. Hypnotics, antidepressants, and non-benzodiazepine sleeping medications may assist elders with sleep problems. Although many of these medications are effective in treating sleep problems, there are a number of side effects that accompany the use of these drugs (Cooke & Ancoli-Israel, 2011). Elders who use these drugs may be at risk for medication dependence or side effects from interactions with other drugs that may also be used for existing diseases or problems. Use of these medications with alcohol can create problems that are potentially life threatening. Additionally, use of these medications may also put older adults at increased risk for falls and accident-related problems. Elders who require these medications require evaluation and consultation from physicians or sleep specialists.

Elders may also consider the use of herbal remedies for sleep problems. Ginseng and valerian are two remedies used by a number of older adults to promote sleep. Melatonin, a hormone synthesized by the pineal gland, may be used to promote sleep. Research indicates that the use of exogenous melatonin may improve sleep in older adults (Miller, 2009). Nutritional supplements, such as L-tryptophan, may also assist in improving sleep. L-tryptophan is an amino acid that aids in serotonin production in the brain. Naturally occurring in proteins and dairy products, use of L-tryptophan shortens sleep latency periods in elders who have difficulty falling asleep (Miller, 2009). L-tryptophan can also be taken in supplement form to enhance sleep.

Assisted living administrators can obtain information about sleep problems and the treatment of sleep problems from clinicians who specialize in sleep disorders, and from other health professionals, including physicians and nurses. Additional information regarding sleep problems can be obtained from a number of online resources, including the National Institute on Aging, the National Institute of Mental Health, and the AARP.

Chronic Pain Issues

A fifth and final issue related to physical aging is chronic pain. Administrators must have an understanding of the importance of chronic pain as they work with elders in assisted living facilities. In addition, administrators must have an understanding of the state regulations that govern administration of medications within assisted living facilities if residents with chronic pain receive these medications as part of a pain management program. Finally, administrators can benefit from information about common causes of chronic pain, as well as some of the age-related changes that affect pain in older adults.

Chronic pain is defined as pain that persists beyond the usual course of a disease or injury, or lasting longer than a minimum 3- to 6-month time period (Miller, 2009). Some experts now recommend the use of persistent pain rather than chronic pain as a label that evokes a more positive description of this condition (Miller, 2009).

Chronic pain is described as a widespread significant problem for older adults who are at risk for pain as a result of many chronic illnesses. Many commonly occurring diseases are accompanied by chronic pain, including arthritis and diabetes. Arthritis is considered to be the most common cause of persistent pain in elders, with 49% to 59% of this population experiencing some form of arthritis-related pain (Miller, 2009). Diabetes is another problem experienced by many older adults that frequently causes chronic pain in the extremities.

There are a number of functional consequences associated with chronic pain, including: (a) problems with walking and mobility; (b) decline in overall functional abilities; (c) psychosocial problems, including sleep disturbances, depression, anxiety, and fatigue; and (d) increased risk for disability and loss of independence (Miller, 2009). Additionally, age-related changes that may be experienced by older adults are not well understood, and elders may not complain of pain but rather confusion, fatigue, aggression, or restlessness (Miller, 2009).

Assessment for chronic pain should be conducted by clinicians, including physicians, nurses, or pain specialists. Assisted living community administrators can benefit from understanding the assessment process as it relates to residents with chronic pain. Although there are a number of pain assessment instruments and scales available for use in evaluation of pain in older adults, basic assessments should focus on a series of questions. Clinicians should focus on questions that provide information about the nature or intensity of the pain, the location of the pain, the duration of the pain, pain frequency, pain movement or radiation, factors that make the pain better or worse, current treatments for the pain, and other problems that may be associated with the pain. Additional assessment questions should be focused on functional changes that are associated with chronic pain. Elders should be questioned about changes in activities of daily living that result from chronic pain such as an inability to clean, bathe, sleep, perform housework, or shop. Changes in exercise patterns, or inability to exercise, along with a decrease in mobility related to chronic pain, should also be noted. Changes in eating patterns, including decreased appetite or weight loss resulting from chronic pain should be noted. Changes in emotional feelings, including depression, anxiety, or other mood changes should be assessed, as well as changes in socialization with family members and friends that result from chronic pain. Changes in mental functioning also resulting from chronic pain or the medications and treatments used to treat it should be assessed Finally, changes in any other aspects of the elder's life that have been altered as a result of chronic pain should be evaluated as part of a comprehensive pain assessment. Factors, such as economic changes, social isolation, or decreased feelings of well-being and life satisfaction as a result of chronic pain, should be explored and discussed.

Administrators can benefit from an understanding of the importance of treating persistent pain, the need to maximize functioning and quality of life while minimizing the adverse effects associated with pain management (Gallioa-Castillo & Weiner, 2019). Understanding both the benefits of nonpharmacologic strategies and some of the challenges associated with pharmacologic pain management strategies is important for assisted living administrators. Exercise is a mainstay of nonpharmacologic pain management. For elders with chronic pain due to arthritis or other musculoskeletal problems, exercise programs, such as swimming or yoga, have been shown to be of benefit, and may serve to reduce pain. Stress management activities, such as relaxation exercises, meditation, aromatherapy, art therapy, music therapy, or guided imagery, can provide benefits in pain modification or reduction. Physical therapy, acupuncture, or acupressure have also been identified as strategies that may be beneficial to elders experiencing chronic pain. Additional benefits may be obtained from the use of herbal or nonprescription treatments. Vitamins and herbal supplements may be used by elders to reduce pain. In addition, the topical use of agents, such as capsaiacin or analgesic ointments or creams, can provide relief for musculoskeletal pain and joint pains from arthritis.

The pharmacologic management of chronic pain should be managed by physicians, advanced practice nurses, or pain management specialists. There are a number of medications available for chronic pain management, including over-the-counter analgesics and a variety of prescription analgesics, including opioids. Specialists in pain management are able to identify medication management programs that are tailored to individual elder needs and are also then qualified to monitor and reassess elders on an on-going basis. Challenges associated with the administration and utilization of opioid medications in assisted living facilities focus on how these drugs are administered and stored. Administrators need to review individual state and local regulations governing medication storage and administration for controlled and regulated medications. Administrators should also review state and local regulations for appropriate disposal strategies when opioids and other controlled pain medications need to be removed from assisted living facilities.

Administrators can access a number of resources to obtain information regarding chronic pain management for elders living in assisted living facilities. Clinical experts in chronic pain management include physicians, nurses, pharmacists, pharmacologists, pain specialists, and psychologists. In addition, administrators can access current and accurate information regarding chronic pain management from a number of online resources, including the National Institute on Aging and the National Institute of Mental Health.

CONCLUSIONS

Assisted living administrators can benefit from an awareness of some of the many physiologic changes that normally occur in the body systems of elders. Changes to the cardiovascular, respiratory, muscular, orthopedic, gastrointestinal, genitourinary, skin and lymphatic, and neurological systems that occur as part of the aging process presented in this chapter can also place older individuals at risk for a number of problems that are both acute and chronic. Staff in assisted living communities need to identify and address functional alterations and problems resulting from normal age-related physical changes. Administrators can facilitate these processes with a basic understanding of some of the age-related physiologic changes. Commonly occurring issues related to nutrition, mobility, fall prevention, sleep, and chronic pain management are identified and briefly discussed. Administrators can work to improve services to elders through an understanding of these important issues. In addition, the best-practice case study highlights the value of measuring ADL as a measurement of functional status and abilities.

REFERENCES

Berman, A., Snyder, S., & Jackson, C. (2009). *Skills in clinical nursing* (6th ed.). Pearson Education.

Burns, E. R., Stevens, J. A., & Lee, R. (2016). The direct costs of fatal and non-fatal falls among older adults—United States. *Journal of Safety Research, 58*, 99–103. https://doi.org/10.1016/j.jsr.2016.05.001

Clegg, M. E., & Williams, E. A. (2018). Optimizing nutrition in older people. *Maturitas, 112*, 34–38. https://doi.org/10.1016/j.maturitas.2018.04.001

Cooke, J. R., & Ancoli-Israel, S. (2011). Normal and abnormal sleep in the elderly. *Handbook of Clinical Neurology, 98*, 653–655. https://doi.org/10.1016/B978-0-444-52006-7.00041-1

Elkin, M. K., Perry, A. G., & Potter, P. A. (2007). *Nursing interventions and clinical skills* (4th ed.). Mosby Elsevier.

Gallioa-Castillo, M.C., & Weiner, D. K. (2019). Treatment of persistent pain in older adults. *UpToDate.* https://www.uptodate.com/contents/treatment-ofpersistnt-pain-in-older-adults

Haddad, Y. K., Bergen, G., & Luo, F. (2018). Reducing fall risk in older adults. *American Journal of Nursing, 118*(7), 21–22. https://doi.org/10.1097/01.NAJ.0000541429.36218.2d

Healthy People 2020. (2019). *Nutrition and weight status.* https://www.healthypeople.gov/2020/topics-objectives/topic/nutrition-and-weight-status

Linton, A. D., & Lach, H. W. (2007). *Concepts and practice. Gerontological nursing* (3rd ed.). Saunders Elsevier.

Mauk, K. L. (2018). *Gerontological nursing. Competencies for care* (4th ed). Jones & Bartlett Publishers.

Miller, C. A. (2009). *Wellness in older adults* (5th ed.). Wolters Kluwer Lippincott Williams & Wilkins.

National Council on Aging. (2017). *Evidence-based falls prevention programs: Saving lives, saving money.* www.ncoa.org/FallsPrevention

Perry, A. G., & Potter, P. A. (2010). *Clinical nursing skills & techniques* (7th ed.). Mosby Elsevier.

Rantanen, T. (2013). Promoting mobility in older people. *Journal of Preventive Medicine & Public Health, 46*(Suppl 1), S50–S54. https://doi.org/10.3961/jpmph.2013.46.S.S50

Rodriguez, J. C., Dzierewski, J. M., & Alessi, C. A. (2015). Sleep problems in the elderly. *Medical Clinics of North America, 99*(2), 431–439. https://doi.org/10.1016/j.mcna.2014.11.013

Suzuki, K., Miyamoto, M., & Hirata, K. (2017). Sleep disorders in the elderly: Diagnosis and management. *Journal of General and Family Medicine, 18*(2), 61–71. https://doi.org/10.1002/jgf2.27

Tabloski, P. A. (2006). *Gerontological nursing.* Pearson Education.

Touhy, T. A. & Jett, K. (2018). *Ebersole & Hess' gerontological nursing and healthy aging* (5th ed). Elsevier.

Wallace, M., & Shelkey, M. (2008). Monitoring functional status in hospitalized older adults. *American Journal of Nursing, 108*(4), 64–71. https://doi.org/10.1097/01.NAJ.0000314811.46029.3d

Webber, S. C., Porter, M. M., & Menec, V. H. (2010). Mobility in older adults: A comprehensive framework. *The Gerontologist, 50*(4), 443–450. https://doi.org/10.1093/geront/gnq013

PSYCHOLOGICAL ASPECTS OF AGING

LEARNING OBJECTIVES

Upon the completion of Chapter 20, the reader will be able to:

- Describe selected normal psychological changes associated with aging.
- Discuss issues related to memory and cognition in aging individuals.
- Describe strategies to maintain memory and cognition.
- Define and describe types of dementia.
- Describe strategies to maintain optimal functioning for aging individuals with dementia.
- Define *depression* and describe strategies for assessment of depression and suicide risks in aging individuals.
- Identify strategies to maintain optimal functioning in aging individuals with depression.
- Define *alcohol and substance abuse* and strategies for assessment of alcohol abuse.
- Describe strategies for dealing with alcohol and substance abuse.
- Identify best practices in addressing dementia and depression.

INTRODUCTION

Although assisted living administrators do not serve as clinicians to older persons within their facility, understanding normal psychological changes related to the aging process allows administrators to perform their work more effectively. Understanding many of the normal aging-related changes in neurological functioning, mental health functioning, memory, and cognition can be important in understanding how elders function in assisted living communities. Furthermore, issues related to memory changes, dementia, depression, suicide risk, alcohol, and substance abuse can be commonly experienced by the elderly. An awareness and understanding of these issues can be beneficial to assisted living administrators and will be discussed further in this chapter. Best practices in selected areas associated with psychological aspects of aging are identified and presented throughout this chapter.

OVERVIEW OF NORMAL PSYCHOLOGICAL CHANGES ASSOCIATED WITH AGING

Neurologic Changes

Overall brain volume remains stable in adults until about age 60, with volume losses of 5% to 10% occurring after age 60. Men have a greater volume of brain loss than women, especially in the temporal and frontal lobes of the brain. Numbers of neurons within the brain decrease with age, and this loss may also be accompanied by the presence of senile plaques within brain tissue (Tabloski, 2006). Lipofuscin, a pigment associated with aging, becomes deposited in nerve cells and amyloid is deposited in brain cells and blood vessels (Touhy & Jett, 2018). In addition, decreased blood flow to the brain may also occur with aging. Each of these chemical and physiologic changes results in changes to the brain and cognitive functioning.

Many of the changes seen in the aging brain are found in the central nervous system, with the older brain described as smaller and weighing less than the younger brain (Touhy & Jett, 2018). There are subtle changes noted in cognitive and motor functions in elders and mild balance difficulties and memory impairments may be viewed as normal aging processes. Despite these changes and overall lengthening of time for task performance, intellectual performance remains constant in elders (Touhy & Jett, 2018). Sensory changes are also seen as part of the aging processes (Touhy & Jett, 2018).

Mental Health Changes Associated With Aging

Some authors note that the prevalence of mental illness is lower in the elderly than in the general population (Mauk, 2018). Depression is one problem that occurs frequently in aging populations due to multiple factors, including medical problems, life transitions, loss of family members and friends, and support systems (Mauk, 2018). Depression in the elderly may also be related to biologic aging factors, sleep changes, and alterations in neuroendocrine substances (Touhy & Jett, 2018). Anxiety, a feeling of distress, fear, or worry may be seen in elders in a number of settings, including assisted living facilities. Presence of generalized anxiety may impact health and quality of life for these elders (Miller, 2009).

Memory and Cognitive Changes Associated With Aging

Mental health and cognition are normally thought to remain stable throughout life with changes in cognition associated with physical or mental illnesses. Tabloski (2006) identifies some of the age-related changes to cognition. Changes in cognition include: (a) the speed neede for information processing, resulting in slower learning rates and an increased need for information repetition; (b) the ability to divide attention between two or more tasks; (c) the ability to switch attention from sources of auditory input; (d) the ability to sustain and maintain attention; (e) the ability to filter out irrelevant information; (f) visual–spatial task abilities; and (g) mental flexibility and abstraction abilities. Short-term, or primary, memory remains unchanged throughout life, whereaslong-term or secondary memory does decline as accumulation of practical experience, or wisdom, continues throughout life.

Gerontologists have developed new theories to understand memory and cognition. Contextual theories explain factors impacting memory, including motivation, expectations, personality, education, learning skills, learning habits, sociocultural background, physical health, emotional health, and style of processing information (Miller, 2009). Psychological developmental theories reveal that the thinking of elders increases in complexity with aging, especially in the area of problem-solving. Mariske and Margrette (2006) have noted: (a) motivation is a strong predictor in decision-making in elders, (b) elders are more selective in the information they use to make decisions, (c) elders need more time for decision-making, (d) task expertise and experience improve decision-making especially for elders, and (e) increased task complexity results in more errors and inconsistencies for both elders and younger individuals.

ISSUES RELATED TO PSYCHOLOGICAL ASPECTS OF AGING

Assisted living administrators will benefit from an understanding of some of the issues related to psychological aspects of aging as they work with elders in their facilities. Although there are a number of psychological problems that administrators must face as they deal with elders residing in assisted living facilities, many problems are commonly seen in a variety of settings. A basic understanding of memory, cognition, and dementia, strategies to assist elders with dementia and depression, and strategies to assist elders with depression and alcohol and substance abuse can provide assisted living administrators with information to enhance services for elderly residents. Each of the issues noted above will be briefly described.

Memory and Cognition Issues

Many individuals associate memory changes and problems as an inherent part of the aging process. As noted earlier, research supports some physiologic changes in memory, but overall learning and remembering abilities are not changed in healthy elders (Miller, 2009). A number of factors may alter overall memory and cognition. These factors include: (a) worry and anxiety; (b) stress; (c) physical illnesses; (d) visual, hearing, and functional impairments that preclude information processing; (e) sadness or depression; and (f) the use of medications or alcohol (Miller, 2009). These factors may cause changes in the way individuals process information.

Assessment of memory and cognition is an important evaluation activity for elders entering and residing in assisted living facilities. Although assisted living administrators will not administer assessment tests, understanding basic testing and how the tests provide information can be of benefit in understanding issues related to changes in memory and cognition. Two tests of memory assessment, the Mini-Mental Status Examination and the clock test, will be briefly explained.

Mini-Mental Status Examination

Touhy and Jett (2018) report on the 1975 development of the Mini-Mental Status Examination (MMSE) by Folstein and others. This assessment consists of 11 items that can be administered within 5 to 10 minutes in an elder's room or hospital room. The MMSE contains questions that are both highly specific and highly sensitive. The MMSE includes questions in five categories. Orientation questions elicit information regarding the ability to understand the day, date, month, year, and season as well as location (room, city, state, and country). *Registration* questions ask elders to name three objects and to continue to repeat these objects. *Attention and calculation* questions elicit information about an elder's ability to count backward from 100 by seven or to spell words backward. *Recall* questions elicit the ability to remember information. Finally, *language* questions ask elders to follow three-stage commands, write a sentence, or copy a picture of two intersecting pentagons. The MMSE is scored by giving a point for each question answered correctly for a total of 30 points. Normal scores are considered from 24 to 30. Scores of 23 or less are indicators of memory and cognitive decline. Very low scores on the MMSE suggest dementia.

The MMSE can also be used to monitor changes in cognition. Re-administration of the test with a decline of four or more points serves as an indicator of cognitive change and decline.

The Clock-Drawing Test

The Clock-Drawing Test is another simple test that can be administered within assisted living facilities. The test requires that the elder draw a clock face on a preprinted circle that is 4 inches in diameter. The ability to draw a correct clock face requires that the elder can follow directions, comprehend language, visualize the proper orientation of objects, and execute normal movements. Clock drawings are normal if the elder has included most of the 12 numbers in the correct clockwise orientation. Changes in the ability to accurately draw a clock face strongly indicate the presence of dementia (Touhy & Jett, 2018).

Strategies to Maintain and Improve Memory in Elders in Assisted Living Facilities

Assisted living administrators can work with staff and elders to maintain and improve memory for elders residing in assisted living facilities. A number of these strategies will be briefly discussed.

Maintaining Memory Through Educational Programs

Miller (2009) noted that the educational process itself serves to maintain memory and cognitive functioning. Cognitive wellness then can be maintained through elder participation in adult education programs. Use of group education programs as well as computer-based educational programs can work to enhance memory. Additionally, elders can be encouraged to participate in local community college and university continuing education programs. The Institute for Learning in Retirement is a community-based organization designed to develop and implement educational programs for retirement-aged workers (Miller, 2009).

Strategies to Improve Memory Skills

There are a number of simple memory enhancement skills that can be used for elders in assisted living communities. Writing down information in journals, calendars, and making lists, assigning specific places for specific items, and placing reminders in specific places can be used to improve memory. Use of auditory cues and visual reminders, as well as rhyming and first letter associations, also help improve memory. Additionally, there is current evidence, which suggests that memory can improve with the regular use of mind-enhancing games and puzzles, including crossword puzzles and computer games.

Maintaining Memory Through Aerobic Exercise

The relationship between physical or aerobic exercise and memory enhancement is well noted (Mauk, 2018). Elders who regularly engage in exercise through formal programs or informal activities, such as walking, have been found to increase overall cognitive functioning.

Music Therapy

Touhy and Jett (2018) note the value of music therapy for elders to improve connections through touch as well as cognitive enhancement. Although music therapy has been used in the treatment of Alzheimer's disease, benefits of improved cognition through exposure to music may also help elders in assisted living communities.

Nutritional Supplements

There is literary information suggesting that memory and cognition can be improved through the use of nutritional supplements and herbal remedies. There are a number of vitamins associated with improved memory, including vitamin B12, along with a number of herbal remedies associated with memory and cognition, one of which is gingko biloba (Tabloski, 2006). Assisted living administrators should work with healthcare professionals and with individual elders to determine whether supplements can be of benefit in memory enhancement.

Best Practices

In addition to the memory enhancement strategies identified in this chapter, many assisted living communities use photos, personal mementos, and communication of resident stories to improve resident interactions. Specific rooms or portable carts containing lights, aromas, music, colors, and specific shapes and textures can also serve to increase sensory stimulation for relaxation and sensory redirection in memory enhancement.

Resources Available to Assisted Living Administrators

As administrators deal with issues related to the maintenance and improvement of memory and cognition in elders, healthcare professionals can provide additional consultation and information. Psychologists, neurologists, gerontologists, social workers, geriatric case managers, and geriatric nurses are some of the specialists whom administrators can consult regarding issues related to memory and cognitive improvement. Consultants serve to initially assess elders in assisted living communities and can also work to provide ongoing evaluation of mental status. Assisted living administrators can also use online resources for memory and cognition information. Up-to-date, research-based resources are available to administrators from a number of organizations, including the AARP, the National Institute on Aging, and the National Institute of Mental Health.

Dementia Issues

Assisted living administrators must have a basic understanding of dementia, how dementia is identified and assessed, and how elders with dementia can be assisted to function optimally in assisted living communities. While each state has specific regulations and requirements for elders with dementia and Alzheimer's disease that assisted living administrators must adhere to, additional information on this problem can be beneficial.

Dementia in Assisted Living Populations

Dementia is a progressive illness that causes impairments in social and occupational functioning. Dementia is characterized by the following: (a) symptoms interference with functioning at work or in completion of usual activities, (b) decline in previous levels of performance and functioning, and (c) symptoms unexplained by major psychiatric disorders or delirium (Mauk, 2018). A common problem experienced by older adults is the increasing likelihood of dementia as one ages. Dementia is characterized by a slow progressive onset, and a continuation of cognitive decline that is not connected to other problems (Tabloski, 2006). A diagnosis of dementia requires the loss of intellectual abilities that impact social and occupational functioning, as well as awareness that delirium is not present (Tabloski, 2006).

Delirium is an acute state of confusion, characterized by diminished attention, clouded state of consciousness, physiologic disturbances, and possible hallucinations (Touhy & Jett, 2018). Delirium is usually reversible, as opposed to dementias, which are progressive and irreversible. Delirium is also viewed as a syndrome of multiple factors, including: (a) disturbances in awareness and attention; (b) disturbances that develop over a short time period of hours to days; (c) disturbances that represent a change from baseline awareness and attention; (d) additional disturbances in cognition, including disorientation and language or perceptual changes; and (e) evidence that the changes are a direct consequence of an existing problem such as toxin exposure or substance abuse (Touhy & Jett, 2018). The risk factors for delirium include advanced age, pain, medications, dementia, surgical procedures, and physiologic problems (Miller, 2009). Because delirium is an acute problem that can be reversed, it is important for administrators and those assessing elders in assisted living facilities to be able to identify and differentiate delirium from dementia.

Dementia Assessment

Although assisted living administrators are not in roles designed to assess for dementia, understanding the components of this assessment process are valuable in facilities with elders who have or are at risk for this syndrome. Regulatory requirements for dementia and Alzheimer's assessment vary by state, but again, an understanding of assessment components can facilitate this important process. Elders being assessed for dementia should complete a comprehensive health history. This information includes a history of prior neurological problems, prior cognitive or memory problems, and prior acute and chronic medical problems such as diabetes, heart disease, stroke, cancer, liver, or kidney disease. Past educational background, past employment history, and past hospitalizations or surgeries should also be obtained. It is also necessary to include information about family and social functioning. Many times, family members serve as important informants and can provide information about changes in memory or cognitive functioning that an elder may miss or be unwilling to disclose. Additional information should be obtained about all medication use, including the use of nutritional supplements, vitamins, and herbal supplements. Use of alcohol or other illegal substances should also be discussed and included as part of the assessment. Mental status tests, such as the Mini-Mental Status Examination or the Clock-Drawing Test, can also be used in dementia assessment.

Because dementia causes changes in life functioning, a functional assessment that includes an ability to adequately perform activities of daily living should also be part of the dementia assessment process. Elders who are unable to provide for daily needs, such as care for face and teeth or grooming needs, may have early signs of dementia.

Types of Dementia

Assisted living administrators may benefit from an understanding of the most common types of dementia that may be present in elders residing in assisted living facilities. Although dementia is a syndrome, or cluster of problems, identifying characteristics of specific dementias, including Alzheimer's disease, Lewy body dementia, vascular dementia, and dementia associated with alcohol or drug use, is helpful. Each of these dementias is briefly discussed.

Alzheimer's Disease

In 2015, the number of individuals living with dementia worldwide was estimated at 47.47 million (Alzheimer's Disease International, 2013). Dementia and cognitive impairment are the leading cause of disability and dependence among elders worldwide (World Health Organization, 2012).

The incidence of dementia from Alzheimer's disease increases significantly with age (World Health Organization, 2012). The hallmark signs of Alzheimer's disease can only be seen on autopsy, and include neuritic plaques and neurofibrillary tangles in the neocortex of the brain (Miller, 2009). Mild cognitive impairments associated with Alzheimer's disease include short-term memory loss, difficulties with complex cognitive skills such as arithmetic, and also impairments in the ability to perform daily activities (Miller, 2009).

Theories about the causes of Alzheimer's disease vary at this time, and include familial or genetic risks for inflammatory disease processes; vascular risk factors, including smoking; prior head trauma; exposure to environmental toxins; and psychological factors such as depression (Morris, 2005). Currently, there are no cures available for Alzheimer's disease.

Lewy Body Dementia

Lewy body dementia is now recognized as the second most common form of dementia in the United States. Formed by proteins in the brain, Lewy body dementia may be a variant of Alzheimer's disease, Parkinson's disease, or a disease that combines elements of both diseases (Morris, 2005). Characteristics of this dementia include: (a) impaired cognition, especially executive functioning; (b) widely fluctuating cognition; (c) recurring visual hallucinations; (d) parkinsonism with motor symptoms; and (e) falls, apathy, sleep problems, and depression (Morris, 2005). Individuals with this dementia are considered to be very medically frail, and may have significant problems with the addition of minor illnesses or environmental changes (Miller, 2009).

Vascular Dementia

Caused by the death of nerve cells that do not receive adequate blood flow, vascular dementia also occurs with other types of dementia such as Alzheimer's disease (Miller, 2009). Causes of vascular dementia include changes to arteries caused by diseases such as diabetes, hypertension, or arteriosclerotic disease, and overall decreases in perfusion from problems such as congestive heart failure, hypotension, or cardiac arrhythmias (Miller, 2009). Elders with vascular dementia often have cognitive impairments such as aphasia and memory loss; behavioral changes, including depression; and changes in sensory motor functions, including changes in gait, sensation, and urinary incontinence (Miller, 2009).

Dementia Related to Alcohol and Drug Use

Chronic abuse of alcohol or drugs may produce symptoms of dementia similar to those seen in early Alzheimer's disease. A comprehensive history of prior alcohol or drug use should serve as an indicator of the cause of this dementia.

Strategies to Provide Optimal Functioning in Elders With Dementia

Assisted living administrators can work with staff to provide a number of services that may be of benefit to elders with dementia. Programs that support exercise include formal classes or informal exercise programs such as walking. Music therapy, the use of music to improve cognition or behavioral functioning, has been used in a number of settings. Researchers have noted an improvement in cognition following 30 minutes of music therapy twice weekly (Linton & Lach, 2007). The use of art therapy, dancing, and social activities can also dementia. The use of therapeutic touch can also be of benefit. Family involvement within the assisted living environment can benefit elders with dementia, as can the use of a number of social services. Environmental strategies to provide orientation for those with dementia are also of potential benefit in an assisted living setting. Calendars and clocks with large, easy to read numbers are visual aids to help orient elders. Environments that incorporate nature and reduce stimulation through the use of quiet sounds, no television, and moderated lighting can be used to assist elders with dementia. Additionally, the implementation of strategies to enhance the sensory environment, such as massage, therapeutic touch, and aromatherapy, can be used in assisted living facilities.

Resources Available to Assisted Living Administrators

As administrators deal with issues related to elders experiencing dementia, various healthcare professionals can provide additional consultation and support to address problems related to dementia. Psychologists, neurologists, gerontologists, social workers, geriatric case managers, and geriatric nurses are some of the specialists whom administrators can consult regarding issues related to dementia. Administrators should plan to work with selected consultants to provide assessment and ongoing services for elders with dementia. Assisted living administrators can also use online resources for current information on dementia. Updated and research-based resources are available to administrators from a number of organizations, including the Alzheimer's Association, AARP, the National Institute on Aging, National Institutes of Health, and National Institute of Mental Health.

Depression Issues

Administrators working in assisted living settings need to understand issues related to depression, a commonly occurring problem in elder populations. Clinical depression is the most commonly occurring mental health problem in older adults, with an increased prevalence in those adults who reside in long-term care or assisted living facilities (Mauk, 2018). According to the American Psychiatric Association (2000), to receive a diagnosis of clinical depression older adults must experience five or more of the following symptoms during a 2-week period, including lack of enjoyment in previously enjoyed activities, sadness, sleep disturbances, restlessness, fatigue, feelings of worthlessness, an inability to think clearly, and suicidal thoughts. Depression can be thought of as a group of disorders with variable severity. It is important for administrators to note that elders who are in the very early stages of dementia may feel that there is something wrong, and begin to experience mild depression along with their dementia (Tabloski, 2006). Depressed elders report more cognitive and physical symptoms, including apathy, as compared to younger adults. Elders with depression also frequently experience anorexia, weight loss, early morning awakening, and withdrawal from social activities (Miller, 2009).

Because clinical depression may co-exist with dementia, it is important for those working with elders who have either depression or dementia to differentiate between the two problems. A number of distinguishing features exist between depression and dementia. According to Miller (2009), the onset of symptoms differs between depression with rapid, abrupt onset, and dementia with a more gradual onset. Memory and attention problems associated with depression are related mainly to a lack of motivation and an inability to concentrate. In individuals with dementia, memory and attention are usually impaired, especially concerning recent events. Emotions in those with depression are usually of sadness while those with dementia may exhibit apathy. Elders with depression have little concern about personal appearance because of a lack of motivation, in contrast to those with dementia who exhibit inappropriate dress and actions. Physical symptoms of anorexia, weight loss, fatigue, insomnia, and constipation may accompany depression along with an exaggerated sense of impending problems.

Assessment of Depression in the Assisted Living Facility

As noted earlier, although administrators may not administer assessment tests or screenings for depression, an understanding of strategies to assess for this problem can be of benefit in the assisted living facility environment. As discussed earlier, a routine, comprehensive health history as well as performing depression screening should be conducted on elders suspected of depression. Many elders with depression have decreased energy, increased dependency, difficulty in activities of daily living resulting in poor grooming, withdrawal from friends, family members, or prior activities, and a preoccupation with death (Touhy & Jett, 2018).

There are a number of screening instruments designed to measure depression that can be used in assisted living facilities. One of the more widely used screenings includes the Beck Depression Inventory, a 13-item questionnaire that inventories mood, self-image, and somatic complaints (Beck & Beck, 1972). A score of 16 or higher on this instrument indicates severe depression. The instrument has been shown to be reliable and valid, measuring changes in depression intensity over time (Beck & Beck, 1972).

The Geriatric Depression Scale is a widely used 15-item self-rated scale designed for use with older adults to assess for depression by reducing an emphasis on physical complaints, lack of appetite, and sex drive (Touhy & Jett, 2018). This depression scale has been shown to be accurate, feasible, and acceptable for use in a number of clinical settings.

Types of Depression

Administrators can benefit from understanding the types of depression that may impact elders, especially those residing in assisted living facilities. Minor, subthreshold, or subclinical depression, occurs with few or minor symptoms. Major depression occurs with a number of serious symptoms, sometimes requiring hospitalization or medication. Current thinking about depression maintains that minor and major depressions are distinguished by symptom severity (Miller, 2009). Suicide is a very serious consequence of late-life depression. Suicide rates are higher in older adults than the national average and are more common among nursing home residents (Substance Abuse and Mental Health Services Administration, 2011). These rates do not reflect unrecognized suicidal acts such as failure to eat, failure to take medications appropriately, and other acts of self-neglect (Miller, 2009). Risk factors for suicide in elders residing in senior living communities include mental illness, substance abuse and substance misuse, physical illness and disabilities, family history of suicide, low self-esteem, social isolation, major life transitions, financial problems, and loss of autonomy (Substance Abuse and Mental Health Services Administration, 2011).

Strategies to Promote Optional Functioning in Depression

Assisted living administrators can work with staff and elders to address depression through a number of strategies. The benefits of exercise to reduce depression are well documented. Educating elders to recognize the benefits of exercise can also serve to prevent depression. In assisted living communities, group exercise programs may be of benefit to those with depression as well for other elders.

Nutrition is another beneficial intervention for elders with depression. Good nutrition has overall positive effects on general health, mental health, and overall functioning. For those with depression, poor eating habits, anorexia, and negative nutritional status, depression may increase as well as create a number of other physical and psychological problems (Miller, 2009). Malnutrition can be a consequence of serious depression in elders, leading to a number of serious or life-threatening problems. Use of nutritional supplements as well as dietary interventions can be used to treat depression. Diets should include foods high in tryptophan and phenylalanine, including meat, poultry, fish, and soybeans (Miller, 2009).

Patient education and counseling services are interventions that can be of benefit to elders with depression. There are a number of therapies that may be used in the treatment of depression. Some of these therapies include behavioral therapy with an emphasis on problem-solving, cognitive therapy that focuses on restructuring negative thoughts, interpersonal therapy with an emphasis on exploring relationships, supportive therapy designed to facilitate choices to improve coping, and bibliotherapy, which focuses on reading and exercises to reduce dysfunctional thought processes (Miller, 2009). Additionally, elders with depression may also benefit from group therapy sessions. Group therapy sessions can provide elders with information on depression, improve social interactions, improve self-esteem, and facilitate personal development (Miller, 2009).

Health promotion interventions can be used to alleviate depression. These interventions include the use of regular exercise and the avoidance of smoking, caffeine, and artificial sweeteners. The consumption of alcohol should also be evaluated and moderate or large quantities should be avoided.

Complementary and alternative therapies may also be of benefit to elders with depression. Bright light therapy used on a daily basis may reduce depression. Aromatherapy, including the use of rose, lavender, sage, bergamot, chamomile, basil, and jasmine, may also serve to reduce depression. Art, yoga, dance, imagery, meditation, relaxation, stress management, and spiritual healing are additional strategies designed to reduce depression (Miller, 2009). Some elders may wish to discuss the use of these therapies, such as taking St John's Wort for the treatment of mild to moderate depression, with their physicians or providers of herbal treatments.

Best Practices

In addition to strategies designed to improve depression, administrators, staff, and residents in a number of assisted living facilities have been recognized for practices that support treatment of aging individuals with depression. Best practices in the area of depression and suicide prevention will be identified and briefly discussed. Depression and suicide are significant problems for many elders. These services are focused specifically on the needs of older adults at risk for these problems. The services provided include counseling, assessment, connections with others, and crisis intervention referrals. The center also provides elders with a number of support groups and telephone hotlines for older individuals experiencing grief or traumatic loss, and for survivors of suicide.

Resources Available to Assisted Living Administrators

Administrators have a number of resources available to assist in the provision of services for depressed elders. Psychologists, gerontologists, registered nurses, social workers, and nutritionists can provide assistance in the assessment and treatment of depression ranging from mild to severe. Online resources can also provide current information on best practices in dealing with depression. Some of these resources include the American Association of Retired Persons, the National Institute of Mental Health, the National Institutes of Health, and the National Institute on Aging.

Alcohol and Substance Abuse Issues

Assisted living administrators need to clearly understand issues related to alcohol and substance abuse in elders residing in assisted living facilities. These are problems that are widespread, poorly understood, and difficult to treat in all age groups, especially in older persons. A number of authors note that problems with alcohol frequently go undetected in the elderly population. Because many elders are not working or spending time in social settings, they are able to drink without observation. Alcoholism is the third most prevalent psychiatric disorder in older men but frequently is unrecognized. In the United States, problems related to alcohol account for 6.7% of elders aged 65 and over have problems related to alcohol (Touhy & Jett, 2018). Older persons are at significant risk for alcohol-related problems because of age-related physiologic changes, in which decreases in lean body mass, higher body water mass, and changes in liver function influence the body's ability to metabolize even small quantities of alcohol. Elders frequently have a number of chronic illnesses, and use a number of medications that also impact alcohol metabolism. Additionally, dietary changes and smaller body size also influence alcohol metabolism.

Physiologic problems related to alcohol use are frequently seen in elders. Specific problems with nutrition include malnutrition due in part to failure to eat nutritious foods on a regular basis. Weight loss and anorexia may be seen in individuals with heavy alcohol use. Decreases in gastric absorption of nutrients and osteomalacia, or thinning of the bones, also occurs with increased alcohol use. Changes in liver function and cirrhosis of the liver are frequently seen as consequences of increased alcohol consumption. A number of neurological changes are associated with increased alcohol use. Changes in gait and motor function increase the risk for accidents, falls, and possible fractures, especially hip fractures. Changes in cognitive functioning may cause significant problems with memory, along with the ability to process information. Elders who abuse alcohol may experience problems with depression and may also exhibit symptoms associated with dementia. Because alcohol has a generalized effect on the central nervous system, learning, judgment, and reasoning are altered, as are social and emotional functioning. When elders consume large quantities of alcohol, they may experience drowsiness and stupor, leading to serious motor coordination problems and risks for serious falls.

Factors Influencing Alcohol and Substance Abuse in Elders

There are a number of factors that influence alcohol and substance abuse in elders. Administrators can assist elders in their facilities by understanding some of the factors that cause or contribute to alcohol and substance abuse. Many researchers note that elders use alcohol and prescription medications to deal with chronic pain. Elders with problems, such as arthritis, myalgia, and prior hip fractures, are at risk for chronic pain. Many of these individuals will use alcohol and other substances in an attempt to reduce and relieve pain. Opioids are increasingly being prescribed for use in the management of both short-term and chronic pain. Use of high-daily-dose opioids increases risks for many adverse events (Musich et al., 2019). Many elders prescribed opioids for chronic pain engage in misuse behaviors by taking more medications than prescribed or by abusing opioids, thereby causing significant social, occupational, or health problems (Chang, 2018). As noted earlier, many elders suffer from depression. The use of alcohol and other medications to self-treat depression are well described in the literature and in fact; depression is considered to be a major risk factor for alcohol abuse (Touhy & Jett, 2018). Social changes experienced by elders are a well-known contributing factor to alcohol and substance abuse. The changes associated with moving into assisted living facilities may contribute to or increase the risk for potential abuse. Social isolation can occur among elders living alone or living in institutional settings such as assisted living facilities, and is a problem that is well described in the literature. Also well described is the use of alcohol and other substances by elders as they attempt to deal with significant and serious problems associated with social isolation. Also well described in the literature are problems associated with grieving and loss. Many elders use alcohol and drugs to cope with losses and the depression that frequently accompanies grief and loss.

Assessment for Alcohol Abuse in Assisted Living Communities

Assessment for alcohol abuse in elders residing in assisted living communities should be performed whenever alcohol abuse is suspected. Descriptions of the criteria for alcohol dependence and alcohol abuse, as well as commonly used assessment strategies, can provide useful information to administrators.

The American Psychiatric Association (2000) criteria for alcohol dependence include three or more of the following problems: (a) tolerance or drinking more alcohol to get the same effects; (b) withdrawal or drinking to prevent withdrawal symptoms; (c) drinking in larger quantities or for longer time periods than expected; (d) unsuccessful efforts to quit drinking; (e) spending a lot of time obtaining or using alcohol, or recovering from the effects of alcohol; (f) giving up social or recreational activities to drink alcohol; and (g) drinking despite the presence of physical or psychological problems. The American Psychological Association (2000) criteria for alcohol abuse include one or more of the following problems: (a) drinking resulting in the failure to complete major obligations; (b) drinking in situations that are physically hazardous for the individual; (c) drinking that results in alcohol-related legal problems; and (d) continued drinking despite social problems that are alcohol-related.

One screening test for alcohol dependency and abuse in widespread use is the CAGE questionnaire. This questionnaire is a self-reported screening instrument that asks respondents to answer four questions. CAGE is a mnemonic formed by first letter of the four questions: (a) Have you ever felt the need to cut down on ycut down, a question that elicits attempts to cut down on drinking (b) Have people annoyed you by criticizing your drinking? (c) Have you ever felt guilty about drinking? and (d) eye opener, a question related to the use of alcohol in the morning to remain functional Have you ever felt the need for an eye-opener first thing in the morning (Ewing, 1984)? One or more positive responses to the CAGE questions is strongly indicative of alcohol-related problems. The CAGE questionnaire has been found to be both sensitive and specific in recognizing problems with alcohol (Mauk, 2018).

Assessment for alcohol and substance abuse should also include information from screening health histories. Health professionals should plan to increase awareness of substance abuse issues to include integration of mental health and sleep management in evaluation and interventions for elders on opioids (Musich et al., 2019). Many assisted living communities require that elders be assessed as they enter the facility and evaluated at regular intervals. Questions about drug use should be focused on the number and types of prescription drugs used on a regular basis, as well as the use of over-the-counter drugs, vitamins, and herbal remedies. Elders should also be questioned about their use of illicit or street drugs, the types of drugs used, and the frequency of drug use. It is also important for elders to indicate their reasons for using drugs, especially if these drugs are used in the treatment of pain, depression, sleep disturbances, or other problems.

Strategies to Deal With Alcohol and Substance Abuse in Assisted Living Communities

Administrators in assisted living communities can benefit from an understanding of strategies that can be used to address alcohol and substance abuse problems. There are a number of steps in the treatment of alcoholism that may be used in assisted living communities. Initially, screening tests should be conducted to identify elders with alcohol problems requiring treatment. Secondly, the individual's willingness and readiness to discuss treatment needs to be identified. Thirdly, individuals who need hospitalization for detoxification from alcohol and/or drugs need to be identified. Finally, care plans should be made for elders following detoxification (Mauk, 2018).

Elders with alcohol and substance abuse should be referred to experts for evaluation and treatment. Referrals to physicians and alcohol treatment specialists are a recommended first step in addressing abuse problems. Psychologists, nurses, social workers, and gerontologists can provide expertise in addressing these problems. Additionally, a number of professional counseling, group counseling, and social support groups have been found to be beneficial. There are a number of local and national alcohol treatment programs that elders can utilize. Of special note is Alcoholics Anonymous, a world-wide self-help group with an established record of services for alcoholics. Elders in assisted living communities can benefit from referrals to this organization.

Most experts agree that hospitalization should be required for elders who are dependent on alcohol. Because elders are frail, have diminished physical and psychological reserves, and frequently have a number of coexisting medical conditions, they are at increased risk for problems during alcohol withdrawal and detoxification. Delirium and seizures are more commonly seen in elders withdrawing from alcohol use (Mauk, 2018). Acute agitation and hallucinations may also accompany alcohol withdrawal. These problems are best managed in a hospital setting. A number of medications can be used to assist elders as they withdraw from alcohol. Drugs, such as benzodiazepines, can be used in the detoxification process. Following the acute detoxification process, elders will need to have supportive counseling services to assist in the recovery process.

Resources Available to Assisted Living Administrators

Assisted living administrators can access a number of resources in dealing with alcohol and substance abuse issues. As noted earlier, there are a number of professionals who can assist in the assessment of alcohol and substance abuse, including physicians, nurses, social workers, and alcohol abuse experts. Evaluation and treatment of elders with alcohol dependence and abuse problems should be conducted by professionals with expertise in this area. Physicians and alcohol abuse experts need to be consulted when elders require detoxification from alcohol. Online resources can provide current and relevant information for administrators. Alcoholics Anonymous and the Council on Alcoholism have websites that provide important information and resources for understanding alcoholism. The National Institute on Aging, the National Institute of Mental Health, and the American Association of Retired Persons also serve as important sites for administrators.

CASE STUDY

SG is a long-term assisted living community resident with many friends among the residents and facility staff. A retired school teacher, SG has participated in many of the facility events and has contributed to several facility educational programs. Several of her friends have noted that SG has become more forgetful in the past 6 months, forgetting the location of her keys, credit cards, and check book on a regular basis. When her friends commented on her increased forgetfulness, SG became very angry, indicating that she was not forgetful but distracted because of the weather and the poor economy. Concerned about SG, her friends asked the staff and the administrator to help resolve her forgetfulness. The administrator worked with staff members to use a best practice to assess SG's mental status. The staff administered the Mini-Cog, a brief screening instrument designed to differentiate individuals with dementia from those without

(continued)

CASE STUDY

dementia. The Mini-Cog consists of two mental status tests: three-item recall and the Clock-Drawing Test (Doerflinger, 2007).

SG agreed to take the Mini-Cog screening exam and the staff determined that her scores on both the three-item recall and the Clock-Drawing Test strongly indicated that SG had dementia. SG was then referred to her physician, who diagnosed SG with early-onset Alzheimer's disease. The administrator and staff were then able to work with SG and to also provide counseling and support for SG's friends. While SG continued with progressively worsening forgetfulness, her friends found the counseling and support from both the administrator and the staff to be extremely helpful.

CONCLUSIONS

Assisted living administrators can improve their work with elders through a comprehensive understanding of normal psychological changes associated with the aging process. As noted in this chapter, an understanding of selected psychological issues, including memory changes, and the assessment of memory, dementia, depression, and alcohol abuse can also provide administrators with valuable information that can be used to enhance services to elderly residents. Best practices can provide administrators with information and examples of strategies for approaching some of the psychological issues present in aging individuals.

REFERENCES

Alzheimer's Disease International. (2013). *Policy brief for G8 heads of government. The global impact of dementia 2013–2050.* Alzheimer's Disease International.

American Psychiatric Association. Committee on Nomenclature and Statistics. (2000). *Diagnostic and statistical manual of mental disorders* (4th ed., text revision). American Psychiatric Association.

Beck, A. T., & Beck, R. W. (1972). Screening depressed patients in family practice: A rapid technique. *Postgraduate Medicine, 52,* 81–85. https://doi.org/10.1080/00325481.1972.11713319

Chang, Y. P. (2018). Factors associated with prescription opioid misuse in adults aged 50 or older. *Nursing Outlook, 66,* 112–120. https://doi.org/10.1016/j.outlook.2017.10.007

Doerflinger, D. M. C. (2007). The Mini-Cog. *American Journal of Nursing, 107*(12), 62–71. https://doi.org/10.1097/01.NAJ.0000301030.81651.66

Ewing, J. A. (1984). Detecting alcoholism: The CAGE questionnaire. *Journal of the American Medical Association, 252,* 1905–1907. https://doi.org/10.1001/jama.1984.03350140051025

Linton, A. D., & Lach, H. W. (2007). *Gerontological nursing. Concepts and practice* (3rd ed.). Saunders Elsevier.

Mariske, M., & Margrett, J. A. (2006). Everyday problem solving and decision making. In J. E. Birrin & K. W. Schaie (Eds.), *Handbook of the psychology of aging* (6th ed., pp. 57–83). Academic Press.

Mauk, K. L. (2018). *Gerontological nursing. Competencies for care.* (4th ed.). Jones & Bartlett.

Miller, C. A. (2009). *Wellness in older adults* (5th ed.). Wolters Kluwer Lippincott Williams & Wilkins.

Morris, J. C. (2005). Dementia update 2005. *Alzheimer Disease and Associated Disorders, 19,* 100–116. https://doi.org/10.1097/01.wad.0000167923.56275.d8

Musich, S., Wang, S. S., Slindee, L., Kraemer, S., & Yeh, C. S. (2019). Prevalence and characteristics associated with high dose opioid users among older adults. *Geriatric Nursing, 40,* 31–36. https://doi.org/10.1016/j.gerinurse.2018.06.001

Substance Abuse and Mental Health Services Administration. (2011). *A guide to promoting emotional health and preventing suicide in senior living communities.* U.S. Department of Health and Human Services.

Tabloski, P. A. (2006). *Gerontological nursing* (3rd ed.). Pearson Education.

Touhy, T. A., & Jett, K. (2018). *Ebersole and Hess' gerontological nursing and healthy aging* (5th ed.). Elsevier.

World Health Organization. (2012). *Dementia: A public health priority.* Author.

MEMORY CARE UNITS IN ASSISTED LIVING: BENEFITS AND CHALLENGES FOR ADMINISTRATORS

LEARNING OBJECTIVES

Upon completion of Chapter 21, the reader will be able to:

- Identify definitions of *neurocognitive disorder.*
- Describe the need for memory care units in assisted living.
- Identify services offered in memory care units in assisted living.
- Describe regulatory requirements for memory care units in assisted living.
- Discuss selected benefits and challenges associated with memory care units in assisted living.
- Apply information about memory care units in a case study.

INTRODUCTION

The number of elders dealing with neurocognitive disorder (also known as *dementia*) is expected to increase on a global level within the next 20 years. The demand for neurocognitive disorder-related care (formerly known as *dementia care*), especially in placement services for elders in the United States, is also expected to sharply increase. Elders residing in assisted living communities will continue to require neurocognitive disorder services across the spectrum of neurocognitive disorder-related disease processes.

Memory care units in assisted living communities offer important care options for affected elders. Administrators need to understand some of the benefits and challenges associated with the management of memory care units. The purpose of this chapter is to briefly define neurocognitive disorder seen in the assisted living setting, identify the need for memory care units, describe important elements of memory care units, review selected regulatory requirements for memory care units, and explore the benefits and challenges faced by assisted living administrators in the management of memory care units. The chapter also includes a memory care unit case study.

DEFINITIONS OF *NEUROCOGNITIVE DISORDER*

In 2013, the American Psychiatric Association's *Diagnostic and Statistical Manual of Mental Disorders* (*DSM-5*) presented a framework for replacing the diagnostic label of dementia with the term *neurocognitive disorder*. Individuals with minor or mild cognitive impairments are now identified as possessing mild neurocognitive disorders and individuals with significant impairments as possessing major neurocognitive disorders (APA, 2013).

Although some reductions in memory or cognitive slowing are considered to be components of normal aging processes, changes compromising either occupational or social functions are suggestive of either mild or major neurocognitive disorders (Hugo & Ganguli, 2014). Clinicians are faced with the challenges of identifying both the nature and extent of cognitive changes.

One of the major neurocognitive impairments seen in elders is Alzheimer's disease. There are more than 5 million individuals in the United States living with Alzheimer's disease, the most common form of neurocognitive disorder in elders. This number is expected to triple by 2050. The specific causes of Alzheimer's disease remain unknown at the present time. In general, the criteria for identifying the neurocognitive disorder associated with Alzheimer's disease include the presence of cognitive or behavioral symptoms associated with: (a) noted decline in prior levels of functioning and performance, (b) interference with an ability to function at usual activities or work, (c) poor judgment, (d) impaired language functions, (e) impaired ability to remember or acquire new information, (f) changes in personality or behavior, and (g) changes that cannot be explained by major psychiatric disorders or delirium (Mauk, 2018). Elders exhibiting symptoms of neurocognitive disorder with additional symptoms may be exhibiting Alzheimer's disease. Additional symptoms include: (a) insidious onset of symptoms over months to years, (b) clearly observed cognitive worsening, (c) impaired reasoning and problem-solving, (d) impaired learning and recall of information, (e) word-finding difficulties, and (f) impaired facial recognition (Mauk, 2018).

Older persons with Alzheimer's disease or neurocognitive disorder are diagnosed by clinicians who conduct routine physical examinations, checking for abnormalities in blood counts, thyroid function, or changes in endocrine function. Neurological testing may also reveal changes associated with neurocognitive disorder. At the present time, there are no specific lab tests or imaging studies available to accurately diagnose Alzheimer's disease or neurocognitive disorder.

The stages of Alzheimer's disease can be identified to aid in the management of elders with this neurocognitive disorder. In the first or mild stage of the disease, the elder has symptoms that are subtle, intermittent, not readily observed by the elder or family members, and frequently attributed to aging. In the second or moderate stage of the disease, the elder has psychological or behavioral symptoms, including short attention span, difficulty with learning new things, agitation, anxiety, increased memory loss, repetitive statements or movements, delusions, paranoia, impulsivity, and an inability to complete activities of daily living (ADL). In the third or most severe stage of Alzheimer's disease, the elder experiences weight loss, seizures, difficulty swallowing, incontinence, contractures, and an inability to recognize family members or friends (Alzheimer's Association, 2016; Mauk, 2018). Current research is focused on strategies to diagnose the risk for developing Alzheimer's disease as well as disease prevention. The development of drugs to treat all stages of Alzheimer's disease is also currently in process.

Although assisted living administrators do not manage or treat elders with neurocognitive disorder or Alzheimer's disease, they can benefit from an understanding of these disease processes. Elders residing in memory care units may have neurocognitive disorder from multiple causes, including vascular disease, traumatic brain injuries, and cognitive problems related to accidents or other illnesses. The majority of elders in memory care units will have a diagnosis of Alzheimer's disease. Management of memory care units requires an understanding of current information regarding the assessment and best approaches to care delivery for patients with cognitive decline.

NEED FOR MEMORY CARE UNITS

As noted, because of increases in the number of elders with neurocognitive disorder and Alzheimer's disease, the need for memory care units is growing. Without known causes or cures, the burdens of caregiving for family members with neurocognitive disorder currently reside with family members, friends, and other unpaid, untrained caregivers. Estimates place the number of Americans providing these unpaid services at 15 million individuals who spent about 18.2 billion care hours at a cost of over $230 billion (Assisted Living Today, 2017). As baby boomers age and the numbers of elders increases annually, estimates for the numbers of elders requiring services and the numbers of individuals required for neurocognitive disorder care delivery will continue to significantly increase.

Currently, assisted living communities provide services and appropriate care delivery for elders with early or mild Alzheimer's disease. Elders with mild neurocognitive disorder symptoms may not have significant cognitive changes or significant numbers of medical problems. Many of these individuals do require more assistance and support with one or more ADL that add to quality of life as well as those activities necessary for daily functioning. Elders who fall into these functional categories are able to do well within assisted living settings and do not require placement in a memory care unit.

The elder with mild or even moderate neurocognitive disorder can benefit from living in an assisted living community where a certain degree of independence can be maintained on a regular basis. Elders with mild or moderate neurocognitive disorder can function more independently in settings with secure areas and care in areas, including medication administration (Assisted Living Today, 2017).

Elders with moderate or severe neurocognitive disorder fall into a category of care requiring closer monitoring. Memory care units provide higher levels of skilled care and professional supervision. Supervision in these special care units is offered on a 24-hour basis by staff members who have the training to assist with the special needs of neurocognitive disorder patients. Services offered to elders in memory care units may also include memory stimulation activities, including puzzles, crafts, and games. Structurally, memory care units offer both shared and private spaces and may be connected to assisted living settings or in independent settings.

ADDITIONAL MEMORY CARE UNIT SERVICES

Assisted living administrators can benefit from an understanding of the additional services offered in memory care units. These services include rehabilitation programs, focused nutritional strategies, and daily activities for patients with moderate to severe Alzheimer's and other neurocognitive disorders. IN addition, administrators need to have an awareness of differences between assisted living settings and memory care units.

Rehabilitation Programs

Rehabilitation is a critical element of care provision in memory care units. The goal of rehabilitation programs for neurocognitive disorder patients is to slow the progression of Alzheimer's disease and other neurodegenerative, neurocognitive disorders. Rehabilitation programs also serve to reduce or alleviate many neurocognitive disorder symptoms, including aggression and agitation (Assisted Living Today, 2017). Physical and occupational therapists work with patients to provide therapies to strengthen muscles, improve balance and reduce falls, increase mobility, facilitate ADL, and promote exercise through gait-training exercises. Sensory stimulation and a number of cognitive therapies administered by physicians, nurses, psychologists, and social workers are also components of rehabilitation programs. Music therapy, art therapy, and group activities are also offered to address and slow neurocognitive disorder progression (Assisted Living Today, 2017).

Nutritional Strategies

Administrators need to understand the strategies necessary to maintain adequate nutrition in Alzheimer's and other neurocognitive disorder patients. Changes in cognition are often accompanied by a lack of appetite or lack of interest in eating. Administrators can employ dieticians to ensure that neurocognitive disorder patients have adequate nutritional intake on a daily basis. The challenges associated with these issues can be met by providing small, frequent meals, offering flexible and varied food choices, and contrasting the color of the foods with serving plates to enhance the appeal of the foods offered at meal sessions.

Daily Activities

Administrators in memory care units have opportunities to increase the activities offered to Alzheimer's and other neurocognitive disorder patients on a regular or daily basis. Recreational specialists can work in these settings to provide activities designed to enhance memory. Some of these activities include physical and cognitive exercises, nature programs, participation in a number of reminiscence activities, including story-telling, letter writing, creating memory books or boxes, or patient and family participation in video or audiotaped family histories. Patients with moderate neurocognitive disorder may benefit from carefully structured field trips, music therapy, and art therapy. Neurocognitive disorder patients may also benefit from participation in pet therapy with regular exposure to therapy animals, including dogs, cats, or birds. Aromatherapy is also used as a daily activity in a number of memory care units.

Differences Between Assisted Living Settings and Memory Care Units

Assisted living administrators should have a clear understanding of identified differences between care delivery in assisted living settings and dedicated memory care units. These differences include: (a) physical structure of settings; (b) security; (c) staff; (d) approach to medication management; and (e) service costs. Each of these differences will be discussed further.

Physical Structure

The physical structure of memory care units differs from units in assisted living communities. The architectural design of many memory care units is circular rather than linear so that patients with moderate neurocognitive disorder do not experience stress or disorientation when walking in hallways that abruptly end. Patients can also move more freely in settings that are circular. Patient safety should limit patient wandering. Painting communal areas in memory care units with bright colors frequently reduces stress and supports relaxation in neurocognitive disorder patients as does the use of natural rather than artificial lighting. Memory care units are frequently smaller in size than other assisted living units and do not have the kitchens that are frequently seen is assisted living units. Memory care units are designed to be inclusive with dining facilities, living areas, and activities all contained within the same space. This keeps neurocognitive disorder patients secure and helps to reduce overall symptoms of stress and anxiety.

Security

Security is an issue for patients with moderate to severe neurocognitive disorder. Although assisted living communities provide security for all patients, memory care units are designed to promote enhanced security and reduce the wandering prevalent in many patients with moderate neurocognitive disorder. Security measures include units that are locked with access controlled by keypads; secure entrances and exits; controlled access to outdoor areas, elevators, and stairs; use of securityncameras in public areas; and around-the-clock supervision (Senior Living Care, n.d.). Door and elevator alarms are designed to alert staff if neurocognitive disorder patients are trying to wander. Staff and visitors access memory care units only with authorization.

Individual security measures are used primarily in memory care units and may include personal bed and wheelchair alarms or electronic alarm bracelets (Senior Living Care, n.d.). An electronic seat alarm alerts patients and staff about patients trying to stand without assistance and electronic bed alarms alert staff about patients trying to get out of bed without help. The use of these alarms is potentially beneficial for patients with neurocognitive disorder who are at risk for falls (Assisted Living Today, 2017).

Staffing

There are differences in the staff employed in assisted living settings and staff working in memory care units. Staffing in both assisted living settings and memory care units primarily includes RNs, licensed vocational nurses (LVNs), and nursing assistants who may be certified (CNA) or uncertified. All staff in assisted living facilities are trained to assist patients with ADL and work to address individual patient needs, especially for patients with mild neurocognitive disorder. Staff members in memory care units are trained to assist neurocognitive disorder patients who have moderate to advanced disease with ADL and to address specific care requirements associated with more advanced disease. Memory care staff have received training in understanding how Alzheimer's disease and other neurocognitive disorders impact behaviors, how to communicate with neurocognitive disorder patients, and how to respond to many of the challenges associated with care of Alzheimer's patients.

Sufficient staff-to-patient care ratios in assisted living communities as well as in memory care units are determined by individual communities or by state regulations. There are no set guidelines for what governs sufficient or adequate staffing ratios in assisted living facilities. The staffing ratios for memory care units are not governed at the national level. Many states have regulations that determine staff-to-patient ratios in these settings. Memory care units are staffed, however, at higher staff-to-patient ratios and in many settings there is one staff member for every five to six patients to reflect increased care requirements for patients with more complex problems and more care needs. Staffing for both of these units is composed primarily of LVNs and CNAs with RNs providing direct patient care services as well as supervising LVNs and unlicensed personnel.

Medication Management

The approach to medication management also differs between assisted living settings and memory care units. Medication management in assisted living communities is governed by state regulations. Some states allow patients to self-administer medications while other states require trained staff to administer all medications. Patients with moderate to severe Alzheimer's disease or other neurocognitive disorders need assistance with all medication administration. The way patients receive medications in memory care units is also regulated in many states.

The use of cannabidiol (CBD) has become popular for Alzheimer's and neurocognitive disorder patients. Patients who can self-administer medications may also be able to use CBD. Patients in memory care units are not be able to independently use CBD. Variability in the legal status of this compound complicates its use in both assisted living and memory care settings and administrators will need to identify the state laws governing use of CBD in specific assisted living or memory care units.

Service Costs

Service costs also differ for assisted living settings and memory care units. The costs of assisted living care are lower than memory care units due to increased staffing and patient care ratios required for patients with more complex problems associated with more advanced neurocognitive disorder. The security measures and physical requirements in memory care units also increase overall monthly costs for these services. Overall costs for both types of service depend on the level of service and the degree of the neurocognitive disorder severity. Variability in the state and geographic location of the facility, the type of room selected, and the level of care required are all factors influencing the costs of care delivery. Because these services are not provided in skilled nursing settings, the overall costs of services in both areas are covered by private patient funds.

REGULATORY REQUIREMENTS FOR MEMORY CARE UNITS

Assisted living administrators responsible for supervision and oversight of memory care units will need to understand and carefully adhere to a number of regulatory requirements for this care delivery model. Regulations and accreditation requirements for memory care units occur at the national, federal, and state levels. The Joint Commission accreditation requirements for memory care units operating in nursing care centers are issued at the national level. Regulations from the Centers for Medicare and Medicaid Services (CMS) are issued at the federal level. Regulations for neurocognitive disorder care are also issued at the state level. Regulatory requirements at the national, federal, and state levels will be reviewed further.

The Joint Commission Accreditation Requirements

The Joint Commission, a national accrediting agency, established memory care unit requirements in 2014 with the overarching purpose of ensuring that patients with neurocognitive disorder are able to function at the highest level possible for the longest time possible and to remain engaged in their immediate environment at the highest cognitive ability level (Joint Commission, 2014). Memory care unit requirements are now a component of nursing care center accreditation processes. Key elements for care provision for patients with Alzheimer's disease or neurocognitive disorder form the basis for accreditation and include the following: (a) care coordination with a focus on staff collaboration to assess, plan, and implement care that is congruent with advances in neurocognitive disorder care; (b) staff competency and knowledge in the area of memory impairment that is consistent with the necessary education, skills, and training for the care of patients with neurocognitive disorder; (c) programming of patient activities that match the patient's memory, cognitive abilities, language, reasoning abilities, and physical abilities; (d) understanding how to use nonpharmacological interventions as alternatives to antipsychotics for behavior management of patients with neurocognitive disorder; and (e) creation of a physical environment that is modified to promote safety, minimize confusion, and prevent overstimulation in patients with neurocognitive disorder (Joint Commission, 2014). All memory care units operating in nursing care centers accredited by the Joint Commission must demonstrate compliance with these five key elements and the administrator of these memory care units must provide the necessary evidence for compliance with these elements.

In addition to the key elements, The Joint Commission also requires that administrators of memory care units in nursing care centers meet a series of accreditation standards. These standards require that (a) organizations have necessary staffing, including RN, licensed vocational nurse, and nursing assistant staff, to meet all of the individual needs of neurocognitive disorder patients; (b) all staff participate in annual training and education that is alignment with current neurocognitive disorder care best practices, including knowledge of symptoms and progression of neurocognitive disorder, communication techniques, approaches to unmet needs, and abuse prevention; (c) all staff are competent to perform their duties and have access to knowledge-based resources; (d) care, treatment, and services provided to residents have medical director oversight; (e) use of psychotropic medications are monitored by the medical director and the organization to minimize misuse; (f) the organization assesses and reassesses all patients and includes the patient and family members in the assessment process as much as possible; (g) patients without an established neurocognitive disorder diagnosis be evaluated by a neurologist, geriatrician, or psychiatrist; (h) the organization provides a personalized approach to care and care planning to include activities that promote quality of life; (i) the organization employs an interdisciplinary team to discuss care, treatment, and family services; (j) direct care staff of neurocognitive disorder patients communicate with each other during shifts; (k) the organization makes food and nutrition products available to patients; (l) patients have opportunities to participate in social and recreational activities; (m) when a patient is transferred or discharged from the memory unit, information is provided to other providers at the time of discharge; and (n) the organization collects data to monitor performance (Joint Commission, 2014). Administrators working in memory care units in nursing care centers must complete comprehensive planning to ensure that the memory care units are in compliance with all of these regulations.

Regulations of the Centers for Medicare & Medicaid Services

The CMS established standards for the provision of Medicaid-reimbursed home- and community-based services (HCBS) in 2014 (Edwards et al., 2018). Memory care units in assisted living communities serve as an alternative to nursing facility care for individuals with Alzheimer's disease or other neurocognitive disorders and may be physically separate from other sections of the assisted living setting. For assisted living facilities to qualify for Medicaid-reimbursed HCBS, memory unit care must be both supported and integrated with full access to the entire assisted living community. Patients must have opportunities to control their personal resources, receive community services, and fully engage in community life. Memory care units must also ensure freedom from coercion and restraints, ensure the autonomy and independence in making life choices, and ensure every individual's rights of privacy, respect, and dignity (Edwards et al., 2018). Memory care units in provider-owned or controlled settings must adhere to additional regulatory requirements. These requirements include requirements for individual privacy in sleeping or living units, units that have entrance doors lockable by the individual and accessed only by appropriate staff, and schedules and activities that individuals have the freedom to control (Edwards et al., 2018).

The HCBS regulations were designed to recognize the need for possible modifications based on variations in medical conditions and assessed patient need justified in the development of a person-centered service plan. Requirements for these plans include documentation of: (a) specific assessed individual needs, (b) clear descriptions of conditions proportionate to specific assessed needs, (c) informed consent of the individual, and (d) assurances that interventions and supports will not cause any harm to the individual (Edwards et al., 2018).

In memory care settings where there is controlled egress, both an HCBS case manager and the manager of the assisted living and memory care settings should follow the person-centered service plan to carefully document each individual's understanding of setting safety features, choices to prevent unsafe wandering, specific services and environmental designs to promote mobility and activity participation, and the continued need for controlled egress based on scheduled data collection and review (Edwards et al., 2018). Adherence to HCBS plan development, implementation, and review assures administrators that modifications are both necessary and of benefit to the individual neurocognitive disorder patient.

The administrator working in the memory care unit can use a number of best practices for neurocognitive disorder patients as they adopt person-centered strategies. The Alzheimer's Association identifies a number of elements in quality neurocognitive disorder care practice. These elements are focused on: (a) fluid and food consumption to promote optimal nutrition and hydration through meals and snacks that are culturally appropriate; (b) pain management strategies that avoid the overutilization of psychotropic medications while accurately assessing and tailoring pain management for each individual; and (c) opportunities for social engagement that represents fun, meaningful interactions (Alzheimer's Association, 2017).

State Requirements and Regulations

The number of assisted living patients in the United States with Alzheimer's disease or other forms of neurocognitive disorder ranges from 40% to 90% (Zimmerman et al., 2014). As noted, patients with mild neurocognitive disorder do well with fewer staff supports, whereas patients with moderate or severe cognitive decline require the more intensive staff services offered in memory care units. Licensure and monitoring of these settings occurs at the state rather than the federal level, and these regulatory requirements vary from state to state (National Center for Assisted Living, 2019).

There were 28 states regulating neurocognitive disorder care in the United States in 2000 (Mollica et al., 2007). This number increased to 49 states in 2015 (Carder et al., 2015). Twenty-two percent of assisted living settings had identified neurocognitive disorder care designations or distinct neurocognitive disorder care units in 2014 (Harris-Kojetin et al., 2016). Because specific regulations are determined by each state, the variability of requirements for neurocognitive disorder care is significant.

Each state (including the District of Columbia) has a minimum of one neurocognitive disorder care assisted living requirement with levels of regulatory control ranging from low to high. A total of 18 states have low levels of regulatory control with the inclusion of one or more neurocognitive disorder care requirements (Carder, 2017). A total of 17 states require agency review for neurocognitive disorder or memory care units or the provision of neurocognitive disorder care, while a total of 16 states license or certify neurocognitive disorder units separate from assisted living regulations (Carder, 2017). A number of states ($N = 14$) require pre-admission assessments to determine which patients would benefit from neurocognitive disorder care services or units. The assessment criteria are variable ranging from a mental status exam to a comprehensive history and physical functioning exam to behavioral screening (Carder, 2017).

Staffing requirements are variable at the state level. There are 17 states indicating minimal staffing levels and ratios for care in memory or neurocognitive disorder units. There are only 14 states that have specific staff designations, including RNs, social workers, and administrators, as required staff in neurocognitive disorder or memory care units (Carder, 2017).

Administrators in every state must operate assisted living policies and activities with requirements for training that may include specific hours of training and continuing education in a number of training topics, such as understanding neurocognitive disorder and general medical problems of elders (Carder, 2017). State requirements are in contrast to the more comprehensive regulations discussed earlier and required by The Joint Commission.

Many states regulate building design requirements for memory or neurocognitive disorder care units. A total of 29 states require that memory care units have a minimum of one or more of the following: (a) devices for control of building egress, (b) access to controlled outdoor areas, and (c) shared common areas (Carder, 2017). Egress features restricting patient movement out of buildings unescorted are required in 25 states. In addition, some states have requirements for encouraging patients to furnish their rooms and that all rooms be individually identified to aid patients in room recognition, but no states have regulations requiring private bathrooms in neurocognitive disorder units (Carder, 2017).

Assisted living administrators must have a comprehensive understanding of their state regulations and how the state regulations interface with federally mandated Medicare regulations and national requirements of The Joint Commission in the administration of assisted living and memory care units. Understanding the similarity and differences between regulations and requirements can be of benefit to administrators, patients, and families who utilize these units.

BENEFITS AND CHALLENGES OF MEMORY CARE UNITS

Benefits

Memory care units within or connected to assisted living communities are beneficial to patients, families, and staff members. Patients with Alzheimer's disease or neurocognitive disorder are faced with a progressive disease with no cure at the present time. Current treatments for patients focus on assisting and supporting patients as they deal with neurocognitive disorder symptoms. Patients with moderate to severe neurocognitive disorder require careful monitoring to promote safety, prevent injury, and support health and active functioning. Memory care units are designed to accomplish these goals through the creation of an environment that keeps patients from wandering and exiting facilities, while decreasing stress and anxiety through the replacement of long hallways with circular units and the use of soothing paint colors and natural lighting. Memory care units also are designed with staffing necessary to provide more individualized neurocognitive disorder care with a focus on rehabilitation, enhanced nutrition, and activities to enhance memory and promote social interactions with other patients. Additional staffing also ensures patient safety and security.

Patients and families benefit from the inclusion of memory care units within assisted living communities, as patients are able to remain at a facility and transition into a memory care unit rather than having to be discharged into a new long-term care facility. The ability to transfer from one section of an assisted living setting into a memory care unit provides security and support for neurocognitive disorder patients who benefit from this approach. Administrators and staff also benefit from the capacity to continue services for patients who are viewed many times as family members.

Challenges

Administrators note there are challenges associated with memory care units in assisted living communities. Regulatory requirements for memory care units present challenges. Unique building requirements and different life safety codes for dedicated memory care units increase both costs and complexity of unit administration (Honn, 2019). Staffing in memory units requires higher staff-to-patient ratios, additional specialized training requirements as well as costs for staff members. Staff retention can present both employment challenges and increased labor-cost pressures (Honn, 2019). The demand for stand-alone memory care units has not grown as quickly as the demand for assisted living units with a range of neurocognitive services (Adler, 2018).

A major challenge within the concept of memory care is focused on the need to balance the critical importance of elder personal freedom with the need to ensure elder safety. In addition to curtailing personal freedom, the rapid growth of memory care units has created a number of potential health and safety risks for elders residing in these units. Elopement, falls, violence, and aggression are examples of serious problems associated with memory care units (Assisted Living/Senior Living, 2019). Memory care resident elopement is a major area of concern for staff and administrators in memory care units. Many report negative outcomes for elders who elope from memory care units (Assisted Living/Senior Living, 2019).

Memory care units also require additional professional services for residents. These services add additional training requirements and additional costs to care as opposed to service costs in assisted living facilities. The care in these specialized units increases service costs for agencies and also significantly increases costs for the elders residing in these units. Additional costs, care delivery complexity, increased regulatory requirements, and an overall reduction in elder personal freedom are many of the challenges associated with memory care units.

CASE STUDY

AH is a 90-year-old male who has been happily living in an assisted living community for the past 6 years. AH is well liked by both the staff and his many friends and he enjoys singing at weekly music sessions to "entertain the old people." Although AH has experienced forgetfulness in the past, his ability to remember and retain new information has decreased in the past 6 months as has his ability to remember the names of staff members who have cared for him during the past 6 years. AH complains of difficulties in sleeping, blaming nearby assisted living residents for large and very loud parties that wake him up at night despite the fact that none of the residents play loud music or hold parties during evening hours.

Over the past 6 months, staff members have noted that AH has stopped singing and spends more time wandering in the halls and trying to walk into patient rooms throughout the assisted living community. When questioned, he states he is not lost, just trying to say hi and talk with his friends. He is adamant that he is not having any problems. On

(continued)

CASE STUDY

multiple occasions in the past 3 months, the night staff found AH at the locked entrance of the facility in the middle of the night. When questioned, AH stated he was just going out to get his cat and would be back to the building very shortly. Although AH once did have a cat in his room at the assisted living community, the cat died of old age 5 years ago. AH became very belligerent when the staff would not allow him to leave the building. When he was not able to exit the locked entrance doors he threatened to call the police and his attorneys and sue the facility. AH's friends in the assisted living facility have begun to notice the changes in his memory, his intermittent confusion, and his anger and bellig- erence. His friends have expressed their concerns to members of the facility staff.

The RN and assisted living staff brought their concerns regarding AH to the attention of the assisted living administrator, who initially requested that AH be evaluated by his physician and by the facility social worker. Assessment of AH revealed a diagnosis of moderate neurocognitive disorder probably due to Alzheimer's disease. Following this diagnosis, the administrator, physician, and social worker scheduled a family meeting with AH's three children. The children were presented with the changes in AH's behavior and his diagnosis of moderate neurocognitive disorder and care options were discussed. The children initially argued that the observed changes in AH's behavior were probably due to poorly trained staff, old age, or a lack of exercise. They all noted that they had not observed any changes in AH's behavior. The administrator then asked the family members to consider moving AH into the facility memory unit for safer and more com- prehensive care. Family members expressed concerns about the increased cost of a move to the memory care unit and asked for more time to consider the change.

Several weeks after the family meeting, two of AH's children took him to a local restaurant for an evening birthday dinner. AH left the dinner table to use the restroom. When he did not return after 20 minutes and he was not located in the restroom, his children became concerned. A member of the restaurant staff located AH in a poorly lit parking lot nearby; he was wandering among the parked cars and nearby street traffic. When questioned, AH stated he was only going to get his cat and would be right back, becoming angry when he could not continue to search for his cat.

AH's children returned to the assisted living facility and met again with the adminis- trator. A tour of the memory care unit connected to the assisted living facility was suc- cessful and the administrator was able to refer the family for financial consultation. AH was moved into the memory care unit where he did well as his moderate neurocognitive disorder progressed to severe neurocognitive disorder. AH was comfortable and well cared for in the memory care unit at the time of his death several years later.

CONCLUSIONS

Increases in the numbers of elders with Alzheimer's disease and other forms of neurocognitive disorder require the creation of more services to assist those with these diseases as well as their family members. Many elders with mild neurocognitive disorder currently reside in assisted living communities. Memory care units in these communities can provide needed services for patients with moderate or severe neurocognitive disorder. These units allow individuals to remain in the same facility through transfer into safer and more secure memory care units. The ability of patients to change units without transferring facilities provides patients with stability and the benefits of aginginplace within an agency.

Memory care units provide enhanced rehabilitation, nutrition, and daily living services for patients with moderate neurocognitive disorder. These units also provide the physical environment, staffing, and safety features required to care for these elders. Services are enhanced for elders in memory care units. The costs of these units are greater than traditional assisted living services. Oversight at the national and state levels led to complex memory care unit requirements and regulations to provide safety for consumers. These regulations present a number of increased challenges for assisted living administrators. The benefits of offering memory care units to elders with neurocognitive disorder must be weighed with the significant challenges associated with these specialized care services.

REFERENCES

Adler, J. (2018). *Investors rethink memory care*. seniorhousingbusiness.com/investors-rethink-memory-care

Alzheimer's Association. (2016). Alzheimer's disease facts and figures. *Alzheimer's and Dementia, 12*(4), 1–80. https://doi.org/10.1016/j.jalz.2016.03.001

Alzheimer's Association. (2017). *Neurocognitive disorder care practice recommendations for assisted living residences and nursing homes*. https://www.alz.org/national/documents/brochure_DCPRphases1n2pdf

American Psychiatric Association. (2013). *Diagnostic and statistical manual of mental disorders* (5th ed). Author.

Assisted Living Today. (2017). *What is memory care and how much should it cost?* https://assisted living today.com

Assisted Living/Senior Living. (2019). *Improving safety for memory care residents starts with understanding risks*. pharmerica.com/improving-safety-for-memory-care-residents-starts-with-understanding-risks

Carder, P. C. (2017). State regulatory approaches for dementia care in residential care and assisted living. *The Gerontologist, 57*(4), 776–786. https://doi.org/10.1093/geront/gnw197

Edwards, B.C, Lewis, S., Patterson, R., & Hummel, L. (2018). Home and community-based services settings rule: An effective person-centered planning process is key for memory care units. *National Center for Assisted Living*. www.ncal.org

Harris-Kojetin, L., Sengupta, M., Park-Lee-E., Valverde, R., Caffrey, C., Rome, V., & Lendon, J. (2016). *Long-term providers and services users in the United States: Data from the National Study of Long-Term Care Providers, 2013–2014*. National Center for Health Statistics. http://www.cdc.gov/pubmed.ncbi-nih/gov/27023287

Honn, C. (2019). *Overcoming key operational and financing challenges in memory care facilities*. modernhealthcare.com/finance/overcoming-key-operational-and-financing-challenges-memory-care-facilities

Hugo, J., & Ganguli, M. (2014). Dementia and cognitive impairment: Epidemiology, diagnosis, and treatment. *Clinical Geriatric Medicine, 30*(3), 421–442. https://doi.org/10.1016/j.cger.2014.04.001

Mauk, K. (2018). *Gerontological nursing. Competencies for care* (4th ed.). Jones & Bartlett Learning.

Mollica, R., Sims-Kasterlein, K., & O'Keefe, J. (2007). *Residential care and assisted living compendium*. Office of the Assistant Secretary for Planning and Evaluation, U.S. Department Health and Human Services.

National Center for Assisted Living. (2019). *Assisted Living 2019 Regulatory Review*. Author.

Senior Living. (n.d.). *Finding the best memory care facility*. https://seniorliving.org/memory-care

The Joint Commission. (2014). *Joint Commission Perspectives, 34*(1), 8–13.

Zimmerman, S., Sloan, P. D., & Reed, D. (2014). Dementia prevalence and care in assisted living. *Health Affairs, 4*, 658–666.

FURTHER READING

Dementia Care Central. (2019). *Residential care for dementia: Assisted living, memory care, nursing homes, & other options*. dementiacarecentral.com/memory-care-vs-assisted-living

PALLIATIVE AND HOSPICE CARE

WITH CONTRIBUTING AUTHOR EDWIN P. CABIGAO

LEARNING OBJECTIVES

Upon the completion of Chapter 22, the reader will be able to:

- Describe the definitions, domains, and importance of palliative care.

- Understand hospice care as one component of palliative care.

- Appreciate the benefits and importance of palliative care practices.

- Identify serious chronic disease processes that may benefit from palliative care interventions.

- Become familiar with the importance of psychosocial support, cultural needs, and spirituality as components of the palliative plan of care.

- Discuss the challenges and barriers faced by the assisted living industry in accessing palliative care programs.

- Read about a successful palliative program and how it serves homebound clients in the community.

INTRODUCTION

The philosophies of assisted living (see Chapter 2) most often include provisions regarding privacy, autonomy, and decision-making. When individuals decide on an assisted living community to move into, it is often their belief that they will be able to age in place, meaning that they expect the community will adapt to their changing needs so that relocation is not necessary. The key to aging in place is the community's ability to adjust the level of care to meet the resident's needs and avoid transfer to a higher level of care or skilled nursing facility.

In the past, older adults often moved out of assisted living communities when they developed life-threatening illnesses or critically progressed from their chronic diseases, going mostly to nursing homes with round-the-clock skilled care. But now, it is possible for residents to stay at their assisted living communities even when they are seriously ill because of palliative care and hospice care programs (Jerant et al., 2006).

Over 800,000 Americans reside in assisted living. The majority of these residents are over the age of 85. Furthermore, more than half of them have high blood pressure and four out of 10 are living with Alzheimer's disease or other dementias (National Center for Health Statistics, 2019). Logically, many of these residents may benefit from palliative care as their disease processes progress. Palliative care is gaining increasing attention by medical and long-term care providers as research continues to identify and validate its usefulness. Most private and public insurance companies, including Medicare, have a palliative and/or hospice benefit.

DEFINING *PALLIATIVE CARE*

Definition

The World Health Organization (n.d.) defines *palliative care* as

> an approach that improves the quality of life of patients and their families facing the problem associated with life-threatening illness, through the prevention and relief of suffering by means of early identification and impeccable assessment and treatment of pain and other problems, physical, psychosocial and spiritual.

Palliative care provides relief from pain and other distressing symptoms; affirms life and regards dying as a normal process; intends neither to hasten or postpone death; integrates the psychological and spiritual aspects of patient care; offers a support system to help patients live as actively as possible until death; offers a support system to help the family cope during the patient's illness and in their own bereavement; uses a team approach to address the needs of patients and their families, including bereavement counseling, if indicated; enhances quality of life and may also positively influence the course of illness; is applicable early in the course of illness, in conjunction with other therapies that are intended to prolong life, such as chemotherapy or radiation therapy, and includes those investigations needed to better understand and manage distressing clinical complications (World Health Organization, n.d.).

The Center to Advance Palliative Care (2019) states "the evidence is clear: palliative care improves quality of life for patients—and quality outcomes for healthcare organizations—resulting in consistent reductions in the costs of care." Palliative care is specialized care for people with serious illnesses. The key to this specialized care is its focus on relieving the symptoms, pain, and stress of a serious illness. It aims to improve quality of life for both the patient and the family and to deliver an extra layer of support at any age and at any stage in a critical illness. Palliative care can be provided along with curative treatment. It supports patient and family, not only by controlling symptoms, but also by helping to educate regarding treatment options and goals.

Hospice Care

Considered the best program for quality, compassionate care for people suffering from life-threatening illness, hospice care provides specialized medical care, pain management, and emotional and spiritual support expertly customized for an individual person's needs and wishes, as well as those of the person's family. Hospice care focuses on caring, not curing. In many cases, care is provided in the person's home, but may also be provided in freestanding hospice facilities, hospitals, nursing homes, and assisted living communities.

Hospice care involves a comprehensive delivery model of palliative care, but it is often limited to terminally ill persons. The Medicare Hospice Benefit (n.d.) defines *hospice eligibility* as appropriate for patients when a doctor certifies a prognosis of 6 months to live and the person agrees to waive Medicare coverage for curative treatment.

An expert panel of hospice professionals develops a care plan that meets each person's individual needs for pain management and symptom control. This interdisciplinary team (IDT) usually consists of the person's physician; hospice physician; nurses; hospice aides; social workers; bereavement counselors; clergy or other spiritual counselors; trained volunteers; and speech, physical, and occupational therapists as needed to provide comfort. The hospice team is tasked to:

- Treat and manage a person's pain and other symptoms.
- Assist the person and family members with the emotional, psychosocial, and spiritual aspects of dying.
- Provide medications and medical supplies and equipment.
- Train family on how to care for the person.
- Provide grief support and counseling.
- Make short-term inpatient care available when pain or other symptoms become too difficult to manage.
- Provide bereavement support and counseling to surviving family and friends.

Palliative Care Versus Hospice Care

Hospice and palliative care both offer compassionate and specialized holistic care to persons with life-limiting illnesses. However, palliative care—which is always a component of hospice care—can be used as a separate medical practice while the person is receiving treatment. Palliative care focuses on relieving symptoms associated with the person's condition while receiving active curative treatment. The objective of both hospice and palliative care is pain and symptom relief.

Hospice care is for people experiencing a terminal illness with a prognosis of six months or less, based on their physician's estimate if the disease runs its course as expected. The definition of *palliative care* is compassionate comfort care that provides relief from the symptoms and physical and mental stress of a serious or life-limiting illness. Palliative care can be pursued at diagnosis, during curative treatment and follow-up, and at the end of life.

Both palliative care and hospice care provide comfort. However, palliative care can begin at diagnosis, and at the same time as treatment. Hospice care begins after treatment of the disease is stopped and when it is clear that the person is not going to survive the illness.

Hospice care is covered by Medicare, Medicaid, the Veteran's Health Administration, and some private health insurance providers. Medicare and Medicaid cover hospice care for people with a terminal illness who meet admission criteria (both disease-specific criteria and a prognosis of 6 months or less) at no cost to the person. In some cases, those covered by private health insurance plans may be responsible for co-pays.

Similarly, palliative care is covered by both public and private insurance plans, including Medicare Part A, which covers aspects of care such as social services, nursing visits, and spiritual care, and Medicare Part B offers palliative care coverage for some medications and supplies. Medicaid may offer palliative care services as well, although coverage may vary from state to state. Likewise, many private health insurance plans offer some form of palliative care coverage as part of their long-term care or chronic care benefits, but specific coverage may vary from insurer to insurer, and even among individual insurance plans. One goal of palliative care programs is to provide safe, effective, timely, efficient and equitable resident/family-centered care focused on optimizing function and the relief of suffering. An organized process for coordinating and communicating about care across settings as well as appropriate and timely transition to hospice care supports aging in place and quality of life.

THE PRACTICE OF PALLIATIVE CARE

Hospital-Based Palliative Care

Hospital-based palliative interdisciplinary care teams either provide consultation to the primary physician or manage necessary palliative care programs for patients. Typically, a hospitalized person is referred to a palliative care team to address intractable pain and symptoms; communicate with persons, families, and other care disciplines in order to meet the person's goals of care; or to assist in developing a plan of care for safe discharge to minimize the risk of readmission. In the consultation model, the palliative care team does not assume primary management of care for the person and the family; rather, they function as additional support to address the needs of the person and family as a whole.

Community-Based Palliative Care

Community-based palliative care includes a range of care delivery models customized to meet the needs of seriously ill individuals and their families, outside of the inpatient or hospital setting. Palliative care is provided in the person's home, a skilled nursing facility, an independent living or assisted living community, or in an outpatient clinic such as a physician's office, dialysis unit, or cancer center unit. Community-based palliative care models include advanced illness management (AIM) programs, supportive care programs typically included in cancer centers, and "post-acute" transitional care programs. These care models are currently becoming popular to meet the needs of the sickest persons with the most expense—who must otherwise resort to emergency room transfers, readmission back to the hospital, and other clinical issues that could and should have been prevented in the community.

Palliative care is usually provided by palliative care specialists, healthcare practitioners who have received special training and/or certification in palliative care. Often, palliative care specialists practice as part of an interdisciplinary team that may include doctors, nurses, registered dieticians, pharmacists, chaplains, psychologists, and social workers. The palliative care team works either in conjunction with the hospital or with the community-based care team to manage the person's care and maintain the best possible quality of life. Palliative care specialists also provide caregiver support, facilitate communication among members of the healthcare team, and help with discussions focusing on goals of care for the person.

Palliative care may be provided at any point along the care continuum, from diagnosis to the end of life. When a person receives palliative care, he or she may continue to receive treatment. Palliative care interventions focus on physical suffering and being free from physical symptoms. In addition, Intensive palliative care practice targets psychological, social, emotional, and spiritual suffering (Ellershaw & Ward, 2003). They provide holistic care to the person and family or caregiver, focusing on not just the physical component of suffering, but also the emotional, social, and spiritual issues persons may face during illness. This aspect of non-physical suffering, however, is much more of a personal matter, and factors in individual's beliefs, preferences, religion, and culture (Walter, 2003).

Palliative care, like hospice care, strives to define each death as a good one: that is, one with symptom control and free from suffering (Singer et al., 1999). Palliative care manages the symptoms of any serious illness, including cancer, diabetes, congestive heart failure, dementia, and chronic obstructive pulmonary disease (COPD). Although more and more people are talking about end-of-life wishes, it is essential that those wishes are properly documented and communicated. This anticipatory guidance, when included in a palliative care program, can help keep people in place and ensure their wishes are being honored. The practice must be centered on the person's wishes and choices (Clark, 2003). Palliative care gives control back to the person, at least at the very end of life.

The physical and emotional effects of debilitating and life-threatening illness and its treatment may be very different from person to person. Palliative care can address a broad range of issues, integrating an individual's specific needs into care. A palliative care specialist will consider the following issues for each person:

- Physical: Common physical symptoms include pain, fatigue, loss of appetite, weight loss, nausea, vomiting, shortness of breath, and insomnia.

- Psychological: Palliative care specialists can provide assistance to help persons and families deal with depression and anxiety related to their illness.

- Spiritual: When dealing with a life-limiting and terminal illness, persons and families often look more deeply for meaning in their lives. Typically, one's illness brings them closer to their faith or spiritual beliefs, whereas others struggle to understand why it happened to them. Palliative care specialists can help people explore their beliefs and faith to help them find a sense of peace and bring them closer to accepting their situation.

- Caregiver support: Family members are an important part of palliative care. Like the person receiving care, they have evolving needs. It is common for family members to feel overwhelmed by the heavy burden of responsibilities placed upon them. It is stressful trying to give care and handle other duties, such as work, household tasks, and caring for other family members. Palliative care specialists can help families and friends cope and give them the support they need.

- Practical needs: Palliative care specialists can also assist with financial and legal worries, insurance questions, and employment concerns.

Domains of Palliative Care: The National Consensus Project

The National Consensus Project for Quality Palliative Care is a consortium of 16 leading U.S.-based palliative care organizations, recognized experts who achieved consensus and developed voluntary, evidence-based guidelines to ensure quality and consistency of care. In 2018, they released the fourth edition of *Clinical Practice Guidelines for Quality Palliative Care,* an updated edition that was endorsed by more than 80 national organizations. One important piece of this work was defining and refining the domains of palliative care. These domains are available from the National Coalition for Hospice and Palliative Care (www.nationalcoalitionhpc.org/wp-content/uploads/2018/10/NCHPC-NCPGuidelines_4thED_web_FINAL.pdf).

Common Diagnoses

Because palliative care aims to improve quality of life, residents with many different diseases and chronic illnesses can benefit from it. Box 22.1 includes a list of many diagnoses that can be helped using a palliative care approach.

IMPLEMENTING PALLIATIVE CARE PROGRAMS IN ASSISTED LIVING COMMUNITIES

Barriers to Implementing Palliative Care Programs in Assisted Living

Although many states allow exceptions to discharge criteria for the provision of hospice care (Carder et al., 2015), palliative care without hospice care has not yet been addressed by most state

---

BOX 22.1:   PALLIATIVE CARE: COMMON DIAGNOSES

Alzheimer's disease	Kidney disease
Amyotrophic lateral sclerosis	Leukemia
Breast cancer	Lymphoma
Bone marrow transplant	Liver disease
Cancer	Lung cancer
Chronic obstructive pulmonary disease	Multiple myeloma
Colon cancer	Multiple sclerosis
Congestive heart failure	Ovarian cancer
Dementia	Pancreatic cancer
Eosinophil-associated disease	Parkinson's disease
Head and neck cancer	Prostate cancer
HIV/AIDS	Pulmonary fibrosis
Huntington's dsease	Sickle cell anemia
	Stroke

Source: From Get Palliative Care. (n.d.). *Disease types and palliative care.* https://getpalliativecare.org/whatis/disease-types

---

regulatory agencies. Therefore, the obstacles identified by Dr. Ethel Mitty in 2004 still exist today. These include, but are not limited to:

- Regulations in some states do not permit retention of a resident who needs skilled nursing care.
- Dying or terminally ill residents (or their families) request transfer to a nursing home or hospital.
- If the resident needs more care than was stipulated in the service contract, the resident cannot remain in the facility if additional services are needed for end-of-life care.
- A nurse (RN or LPN) is not available on a 24-hour basis.
- If "risk of death" was not in the service contract, the facility could be liable for failure to respond appropriately.
- The assisted living residence is legally liable if a dying resident is not transferred to a nursing home or hospital unless the resident is a hospice patient.
- There is insufficient reimbursement to the facility if it provides additional personal care.
- The components, standards, or requirements of end-of-life care are unknown.
- The facility has inadequate safe storage for pain-management drugs.
- Staff are uncomfortable being with a resident who is dying.
- Physicians do not want their patients to die in an assisted living residence.

Dr. Pippa Hawley (2017, p. 1) wrote,

Despite significant advances in understanding the benefits of early integration of palliative care with disease management, many people living with a chronic life-threatening illness either do not receive any palliative care service or receive services only in the last phase of their illness.

Furthermore, she identified some barriers to accessing palliative care, including:

- Lack of resources to refer to,
- Not knowing that resources exist,

- Ignorance regarding what palliative care is,
- Reluctance to refer patients to healthcare providers,
- Reluctance of patient and/or family to be referred,
- Restrictive program eligibility: rationing of services according to patient characteristics.

On the Horizon: Medicare Care Choices Model

The Centers for Medicare & Medicaid Services is currently testing new options relative to palliative care. This innovative model is described in Exhibit 22.1.

An Award-Winning Model Program

Many private health insurance plans provide some coverage for palliative care as part of their hospice or chronic care benefits. Furthermore, many health maintenance organizations (HMOs) have added palliative care to their list of benefits. Keeping their members at home (or in their assisted living community) is beneficial both for quality of life and cost-effectiveness.

Kaiser Permanente is one of the largest managed care organizations in the United States. Kaiser has implemented palliative care programs throughout its systems (i.e., both inpatient and out-patient care settings). An example of one of their successful programs is the Kaiser Permanente South San Francisco's Home Palliative Care Program. Their work was recognized in 2018 by the California Coalition for Compassionate Care' s Leadership Award (Wolfe, 2018). This prestigious award is given to an organization that has developed innovative programs to improve services for palliative care patients while making significant contributions in advocacy, education, and out-reach to patients, their family members, and the wider medical community (California Coalition for Compassionate Care, n.d.).

This Kaiser program is unique as it follows a primary care model (versus a consultative model) that includes nurse practitioners as primary care providers on the home-care team. Medical social

EXHIBIT 22.1

MEDICARE CARE CHOICES MODEL

Through the Medicare Care Choices Model (MCCM), the Centers for Medicare & Medicaid Services (CMS) will test a new option for Medicare beneficiaries to receive supported care services from selected hospice providers, while continuing to receive services provided by other Medicare providers, including care for their terminal condition. CMS evaluates whether providing these supportive services can improve the quality of life and care received by Medicare beneficiaries, increase patient satisfaction, and reduce Medicare expenditures. Under current payment rules, Medicare and dually eligible beneficiaries are required to forgo Medicare payment for care related to their terminal condition in order to receive services under the Medicare or Medicaid hospice benefit.

The model is designed to:
1. Increase access to supportive care services provided by hospice.
2. Improve quality of life and patient/family satisfaction.
3. Inform new payment systems for the Medicare and Medicaid programs.

Source: From Centers for Medicare & Medicaid Services. (n.d.). *Medicare choices model*. https://innovation.cms .gov/initiatives/Medicare-Care-Choices

workers are also included on the team. Many of the clients in the program are homebound and unable to access palliative care in outpatient clinics. Dementia is a common primary diagnosis. This ideal program began is 2004 and continues to grow. Advanced healthcare planning is a primary focus and many persons (including those living in assisted living communities) avoid hospitalization and transition to hospice when appropriate.

CONCLUSIONS

This chapter defines, describes, and discusses many concepts relative to palliative care, specifically focusing on the need for palliative care approaches for residents in assisted living communities. Key terminology and best practices are described. Furthermore, hospice care is discussed as a form of palliative care and distinctions between hospice and palliative care are identified. Although barriers exist to accessing palliative care within assisted living, education is a key part of moving forward to remove them. Palliative care logically goes hand in hand with many concepts of assisted living, especially as many residents desire to age in place.

REFERENCES

California Coalition for Compassionate Care. (n.d.). *Compassionate care leadership and innovator awards.* https://coalitionccc.org/training-events/compassionate-care-leadership-awards

Carder, P., O'Keeffe, J., & O'Keeffe, C. (2015). *Compendium of residential care and assisted living regulations and policy: 2015 edition.* U.S. Department of Health and Human Services, Office of the Assistant Secretary for Planning and Evaluation, Office of Disability, Aging and Long-Term Care Policy and Research Triangle Institute. https://aspe.hhs.gov/basic-report/compendium-residential-care-and-assisted-living-regulations-and-policy-2015-edition

Center to Advance Palliative Care. (2019). *Downloadable tools for making the case.* https://www.capc.org/tools-for-making-the-case/downloadable-tools

Centers for Medicare & Medicaid Services. (n.d.). *Medicare choices model.* https://innovation.cms.gov/initiatives/Medicare-Care-Choices

Clark, J. (2003). Patient centered death. *BMJ, 327*(7408), 174–175. https://doi.org/10.1136/bmj.327.7408.174

Ellershaw, J., & Ward, C. (2003). Care of the dying patient: The last hours or days of life. *BMJ, 326*(7379), 30–34. https://doi.org/10.1136/bmj.326.7379.30

Get Palliative Care. (n.d.). *Disease types and palliative care.* https://getpalliativecare.org/whatis/disease-types

Hawley, P. (2017). Barriers to access to palliative care. *Palliative Care, 10,* 117822421668888. https://doi.org/10.1177/1178224216688887

Jerant, A., Rahan S., Nesbitt, T., Edwards-Goodbee, A., & Meyers, F. (2006). The palliative care in assisted living (PCAL) pilot study: Successes, shortfalls and methodological implications. *Social Science and Medicine, 62,* 199–207. https://doi.org/10.1016/j.socscimed.2005.05.010

Medicare Hospice Benefit. (n.d.). *Medicare hospice benefit definition.* https://www.medicare.gov/pubs/pdf/02154-medicare-hospice-benefits.pdf

Mitty, E. (2004). Assisted living: Aging in place and palliative care. *Geriatric Nursing, 25,* 149–163. https://doi.org/10.1016/j.gerinurse.2004.04.019

National Center for Health Statistics. (2019). *Long-term care providers and service users in the United States: Data from the national study of long-term care providers 2015-2016.* https://www.cdc.gov/nchs/data/series/sr_03/sr03_43-508.pdf

National Coalition for Hospice and Palliative Care. (2018). *Clinical practice guidelines for quality palliative care.* https://www.nationalcoalitionhpc.org/wp-content/uploads/2018/10/NCHPC-NCPGuidelines_4thED_web_FINAL.pdf

Singer, P., Martin, D., & Kelner, M. (1999) Quality end-of-life care: Patients' perspectives. *Journal of the American Medical Association, 2,* 163–168. https://doi.org/10.1001/jama.281.2.163

Walter, T. (2003). Historical and cultural variants on the good death. *BMJ, 327*, 219. https://doi.org/10.1136/bmj.327.7408.218

Wolfe, K. (2018). *Kaiser Permanente South San Francisco's groundbreaking home palliative care program receives prestigious honor.* https://everythingsouthcity.com/2018/04/kaiser-permanente-south-san-franciscos-groundbreaking-home-palliative-care-program-receives-prestigious-honor

World Health Organization. (n.d.). *WHO definition of palliative care.* http://www.who.int/cancer/palliative/definition/en

RESIDENTS' RIGHTS

Upon the completion of Chapter 23, the reader will be able to:

- Identify federal legislation designed to protect the civil rights of residents in assisted living communities.
- Describe selected state statutes enacted to protect the rights of residents in assisted living communities.
- Understand the importance of protecting the social and ethical rights of residents.
- Identify rights of elderly residents, including:

  Religious liberties

  Communication

  Medical care

  Facility transfer

  Complaints

  Receive visits from spouses, family members, and friends

  Respectful treatment

  Privacy

  Dignity, respect, and freedom
- Identify professional resources available to address resident rights in assisted living communities.
- Explain the role of the ombudsman in assisted living facilities.
- Identify issues related to the role of the ombudsman in assisted living communities.

INTRODUCTION

Administrators working in assisted living communities must have a comprehensive understanding of the civil, legal, social, and ethical rights of all assisted living facility residents. Older persons residing in assisted living communities may be vulnerable because of multiple physical and psychosocial comorbidities. Therefore they must be assured that protections are in place, not only for basic safety, but also to enable residents to enjoy quality of life and well-being as they age. A brief description of major federal legislation and state regulations required for assisted living communities so as to protect legal rights of older adults is presented. A discussion of the social and ethical rights of older adults, including those residing in assisted living communities, is addressed alongside a brief discussion of the issues related to resident rights. Finally, a discussion of professional resources, including the role of the ombudsman in protecting residents' rights, concludes the chapter. Selected best practices in areas associated with resident rights are presented throughout.

PROTECTION OF CIVIL RIGHTS

Federal legislation was enacted during the latter part of the 20th century to protect the civil rights of all Americans. Passage of the 1964 Civil Rights Act made discrimination on the basis of race, color, gender, religion, or national origin unlawful (U.S. National Archives & Records Administration, 2009). This legislation set precedence for banning discrimination in the admissions process of residents into assisted living facilities.

The Omnibus Budget Reconciliation Act (OBRA) of 1987 included the Nursing Home Reform Act, emphasizing in part regulations focusing on the rights and quality of life of nursing home residents (Miller, 2009). OBRA identified the importance of long-term care facilities promoting resident rights to ensure the highest possible levels of physical, psychosocial, and mental functioning (Miller, 2009).

The Nursing Home Residents' Bill of Rights was also included in OBRA. The legislation stated in part that long-term care facility residents have the right to self-determination, a dignified existence, and to access and communicate with others and with services both inside and outside of their facility (Code of Federal Regulations, Title 42, § 483.10). This legislation requires the following resident rights: (a) full information, including the right to daily communication in the resident's own language; the right for assistance as needed; and the right to be informed of all available services and the costs associated with each service; (b) participation in the resident's care, including the rights to receive and participate in appropriate care and care planning; (c) ability to make independent choices, including the right to make personal choices and participate in activities; (d) treatment with dignity, respect, and freedom, including the right of self-determination; (e) security of possessions, including the right to manage all financial affairs; (f) transfers and discharges, including the ability to initiate transfers; (g) privacy and confidentiality, including the right to confidentiality regarding medical, personal, and financial affairs; (h) ability to have complaints heard, including the right to bring grievances forward for review; and (i) visits, including the right to immediate familial access, as well as organizations that promote health, social, and legal services.

In addition, this legislation ensures the rights of elders in nursing homes to vote, file lawsuits, practice religion, marry, enter into contracts, make a will, and dispose of property (Tabloski, 2006). Although the Nursing Home Residents' Bill of Rights was designed to promote the rights of residents in long-term care facilities, these rights are also relevant and applicable to residents in assisted living facilities. A copy of the Residents' Bill of Rights is required in all assisted living facilities and must be posted in locations where residents, visitors, and other individuals working or entering the facility are able to easily read the information.

The Patient Self-Determination Act of 1990 details the responsibilities of healthcare providers. It was developed to ensure that healthcare providers in a variety of settings, including assisted living facilities, protect the rights of all individuals. This was accomplished by providing residents the following services at the time of admission: (a) maintaining written policies and procedures for all adults receiving medical services; (b) providing written information to residents regarding the individual's rights under state law to make decisions regarding medical care, including the right to accept or refuse medical or surgical treatments; (c) ensuring compliance with state laws regarding advanced directives; and (d) providing staff and community education on issues concerning advanced directives (Burke & Walsh, 1997).

State regulations for assisted living communities serve in part to protect the rights of all residents. Although there are federal laws that impact assisted living communities, state regulations provide oversight for the approximately 812,000 Americans who reside in assisted living communities (National Center for Assisted Living, 2019). Each of the 50 states and the District of Columbia have enacted regulations governing assisted living community functions. There is variability in each set of state regulations. The Assisted Living State Regulatory Review for 2019 summarizes information from each state's regulations in a number of categories. A number of these categories describe regulations that serve to protect the civil rights of assisted living residents. Disclosure items include specific information that must be provided to residents before they sign any residence or service contracts. This area of state regulation protects the rights of residents to obtain full information, and to have appropriate communication regarding available services and the costs of such services. Many states do not specify disclosure items, whereas some states, including Idaho, have disclosure statements indicating that each facility must have written admission policies made available to residents and the public.

State regulations specify that the facility scope of care, which is a summary of the personal care and nursing services provided by the facility, be readily available. Third-party scope of care describes whether third parties, such as hospice care providers, are able to provide services in the assisted living facility (National Center for Assisted Living, 2019). Information provided in these regulations serves to protect the rights of residents and ensure they receive appropriate communication regarding their care, and the ability to participate in their care. Again, variations in how these regulations are interpreted are noted across states. For example, in Colorado *facility scope of care* is defined as the provision of services to meet the needs of residents, including room and board, a physically safe and sanitary environment, protective oversight, and social care, and third-party scope of care allows facilities or residents to contract with external service providers, including home health agencies or hospice for additional services (National Center for Assisted Living, 2019).

A resident's right to information regarding facility transfers and discharges is addressed in assisted living facility state regulations for move-in and move-out requirements. These regulations specify the types of conditions mandating that residents move out of facilities, as well as conditions that would prevent individuals from moving into facilities (National Center for Assisted Living, 2019). Variation among state regulations is again noted, with some states providing minimal information regarding move-in and move-out requirements. The regulations in Delaware, on the other hand, are comprehensive, listing a number of conditions that would prevent individuals from moving into facilities. These conditions include a need for extensive nursing services, the presence of stage-three or stage-four pressure ulcers, the use of medical equipment such as mechanical ventilators and central lines, and the presence of behaviors that pose a threat to the individual or to others (National Center for Assisted Living, 2019).

State regulations regarding resident assessment include provisions for assessment data collection to identify if an individual's needs can be met by providers, as well as to identify the services required by each individual (National Center for Assisted Living, 2019). This regulation serves to protect the rights of residents to participate in their own care, to receive appropriate care, and to participate in care planning activities. Once again, states broadly interpret this regulation, with some providing minimal information, whereas other states provide specific data. In New York, for example, regulations require that each assisted living facility resident have an individualized service plan (ISP) that is developed jointly by the resident, the resident's representative if indicated, the assisted living facility operator, and the resident's physician. The state of New York also requires that each ISP assess the medical, functional, cognitive, nutritional, rehabilitative, and other needs for each resident, and that each plan must be reviewed every six months or when resident care needs change (National Center for Assisted Living, 2019). Again, the state regulations noted here serve in part to protect the civil rights of all assisted living residents.

PROTECTION OF SOCIAL AND ETHICAL RIGHTS

Administrators in assisted living communities must have an awareness of the social and ethical rights of residents. Although many resident rights are guaranteed through federal legislation and state regulations, social and ethical rights must be protected as well. An understanding of autonomy and individual rights, competency, and decision-making capacities can provide administrators with information regarding residents' social and ethical rights.

Autonomy refers to the personal freedom to take control of one's life without interfering or infringing on the rights of other individuals (Miller, 2009). The autonomous person is able to solve problems through a thought process that is both rational and organized, and thus control many important life decisions. Residents in assisted living facilities have the right to self-determination and to make independent choices, in essence, to take control of their care as autonomous individuals. When residents experience confusion or dementia, they lose not only their autonomy, but also their ability to make reasoned choices regarding their care; many lose independence as well. For many older adults, the loss of independence that accompanies a reduction in autonomy creates great difficulties, and may create problems in ensuring that their rights remain protected.

Competency is defined as the ability to fulfill one's roles and handle all of one's affairs in ways that are both adequate and appropriate (Miller, 2009). Legally, all competent adults are ensured rights guaranteed by the U.S. Constitution, as well as by state laws and regulations, and have the legal right to make all decisions regarding healthcare and medical treatments. Residents in assisted living facilities who are competent have the right to make independent choices, to manage all of their financial affairs, and to participate in and make decisions regarding their medical care, including the right to refuse medications or treatments. For those residents who have cognitive problems or dementia, competency becomes an important issue. Protection of competency is important for individuals with cognitive problems. If residents are evaluated and declared incompetent or unable to participate in their own decision-making, then a legally appointed decision maker can be obtained for the individual. Legally appointed guardians or conservators make either some decisions for residents who have limited abilities in appropriate decision-making, or all decisions for those residents with significant cognitive problems (Miller, 2009). Court monitoring accompanies the appointment of legal guardians or conservators, and reflects the compounding of legal, social, and ethical considerations associated with the removal of an individual resident's rights.

Decision-making capacity refers to an individual's ability to consent or to refuse specific medical procedures or treatments, and is usually determined by healthcare professionals or by members of a healthcare professional team (Miller, 2009). Decision-making capacity is viewed as the ability to both understand and communicate issues related to a specific decision-making situation, and is not related to a resident's age or specific medical diagnoses (Miller, 2009). The concept of capacity is based on a resident's ability to: (a) appreciate the right to make choices; (b) understand the benefits and the risks of proposed medical interventions, as well as the results of no medical interventions; (c) communicate with others about decisions; (d) be stable over time; and (e) be consistent in their values and beliefs (Miller, 2009). Residents with cognitive impairments or mild dementia may be able to participate in decision-making regarding medical procedures if they are able to understand the issues related to proposed treatments. The residents' rights to participate in their own care, as well as to participate in care planning, are linked to decision-making capacity. These rights remain important for residents in assisted living communities.

ISSUES RELATED TO RESIDENTS' RIGHTS

There are a number of issues related to the rights of all residents in assisted living communities. The Nursing Home Residents' Bill of Rights included in the OBRA of 1987 (Code of Federal Regulations, Title 42, § 483.10) identifies rights guaranteed to all residents in long-term care facilities. Individual states have also passed regulations to ensure the rights of residents in assisted living and long-term care facilities. Although state regulations differ among all 50 states and the District of Columbia, basic concepts regarding individual rights remain similar throughout the country. Issues related to these and other rights include rights associated with religious liberties, communication, medical care, transfers, financial affairs, complaints, spousal and family visits, and respectful treatment. The right to privacy includes a discussion of legislation to protect privacy and communication of medical information. Avoiding the use of restraints on residents within assisted living facilities is of additional importance.

The rights of assisted living facility residents to have religious liberties are guaranteed by the U.S. Constitution. Next, residents are ensured under the Nursing Home Residents' Bill of Rights (Code of Federal Regulations, Title 42, § 483.10) the ability to make independent choices, and to participate in activities both in and outside of the facility. Although residents are entitled to the right to religious liberties, assisted living facility regulations do not require the provision of religious services. Although many administrators and facilities work to provide residents with access to religious services, there are no regulatory requirements for this other than the right for residents to participate in unspecified activities.

The right to communication is well identified in the Nursing Home Residents' Bill of Rights (Code of Federal Regulations, Title 42, § 483.10). Residents in assisted living communities are entitled to daily communication, as well as the right to privacy and unrestricted communication with any individual. Issues related to communication may include problems associated with language barriers. The federal legislation was written to ensure that residents have the right to communicate daily in their own language. For administrators in assisted living communities, this means staffing to provide all residents with information in their language. Ensuring the rights of residents to receive clear communication may in fact create challenges and additional costs for administrators. Residents are also ensured the right to be fully informed if they have any sensory problems. Administrators must ensure that those communicating with residents who have visual or auditory problems are able to use appropriate strategies, such as the use of materials with pictures rather than text, or to ensure that residents have functional glasses and hearing aids to facilitate the communication process. Although residents have the right to private and unrestricted communication, certain issues may create challenges in ensuring that resident rights are met. For example, for those residents with roommates, obtaining privacy for communication may be an issue. Some states and facilities impose restrictions on the times that phone calls may be placed, creating potential barriers to the right to unrestricted communication. Administrators must work with residents as needed to make sure that these important rights are maintained.

The rights to medical care are also guaranteed in the Nursing Home Residents' Bill of Rights (Code of Federal Regulations, Title 42, § 483.10). Residents in assisted living facilities are entitled to receive medical care that is both adequate and appropriate, and to participate in the planning and evaluation of care. Although there is agreement on the concept of residents' rights to medical care, state assisted living facility regulations differ among each of the 50 states and the District of Columbia. Variance exists, for example, in the regulations regarding resident assessment designed to identify services required by residents and medication management, identifying the extent to which medication assistance is possible. Administrators need to identify regulations specific to their state in order to ensure that all resident rights are upheld.

Residents in assisted living communities are entitled to rights related to transfer from their facility. Residents are entitled to at least a 30-day notice if they will be required to relocate or to transfer to another facility. It is important to note that there are differences among state regulations for assisted living communities. Although the regulations include a section on the move-in and move-out requirements for assisted living facility conditions, each state has a different interpretation of the regulations. Administrators need to consult their state regulations to ensure that the rights of residents to facility transfer are maintained.

Residents in assisted living communities are entitled to rights related to financial affairs. As noted in the Nursing Home Residents' Bill of Rights (Code of Federal Regulations, Title 42, § 483.10), residents have the right to secure possessions, including the right to manage their own financial affairs and to not have to pay for services that are covered by Medicare or Medicaid. Again, an issue facing assisted living administrators involves strategies to ensure that these resident rights are protected. State regulations governing assisted living facilities differ in each state. The regulations do not specifically address rights related to financial affairs, meaning that facilities must develop their own policies regarding financial rights for residents. This results in a wide variation in approaches to these important rights.

The right to file a complaint is also guaranteed for residents in long-term care communities. This includes the ability to file grievances without reprisals, and to have nursing homes promptly address complaints. For residents of assisted living facilities, these rights are important but are not covered in all state regulations. Although many facilities have developed individual policies regarding residents' ability to file complaints, there are no national standards currently available for review. An example of a best practice to improve elder rights in assisted living communities includes the creation of improved communication through regular resident- coordinated and attended meetings to enhance resident satisfaction and resident participation in decisions regarding living arrangements and resident rights.

Residents in assisted living communities have the right to receive visits from spouses, family members, and friends. As noted in the Nursing Home Residents' Bill of Rights (Code of Federal Regulations, Title 42, § 483.10), residents in nursing homes are entitled to immediate access to relatives and reasonable visits by organizations, in addition to individuals providing health, social, or legal services. Issues may arise for those residents who do not have private rooms, or who have family members wishing to visit at times that may not be convenient for other residents. Again, administrators need to work flexibly with residents and with spouses, family members, and friends to promote these important visits. Many facilities may have their own policies regarding visits. Without state or national standards, individual regulations have the potential to create confusion for both administrators and consumers.

The right to respectful treatment is a right afforded to residents in long-term care facilities along with the rights to dignity, respect, and freedom. Residents in assisted living facilities have the same need for this important right. Although some (National Center for Assisted Living, 2019) report that the right for respectful treatment is implicit in the services that are provided in assisted living facilities, state regulations do not specifically identify respectful treatment for residents within their documents. Many administrators must abide by facility policies, and create a bill of rights for residents to ensure that residents are afforded care that is both dignified and respectful.

Residents in assisted living communities have the right to privacy as do residents in long-term care facilities. Residents have the right to privacy concerning the receipt of treatment and in regard to personal care. Again, this right is identified in the Nursing Home Residents' Bill of Rights (Code of Federal Regulations, Title 42, § 483.10) and should be implemented in all assisted living communities. State assisted living regulations address privacy in terms of physical plant requirements; the square footage requirements for resident rooms; the maximum number of residents allowed per resident room; bathroom requirements, which detail whether bathrooms may be shared, as well as specifying the number of bathing units required per resident (National Center for Assisted Living, 2019). Again, issues related to variability in state regulations must be addressed by assisted living facility administrators, who may augment state assisted living facility regulations with their own policies regarding privacy.

Residents in assisted living communities also have their privacy protected through implementation of the Health Insurance Portability and Accountability Act (HIPPA) of 1996 (Public Law 104–191). Designed to recognize that privacy and confidentiality are considered to be basic rights for all Americans, this is the first federal legislation designed to protect the privacy of patient health information through the development of requirements and standards for the electronic transmission of patient health records (Tabloski, 2006). There is specific healthcare information that is considered to be confidential. This information includes the following: (a) information that identifies residents, including resident name and medical record number or record identification information; (b) health information that is related to the past, present, or future health status or health concerns of the resident; (c) all documentation related to the provision of healthcare services to residents; and (d) any payments for healthcare that may be in the past, present, or future (Tabloski, 2006). In addition, residents in assisted living facilities have the right to review their medical records and to ask questions regarding any of the information contained within those documents.

Residents in assisted living facilities have the right to dignity, respect, and freedom, including the right to be free from both mental and physical abuse (Code of Federal Regulations, Title 42, § 483.10). Although much attention has been paid to the rights of residents in long-term care communities to avoid the use of physical and chemical restraints, which create increased risks for injury as well as physical and emotional problems, current practice encourages changes in a resident's environment to minimize the need for restraints, and careful monitoring of residents who otherwise may be candidates for restraints. The autonomy of residents can best be protected by avoiding the use of physical and chemical restraints, and by administrators recognizing that the use of these devices impedes upon the rights of residents.

PROFESSIONAL RESOURCES TO ADDRESS RESIDENT RIGHTS

Administrators in assisted living communities can ensure that residents and resident rights are protected in part by interested professionals. Chief among these professionals is the ombudsman. Other professionals, including nurses, geriatric specialists, and social workers, also assume a role in protecting resident rights. The roles of these professionals is briefly discussed.

The ombudsman serves as an advocate for the rights of residents and also investigates resident complaints in a number of settings, including long-term care facilities, assisted living facilities, and board-and-care homes. Established under the auspices of the Older American Act

Amendment, the National Long-Term Care Ombudsman Program was granted the authority to investigate safety, welfare, and health of residents. Developed as a federally mandated response to substandard conditions in American nursing homes, the ombudsman model is now established in 53 state ombudsman programs (Colello, 2008). In 1992, the Older Americans Act (OAA) was amended (PL-102–375) and merged the ombudsman, legal services, and elder abuse programs into Title VII, the Vulnerable Elder Rights Protection Activities, a federally legislated addition to the patient and consumer rights movement (Baker et al., 2014).

The role of the ombudsman consists of a number of advocacy and problem-solving functions, including : to (a) identify, investigate, and resolve resident complaints; (b) provide information to residents about long-term care services; (c) protect resident rights through advocacy at governmental agency levels; (d) analyze and recommend changes in laws and regulations that relate to the health, safety, welfare, and rights of residents; (e) educate both consumers and the general public about issues and concerns related to long-term care; (f) promote the development of citizen organizations; (g) provide technical support for the development of family and resident councils to protect the well-being and rights of residents; and (h) advocate for improvements in residents' quality of life and care (State Long-Term Care Ombudsman Program Final Rule, 2015).

Ombudsmen face issues in their current roles. Although ombudsman programs are mandated through the Older Americans Act, implementation of programs occurs at both the state and local level. Because state implementation of programs differs even within the state, data collection and reporting systems are not standardized, making reporting more arduous and the quality of data variable from state to state. In addition, some ombudsmen have experienced problems obtaining data from long-term care and assisted living facilities despite federal legislation guaranteeing access to resident medical records (Netting et al., 1995). Challenges in the collection and dissemination of data required for role completion mean that ombudsmen are less effective in their advocacy efforts on behalf of residents. Volunteers are hired to fill many of the ombudsman positions and their roles are defined at either the state or the local level. Training, certification, and continuing education for these individuals are all determined at the state level. Additionally, volunteers must be recruited, trained, supervised, and supported by professional staff working to maintain the quality of ombudsmen programs (Netting et al., 1995). Despite these and other issues that ombudsmen must deal with, the services that they perform for elders, especially elders in assisted living facilities, are critical to ensuring the rights of these vulnerable individuals.

Many healthcare professionals serve in roles designed to advocate and protect the rights of residents in facilities, including assisted living facilities. Some nurses specialize in gerontological nursing work to protect the rights of older adults. Additionally, nurses involved in the care of elders provide ethical nursing care by: (a) actively listening and using good communication skills; (b) respecting the rights and values of all elders; and (c) providing quality care to all elders (Touhy & Jett, 2018). Geriatric specialists can advocate and protect the rights of assisted living facility residents through their comprehensive understanding of the needs and rights of assisted living facility residents. Social workers provide services that support rights of residents through a number of resident advocacy roles, and frequently work with ombudsmen to provide educational, advisory, and support roles.

Administrators in assisted living facilities can obtain additional information regarding the rights of residents from a number of websites and online resources. The National Institute on Aging, the American Geriatrics Society, and AARP are examples of resources that may be of benefit to assisted living facility administrators.

CASE STUDY

The staff in an assisted living facility located in an affluent community expressed concerns to the administrator about SG, an 80-year-old resident. SG has been seen to have facial and upper arm bruising over the past several months. When questioned, SG stated that her vision is failing; she has been walking into her bathroom door and that is why she has some bruises that do not hurt or cause her any problems. The administrator decided to follow a best practice in the screening of elders for mistreatment through the implementation of the Elder Assessment Instrument, a 41-item assessment designed to identify signs, symptoms, and complaints of elder abuse, neglect, abandonment, and exploitation (Fulmer, 2008). Elders are referred for assistance if data obtained from administration of the instrument reveals evidence of mistreatment, elder complaints of abuse, or if a high risk of abuse exists.

When assisted living staff administered the Elder Assessment Instrument to SG, they found the presence of new and healing bruises on SG's face, arms, and chest. Evidence of financial exploitation and misuse of SG's money were also noted. Further questioning revealed that the bruises occurred following visits by SG's daughter, who had been taking money from SG's checking account and was also trying to access SG's savings accounts. SG stated that her daughter was really a "good girl with a little drug problem" and she was ashamed to admit that her daughter was abusing her and spending money from her checking account. SG finally revealed that her daughter had recently been physically abusive in attempts to get additional money from SG's saving account.

The administrator was able to use the information collected from the Elder Assessment Instrument to contact SG's other family members and local authorities regarding SG's mistreatment and the misuse of SG's funds. The daughter was arrested for both elder abuse and drug abuse and SG's other family members worked on strategies to protect SG's financial assets. SG also spent time with members of the social services staff to address the problems related to the abuse. The staff reported to the administrator that no new bruising was noted following these interventions.

CONCLUSIONS

Protecting the rights of elders residing in assisted living communities is critical, and is the responsibility, in part, of administrators. Comprehension of federal legislation, including the Civil Rights Act, the Nursing Home Reform Act, and the Patient Self-Determination Act, as well as state legislation as described earlier, augments important care provided to residents. Understanding social and ethical rights, and the issues related to the protection of elder's rights as presented in this chapter, also serves to enhance the services that are provided by administrators in assisted living communities.

REFERENCES

Baker, N. R., Jablonski, R. A., & Moss, J. A. (2014). A nurse developed toolkit for long-term care ombudsmen. *Geriatric Nursing, 35*(2), 111–113. https://doi.org/10.1016/j.gerinurse.2013.10.014

Burke, M. M., & Walsh, M. B. (1997). *Gerontologic nursing. Holistic care of the older adult.* Mosby.

Colello, K. J. (2008). *Older Americans Act: Long-Term Care Ombudsman Program*. https://www.amazon
.com/OlderAmericans-Act-Long-Term-Ombudsman-ebook/dp/B005v5B285

Fulmer, T. (2008). Screening for mistreatment of older adults. *American Journal of Nursing, 108*(12), 52–59.
https://doi.org/10.1097/01.NAJ.0000341885.07694.48

Health Insurance Portability and Accountability Act of 1996, Pub.L. No 104–191, 1171 (1996).

Miller, C. A. (2009). *Wellness in older adults* (5th ed.). Wolters Kluwer Lippincott Williams & Wilkins.

National Center for Assisted Living. (2019). *Assisted living state regulatory review.* Author.

Netting, E. F., Huber, R., Paton, R. N., & Kautz III, J. R. (1995). Elder rights and the long-term care
ombudsman program. *Social Work, 40*(3), 351–357.

Nursing Home Residents' Bill of Rights in the Omnibus Budget Reconciliation Act of 1987 42, CFR, 483.10
(1987).

State Long-Term Care Ombudsman Programs. (2015). Final rule. *Federal Register, 80*(28), 7703–7767.

Tabloski, P. A. (2006). *Gerontological nursing.* Pearson Education.

Touhy, T. A., & Jett, K. (2018). *Ebersole and Hess' gerontological nursing.* Elsevier.

U.S. National Archives & Records Administration. (2009). *Teaching with documents: The Civil Rights Act of
1964 and the Equal Employment Opportunity Commission*. http://www.archives.gov/education/lessons/
civil-rights-act/index.html?template=print

FURTHER READING

Nelson, H. W. (1995). Long-term care volunteer roles on trial: Ombudsman effectiveness revisited. *Journal of
Gerontological Social Work, 23*(3–4), 25–46. https://doi.org/10.1300/J083V23N03_03

AFTERWORD: A CALL TO ACTION ON COVID-19 RESPONSE IN ASSISTED LIVING/RESIDENTIAL CARE COMMUNITIES

The year of publication, 2020, for this second edition of *Assisted Living Administration and Management: Effective Practices and Model Programs in Elder Care* will be remembered as one influenced by an unrelenting coronavirus and social unrest. Despite statewide shelter-in-place, social distancing, face mask and handwashing guidelines, the unprecedented COVID-19 global pandemic has disproportionately affected older Americans, who have higher rates of chronic health conditions, which has led to severe illness and death. During the COVID-19 public health crisis, the social unrest did *not* focus on the plight of the elderly, who suffered from not-so-subtle discrimination stemming from ageism (bias based solely on advanced age), double jeopardy (ageism and racial bias) or multiple jeopardy (double jeopardy and additional bias). Instead, the social unrest has focused mainly on multiple reluctant parties who have failed to social distance properly; the Black Lives Matter and "my body, my choice" demonstrations among other community protests and social events potentially have added to COVID-19 cases and deaths.

In May 2020, the Associated Press reported that a Northern California city official, Ken Turnage, was ousted after he posted on social media that sick, old, and injured people should be left to meet their "natural course in nature" during the coronavirus pandemic (https://www
.nbcnews.com/politics/politics-news/california-city-official-ousted-over-his-pandemic-
remarks-n1198716). Although Turnage is entitled to his freedom of speech, his comments proposed that the elderly are expendable for the good of younger people. This misguided thinking was alluded to in a conversation about "Out With the Old: Coronavirus Highlights Why We Need New Names for Aging" with Caroline Cicero and Paul Nash, instructional associate professors of gerontology at the University of Southern California (https://theconversation.com/
out-with-the-old-coronavirus-highlights-why-we-need-new-names-for-aging-131380).

Cicero and Nash talked about the marginalization of older Americans with the rise of COVID-19. Some blame the elderly for the shelter-in-place guidelines, and some even say the elderly should be sacrificed for the good of the country. Nevertheless, the coronavirus affects young and old alike. Although hospitalization and mortality rates increase with age, the Centers for Disease Control and Prevention report that young adults take up more ICU beds than the very old. Optimistically, aging is something we will all experience. Yet ageism is possibly the last widely accepted form of social prejudice. Certainly, the World Health Organization (WHO) believes ageism may be more pervasive than sexism or racism. Research clearly shows negative attitudes about aging when being older can harm your health and well-being, even impact your mortality.

It is very disconcerting that the elderly experienced such prejudicial treatment during the COVID-19 pandemic without redress. Both the lack of compassion for, and ignorance about, the elderly population expressed by the actions of many (but not all) younger adults, who deliberately chose not to shelter-in-place, speak volumes. Making it worse, given the enhanced longevity of our aging society, seniors living in assisted living/residential care communities (skilled nursing facilities) feared that their lives were seen as expendable in the rush to reopen the country. Clearly, as a nation, we can do better to help educate and train younger Americans to better appreciate and care for our aging population. Studies have found that students benefit academically as well as socially from taking gerontology courses. Gerontology courses play an important role in building an *inclusive intergenerational and multicultural society.*

Yet, in order to educate and train people for meaningful advocacy and careers in aging, more colleges and universities must offer and require courses and programs in gerontology so that students may have opportunities to learn about the aged, aging processes, and elder care workforce needs for an aging world. These innovative gerontology courses and programs could help to: (a) emphasize the broad, interdisciplinary nature of issues that relate to and influence older adults; (b) provide students with the academic background, professional experience, and research capabilities necessary to pursue advanced and professional study pertaining to an aging population; and (c) prepare students for professional practice and leadership positions in the public and private sectors where gerontological knowledge is required. We urgently need to educate younger adults about aging and long-term care so that they may contribute to "age-friendly communities" that will better address health and social needs as well as individualized and coordinated services that promote independence and maximize "quality of life" for young and old alike.

In some states, such as California, there have been early legislative attempts to include gerontology education and geriatric training in the college curriculum. One such legislative bill was the California Integrated Elder Care and Involvement Act of 2002 (Senate Bill [SB] 953; Vasconcellos, Chapter 541, Statutes of 2002), which called for: (a) gerontology and geriatric training; (b) academic standards (Requested the California State University [CSU], University of California [UC] and California Community College [CC] systems to develop standards and guidelines for the biological, social, and psychological aspects of aging for professional degree programs at both the bachelor and graduate level, in which the health and welfare of older adults is paramount); and (c) professional licensure requirements. Another legislative bill was Gerontology Service Delivery Personnel: Training (Assembly Bill [AB] 2202; Alquist, Chapter 51, Statutes of 2002), which required the CSU to provide courses and training in gerontology for professional service delivery personnel providing services to the senior population. These professional service delivery personnel included gerontologists, nurses, physical therapists, psychologists, and social workers. Perhaps the call for a new legislative bill might extend the intent of these prior bills to include the education and training of long-term care administrators (such as assisted living administrators and/or nursing home administrators) as well as their "interprofessional team" members, described in Chapter 8.

Collaboration and partnerships are key in the successful education and training of students who will be competent and skilled in working for, and with, the elderly residing in assisted living/residential care communities. Academic programs in gerontology, such as the one at San Francisco State University (https://pace.sfsu.edu/gerontology), have collaborated with a variety of community partners in the assisted living/residential care industry. Moreover, in working together, it is apparent that the assisted living/residential care profession is on a trajectory for significant job growth. For example, the California Assisted Living Association (CALA) website has an informative section on workforce development (https://caassistedliving.org/workforce/) where you will find tools and resources to help assisted living, memory care, and continuing care retirement community (CCRC) practitioners develop and sustain a workforce ready to meet these escalating needs. Whether through community partners serving as guest lecturers, internship preceptors, and/or participation in a careers-in-aging job fair, building relationships by offering student-learning opportunities can help develop the much-needed workforce in assisted living/residential care communities.

Students interested in learning more about the assisted living/residential care profession can apply for scholarship support, through organizations like CALA, to attend a professional conference. Participation at a professional conference enables students to: (a) gain a greater understanding of the assisted living/residential care profession, (b) meet face-to-face with prospective employers online or onsite at the professional conference, (c) attend cutting-edge educational sessions and network with assisted living/residential care professionals, and (d) hear from an assisted living/residential care professional who can share strategies for navigating a career path. Furthermore, from the assisted living/residential care professional perspective, research shows building a team of quality student interns—who are then employed as staff members—leads to a high quality of life for residents.

In addition to academic courses/degrees in gerontology, state certification in assisted living/residential care administration is imperative. Each state sets its own assisted living/residential care regulations and administers its own certification examination. Furthermore, an optional Certified Director of Assisted Living (CDAL) program may be used as a means of promoting professionalism within the senior living industry. The CDAL program is administered under the authority of the Senior Living Certification Commission (SLCC), which is part of Argentum (https://www.argentum.org/assisted-living-executive-director-certification-program).

Ongoing and continuing education for assisted living/residential care administrators and their interprofessional team members remains a cornerstone for continued excellence in elder care delivery. Mandated institutional trainings, professional continuing education, specialty care training, and disaster management trainings addressing natural disasters and the recent COVID-19 pandemic represent educational areas of importance for administrators, practitioners, staff, and residents.

As noted throughout this second edition, assisted living administrators are required to stay current with state-mandated regulations and national recommendations and guidelines. Education for assisted living administrators and interprofessional team members includes state-mandated core trainings and program trainings focused on the domains of practice. These domains of practice include organizational management, human resource management, business and financial management, environmental management, and resident care management. Requirements for mandated institutional trainings in each state are described in reviews of assisted living regulations (National Center for Assisted Living, 2019) and should be a major component of required educational programs. Comprehensive information about mandated trainings is well described in Chapter 5.

Practitioners working in assisted living/residential care communities update their understanding of elder care delivery for residents through a number of formal professional continuing-education programs. Updated information for content on physical aspects of aging, such as memory care, nutrition, medication administration, management of illnesses, including heart disease and strokes, are examples of areas in which professionals regularly improve their education. Continuing-education programs are offered through professional organizations, universities, state licensing boards, and private companies. One example of a state-level organization is the Florida Senior Living Association (FSLA), whose annual conferences, continuing-education courses, and certification exam review questions enable assisted living administrators, practitioners, and staff to remain current through broad-based educational offerings (https://floridaseniorliving.org/). In addition, Chapter 7 offers a comprehensive review of effective practices.

Assisted living community members must remain current in understanding and management of emergencies and disasters. The COVID-19 pandemic presents a new and growing national challenge for administrators, practitioners, staff, and residents as well as for family and friends of assisted living residents. Members of assisted living communities, especially residents and staff members from at-risk demographic groups, remain at significant risk for morbidity and mortality associated with COVID-19. Current and ongoing education is critical in providing administrators and practitioners with effective practices to keep vulnerable assisted living community members safe through the diagnosis, assessment, and management of COVID-19 by offering coronavirus testing, contact tracing, quarantine, and current medical treatments. Federal and state guidelines from the Centers of Disease Control and Prevention, the U.S. Public Health Department, state and local public health departments, and public health and medical and elder organization trainings are examples of educational efforts to provide necessary information during the current healthcare crisis. Chapter 12 of this second edition offers a beneficial review of basic information on disaster-preparedness issues.

As we reflect on the second edition of *Assisted Living Administration and Management: Effective Practices and Model Programs in Elder Care* during what appears to be a marginalization of older Americans (especially those residing in assisted living/residential care communities) with the rise of COVID-19, we offer the following five-step call to action:

1. Call attention to the need to require education about aging, aging processes, and elder care workforce needs and its contribution to individual, family, community, and societal health and well-being.

2. Call attention to the need to cultivate collaboration and partnerships between colleges/universities and assisted living/residential care communities to provide student-learning opportunities such as internship placements.

3. Call attention to the need to implement effective state regulations, state certification, and continuing education in assisted living/residential care administration.

4. Call attention to the benefit of facilitating workforce development and careers-in-aging in assisted living/residential care communities to meet the growing needs of the elderly who age in place and are cared for in place.

5. Last, call attention to actions that may help to save lives of residents of assisted living/residential care communities during the COVID-19 pandemic.

A comprehensive COVID-19 action plan to save lives of residents of California nursing homes and assisted living communities was developed by the California Advocates for Nursing Home Reform* (CANHR; https://canhrnews.com/wp-content/uploads/2020/04/CANHR_COVID-19_Emergency_Action_Plan.pdf). CANHR's action plan includes the following details, which can be adapted and considered for implementation in other states:

---

* Reproduced with permission of California Advocates for Nursing Home Reform.

■   *End the ban on visitation.*

The visitation ban has harmed residents by isolating them and contributing to unmet needs and neglect. Give every resident the right to at least one support-person visitor who can visit in person until the time when full visitation rights can be restored. Establish reasonable infection control precautions for support-person visitors and provide training on safe visitation. Visitation saves lives.

■   *Stop COVID-19 from being introduced into long-term care facilities.*

Order facilities with no known or suspected COVID-19 outbreaks to refuse admission to any outside patients who have tested positive for COVID-19. When COVID-19 enters long-term care facilities, it is highly likely it will spread and kill residents despite precautions.

■   *Designate facilities to provide care to COVID-19 patients after they are discharged from hospitals.*

Establish COVID-19 dedicated postacute care facilities in counties and require all hospital post-discharge patients to be tested for COVID-19 and, if positive, to be transferred to such facilities. Current facility residents should not be displaced to create COVID-19-dedicated facilities; rather, available empty spaces should be used. Set strong standards for dedicated facilities. Ban operators and facilities with poor track records or histories of outbreaks or noncompliance from designation. Post information on designated facilities.

■   *Monitor on a daily basis facilities residents or staff who have COVID-19.*

Assign an inspector to conduct daily onsite monitoring visits at each facility with residents or staff who have active COVID-19 and at facilities with poor compliance histories, to ensure infection control practices and staffing levels are safe and to sound the alarm on the need for immediate intervention if they are not.

■   *Deploy strike teams to intervene at facilities when residents are endangered.*

At the earliest sign of a facility crisis related to COVID-19 that endangers the lives of residents, send strike teams composed of state and local health departments, local health systems, emergency medical services (EMS), the National Guard, ombudsman programs, and Centers for Medicare & Medicaid Services (CMS) Region 9 personnel to provide emergency leadership, medical treatment, care, testing, supplies, and equipment to save the lives of residents in overburdened facilities. Each strike team should give daily public reports describing its actions, findings, resources needed, and the status of residents and staff in the facility.

■   *Ensure staffing is sufficient to keep residents safe.*

Require all long-term care facilities to maintain safe staffing levels; to submit daily staffing reports to California Department of Public Health (CDPH) or Community Care Licensing Division (CCLD), local health departments, ombudsman programs, and CMS; and to post the daily reports on facility, state, and local health department websites.

■   *Provide "hazard pay" and paid sick leave to workers so they do not need to work in multiple long-term care facilities simultaneously or need to work while sick.*

To help address understaffing and prevent cross-transmission of the virus during the pandemic, require long-term care facilities to pay double-time to health care workers during the crisis, and to provide at least 2 weeks of paid sick leave.

■ *Restore full inspections and investigate all complaints at long-term care facilities.*

Inspectors and investigators are the last line of defense for facility residents who are being mistreated, neglected, or abused. Require regulatory agencies to carry out comprehensive inspections and to investigate all complaints in accordance with the law.

■ *Enforce infection control standards and residents' rights.*

Impose immediate sanctions on facilities that jeopardize residents' lives through poor infection control or other substandard care, illegal evictions, or other violations of the law. Direct inspectors to identify and document violations. Post inspection findings and sanctions on existing state websites.

■ *Mandate transparency on infection levels.*

Require facilities to inform residents, families, staff members, state and local health departments, and the local long-term care ombudsman when residents or staff test positive for COVID-19 and when residents or transferred residents die due to confirmed or suspected cases of COVID-19, along with the steps the facility is taking to treat infected residents and to protect other residents. Impose strong penalties on facilities that fail to report or submit false data.

■ *Fully inform the public on outbreaks at long-term care facilities.*

Direct state and local health departments to identify long-term care facilities that have residents or staff members with positive COVID-19 test results, to fully track and report deaths of residents at each facility or following transfers, and to publicly report and update the status of facility infections and deaths on a daily basis.

■ *Test all staff and residents frequently.*

Ensure availability of testing with rapid results at all long-term care facilities statewide. Impose strong penalties against facilities that fail to comply with testing requirements. Report facility-specific findings publicly and update data daily. Implement contact tracing procedures when a positive result is discovered.

■ *Ensure availability of personal protective equipment (PPE) at long-term care facilities.*

Give long-term care facilities high priority for distribution of PPE.

■ *Enable residents to go home temporarily if they are able to do so.*

Give residents who wish to return home temporarily the means to do so by expediting assistance to provide home caregivers, make testing readily available, and give residents the right to return to their long-term care facilities once the crisis recedes or if their stays at home become unsafe or unmanageable.

■ *Suspend nursing home and assisted living evictions.*

During the COVID-19 crisis, it is nearly impossible for vulnerable people being evicted from nursing homes and assisted living facilities to find new places to live. Prevent homelessness by temporarily suspending evictions from these facilities during the pandemic.

The five suggestions in the preceding call to action have one common denominator: this second edition of *Assisted Living Administration and Management: Effective Practices and Model Programs in Elder Care.* This book provides an informative and useful resource for both students and practitioners alike, as they navigate effective practices and model programs for those they serve successfully in assisted living/residential care communities.

Darlene Yee-Melichar, EdD, FGSA, FAGHE
Andrea Renwanz Boyle, PhD, RN, FNAP
Cristina Flores, PhD, RN, FGSA

REFERENCES

California Integrated Elder Care and Involvement Act of 2002. https://leginfo.legislature.ca.gov/faces/billSearchClient.xhtml?session_year=20192020&house=Both&author=All&lawCode=All

National Center for Assisted Living. (2019). *2019 assisted living state regulatory review.* https://www.ahcancal.org/Assisted-Living/Policy/Documents/2019_reg_review.pdf

Appendix A

GLOSSARY OF FINANCIAL MANAGEMENT TERMS

- **Absorption**: the sharing of the costs of a cost center among the products that use the cost center

- **Accelerating depreciation**: a method of computing depreciation, such as the "sum of the year's digits" or "double declining balance," in which the asset loses value more rapidly than would occur by the "straight line" depreciation method

- **Account**: a record in a double-entry system that is kept for each (or each class) asset, liability, revenue, and expense

- **Accounting**: the field that comprises accurate bookkeeping, financial report preparation, as well as the proper interpretation of the financial data and reports of a business

- **Accounting equation**: an expression of the equivalence, in total, assets = liabilities + ALF stockholder's equity; this is the basic foundation for the balance sheet and income statement that comprises "double-entry accounting"

- **Accounting period**: that time period, typically 1 year, to which financial statements are related; it can also refer to a month or a quarter of the year (3 months)

- **Accounting policies**: the specific accounting bases selected and followed by a business enterprise (e.g., straight-line or reducing balance depreciation)

- **Accounting rate of return**: a ratio sometimes used in investment appraisal based on profits, not cash flows

- **Accounting standards**: prescribed methods of accounting using the accounting standards or financial reporting standards regulation body in your jurisdiction; it is also considered to be a standard collection or rules, laws, and conventions that determine how accounting transactions are recorded as well as how they are presented in the financial statements

- **Accounts payable**: the amount of monies owed to vendors for either physical goods or services purchased on credit

- **Accounts receivable collection report**: a table or spreadsheet that depicts the assisted living community's outstanding accounts receivables by the length of time (days, months) that have not been paid and need to be collected

- **Accounts receivable turnover ratio**: used in ratio analysis to determine the efficiency of how the assisted living facility utilizes its assets; here, the receivables turnover is an indication of how quickly the facility collects on its resident's rent owed; it can be expressed as rent charges to resident's accounts during a given period divided by the amount of accounts receivables

- **Accruals**: that which has accrued, accumulated, grown; refers to expenses that have been consumed or enjoyed but that have not been paid for at the accounting date

■ **Accruals convention**: the convention that revenues and costs are matched with one another and dealt with in the profit and loss (P&L) account of the period to which they relate irrespective of the period of receipt or payment

■ **Accumulated depreciation**: that part of the original cost of a fixed asset that has been regarded as a depreciation expense in successive profit and loss (P&L) accounts: cost less accumulated depreciation = net book value; this is also considered the cumulative depreciation expense to date, or the total portion of the original cost of the ALC depreciable assets that have already been allocated to depreciation expense in the prior and current period

■ **Acid test**: the ratio of current assets (excluding stock) to current liabilities; also known as the "quick rate or quick current ratio" and measures the immediate solvency or debt-paying ability of a company

■ **Acquisitions**: operations of a reporting entity that are acquired in a period; separate disclosure of turnover, profits, etc., must be made

■ **Adjusting entry**: a journal entry to the general ledger that is necessary to adjust the book account balances to conform with the actual balances and accrual basis at the end of accounting periods

■ **Aging schedule**: table that separates and categorizes resident accounts according to the length of time (days, weeks, months) they are outstanding

■ **Allocation**: the charging of discrete, identifiable costs to cost centers or cost units; a cost is allocated when it is unique to a particular cost center

■ **Allowable charge**: the maximum fee that a third-party payer (state Medicaid and a long-term care insurer) has negotiated with the facility to reimburse for resident care

■ **Amortization of debts**: the repayment of a debt (e.g., bank loan, mortgage) by the facility over a period of time by making regular payments of the principal and interest; this is another word for *depreciation;* commonly used for depreciation of the capital cost of acquiring leasehold property

■ **Apportionment**: the division of costs among two or more cost centers in proportion to estimated benefit on some sensible basis; apportionment is used for shared costs

■ **Asset value**: a term that expresses the money amount of assets less liabilities of a company attributable to one ordinary share

■ **Assets**: resources of value owned by a business entity

■ **Assets turnover ratio**: a ratio that purports to measure the intensity of use of business assets; calculated as sales over net operating assets; can be expressed as sales as a percentage of net operating assets; asset turnover ratios also provide information on how efficiently the assisted living facility utilizes its assets; they are sometimes referred to as *efficiency ratios, asset utilization ratios,* or *asset management ratios;* two commonly used asset turnover ratios are the accounts receivable turnover ratio and the inventory turnover

■ **Auditing**: the independent examination of, and expression of an opinion on, the financial statements of an enterprise by an appointed auditor or accountant in pursuance of that appointment and in compliance with any relevant statutory obligation

■ **Auditors**: outside independent accountants that are either an outside independent accounting firm (e.g., Ernst & Young, LLP) or certified professional accountants (CPAs) hired by the assisted living facility in order to cross-check the accuracy of the facility's bookkeepers to ensure that the ALC's financial statements are accurate

- **Avoidable costs**: the specific costs of an activity or sector of a business that would be avoided if that activity or sector did not exist

- **Bad debts**: debts known to be irrecoverable and therefore treated as losses by inclusion in the profit and loss (P&L) account as an expense

- **Balance sheet**: a financial statement showing the financial position of a business entity in terms of assets, liabilities, and capital at a specified date

- **Bank statement**: financial statement produced by bank to checking and savings accounts depicting deposits, expenses, balances, interest earned, and any service fees

- **Bankruptcy**: a legal status imposed by a court; usually a trustee is appointed to receive and realize the assets of the bankrupt and to distribute the proceeds to his creditors according to the law

- **Benefits in kind**: things or services supplied by a company to its directors and others in addition to cash remuneration; a good example is the provision of and free use of a motor vehicle; the value of benefits in kind is taxable

- **Bidding**: the facility requesting responses from vendors to their written specifications for goods (e.g., cleaning supplies) or services (e.g., outside auditor)

- **Bill of lading**: a document issued by a carrier to a shipper upon acceptance of goods for shipment that represents a receipt for the goods and the contract stating the terms of carriage

- **Board-designated funds**: unrestricted funds set aside by the facility's governing board (e.g., corporation's board of directors) for specific purposes

- **Bond**: a formal written document that provides evidence of a loan; it is a written promise by issuing entity (e.g., United States, state and local governments, corporations like assisted living company, etc.) under legal seal to repay a sum of monies (principal and interest) at some specific time in the future

- **Book value**: the amount at which an asset is carried on the accounting records and balance sheet; the usual book value for fixed assets is cost less accumulated depreciation; alternative terms include written-down value, net book value, and carrying value; book value rarely if ever corresponds to sellable value

- **Break-even chart**: a chart that illustrates costs, revenues, profit, and loss at various levels of activity within a relevant range

- **Break-even point**: the level of activity (e.g., level of sales) at which the business makes neither a profit nor a loss (i.e., where total revenues exactly equal total costs)

- **Budget**: a formal quantitative expression of management's plans or expectations; master budgets are the forecast or planned profit and loss account and balance sheet; subsidiary budgets include those for sales, output, purchases, labor, cash, etc.

- **Capital**: an imprecise term meaning the "whole quantity of assets less liabilities owned by a person or a business"; it refers to the funds used in a business

- **Capital allowances**: deductions from profit for fixed asset purchases; in effect, capital allowances are a standard system of depreciation used instead of depreciation for tax purposes only

- **Capital budgeting**: the process of planning or appraising possible fixed asset acquisitions

- **Capital employed**: a term describing the total net assets employed in a business; various definitions are used, so beware when talking at cross-purposes

- **Capital expenditure**: expenditure on fixed assets that is chargeable to an asset account when the asset acquired has an estimated life in excess of 1 year and is not intended for sale in the normal running of the business operations

- **Capital structure ratios**: financial ratios showing the relationship of long-term debt to total assets or to capital/equity

- **Cash**: strictly coins and notes but used also to mean all forms of ready money, including bank balances

- **Cash disbursement journal**: records the expenditures of cash

- **Cash discount**: a reduction in the amount payable by a debtor to induce prompt payment (equivalent to settlement discount)

- **Cash flow**: a vague term (compare cash flow difficulties) used for the difference between total cash in and total cash out in a period

- **Cash-flow forecast**: a document detailing expected or planned cash receipts and outgoings for a future period

- **Cash-flow statement**: a formal financial statement showing a summary of cash inflows and outflows under certain required headings

- **Chart of accounts**: the complete listing of names of the accounts in the general ledger

- **Coinsurance clause:** an insurance policy clause that limits the liability of the insurance company to a determinable percentage of the medical loss suffered by the resident (insured)

- **Committed costs**: those fixed costs that cannot be eliminated or even cut back without having a major effect on the enterprise's activities (e.g., rent)

- **Composition ratios:** indicate the relationships between various types of assets and current or total assets

- **Conservatism**: (also known *prudence*) the convention whereby revenue and profits are not anticipated, but provision is made for all known liabilities (expenses and losses) whether the amount of these is known with certainty or is a best estimate; sssentially:future profit, wait until it happens—future loss, count it

- **Consideration**: the amount to be paid for anything sold, including businesses; may be cash, shares or other securities

- **Consistency**: convention that there is consistency of accounting treatment of like items within each year and from year to year

- **Consolidation**: the aggregation of the financial statements of the separate companies of a group as if they were a single entity

- **Contingent liabilities**: possible future debts that may arise due to some future event that is considered possible but not probable

- **Contra account:** an auxiliary account that is an offset to a related account (i.e., allowance for uncollectable accounts offset resident accounts receivable)

- **Contractual discount:** the uncollectable difference between the amount the facility charges for its services and the reduced/lower amount the facility has agreed to accept as reimbursement for either Medicaid/long-term care insurer

- **Contributed capital:** amounts paid into the assisted living facility by investors

- **Contribution**: a term used in marginal costing-the difference between sale price and associated variable costs

- **Contribution clause**: an insurance policy clause that limits the liability of the issuer to a pro rata portion of a loss of property insured by more than one company

- **Control account:** a general ledger account, the detail of which is contained in a subsidiary ledger (e.g., accounts receivable)

- **Controllable costs** (also known as **managed costs**): costs, chargeable to a budget or cost center, which can be influenced by the actions of the persons in whom control is vested

- **Controller:** the title usually given to the financial management executive responsible for the accounting function within the facility; this position usually reports to the chief financial officer (CFO) of the assisted living facility

- **Conversion cost**: the cost of bringing a product or service into its present location or condition; may include a share of production overhead

- **Convertible loan stock**: loans that, at the option of the lender, can be converted into ordinary shares at specified times and specified rates of conversion

- **Corporation:** business concern formed by a group of individuals, using a legal structure provided by law, possessing a "life of its own" so to speak, independent of the individual owners or investors

- **Cost basis**: the use of historical, objectively determined cost as the basis of accounting for most assets

- **Cost behavior**: the change in a cost when the level of output changes

- **Cost center**: a location, function, or item of equipment in respect of which costs may be ascertained and related to cost units

- **Cost control**: the attempt to maintain actual costs at, or below, budgeted levels

- **Cost convention**: the accounting convention whereby balance sheet assets are mostly valued at input cost or by reference to input cost

- **Credit**: commonly used to refer to a benefit or gain, also the practice of selling goods and expecting payment later

- **Credit control**: those measures and procedures adopted by a firm to ensure that its credit customers pay their accounts

- **Creditors**: those persons, firms, or organizations to whom the enterprise owes money

- **Creditors payment or settlement period**: a ratio (usually creditors/ inputs on credit in a year x 365) that measures how long it takes the firm to pay its creditors

- **Current assets**: cash plus those assets (stock, debtors, prepayments, bank accounts) that the management intend to convert into cash or consume in the normal course of business within 1 year or within the operating cycle

- **Current cost accounting (CCA)**: a system of accounting that recognizes the fluctuating value of money by measuring current value by applying specific indices and other devices to historical costs

- **Current liabilities**: debts or obligations that will be paid within 1 year of the accounting date; another term used to describe this is *creditors*: the amount falling due within 1 year

- **Current ratio**: the ratio of current assets to current liabilities

- **Cut-off**: the difficulties encountered by accountants in ensuring all items of income and expense are correctly ascribed to the right annual profit statement

- **Day's revenue in receivable**: the average number of days of billings in accounts receivable and uncollected at a given point in time

- **Debenture**: a document that creates or acknowledges a debt; commonly used for the debt itself

- **Debit**: amount shown in the left side of a T-account, increasing assets and expense accounts and decreasing owner's equity and liability

- **Debt**: a sum due by a debtor to his creditor; commonly used also as a generic term for *borrowings*

- **Debt-to-equity ratio**: long-term liabilities divided by total assets; it should be noted that debt-to-equity ratio of 0.5 or better is considered good

- **Debtors**: those who owe money

- **Debtors payment (settlement) Period**: a calculation of the average time taken by credit customers to pay for their goods; calculated by debtors/credit sales in a year x 365

- **Depletion method**: a method of depreciation applicable to wasting assets such as mines and quarries; the amount of depreciation in a year is a function of the quantity extracted in the year compared to the total resource

- **Depreciation**: a measure of the wearing out, consumption, or other loss of value whether arising from use, passage of time or obsolescence through technology and market changes; depreciation should be allocated to an accounting period so as to charge a fair proportion to each accounting period during the expected useful life of the asset

- **Direct costs**: those costs comprising direct materials, direct labor, and direct expenses which can be traced directly to specific jobs, products, or services

- **Discontinued operations**: operations of the reporting entity that are sold or terminated in a period; turnover and results must be separately disclosed

- **Discount**: a monetary deduction or reduction. Settlement discount (also known as *cash discount*) is given for early settlement of debts; debentures can be redeemed at a discount; trade discount is a simple reduction in price given to favored customers for reasons such as status or bulk purchase

- **Discounted cash flow**: an evaluation of the future cash flows generated by a capital investment project, by discounting them to their present value

- **Discounting of receivables**: a method of short-term financing in which resident receivables are used to secure a loan (which is less than the face amount of the receivables) from a financial institution; also known as *factoring*

- **Discretionary costs:** expenses such as advertisement, sales promotions, donations, etc.

- **Dividend**: a distribution of earnings to its shareholders by a company

- **Dividend cover**: a measure of the extent to which the dividend paid by a company covered by its earnings (profits)

- **Dividend policy ratios**: this provides insight into the dividend policy of the assisted living facility as well as its prospects for future growth; two commonly used ratios are the dividend yield ratioand the payout ratio

- **Dividend yield**: a measure of the revenue earning capacity of an ordinary share to its holder; calculated by dividend per share as a percentage of the quoted share price

- **Double-entry accounting**: a system of recording both the debit and credit aspect of each transaction

- **Earnings**: another word for *profits*, particularly, company profits

- **Earnings per share**: an investor ratio, calculated as after tax profits from ordinary activities/ number of shares
- **Equity**: the ordinary shares or risk capital of an enterprise
- **Equity convention**: the convention that a business can be viewed as a unit that is a separate entity and apart from its owners and from other firms
- **Equity financing**: raising funds by issuing capital stock, or ownership shares in the assisted living facility
- **Exceptional items**: material items that derive from events or transactions that fall within the ordinary activities of the reporting entity and that need to be disclosed by virtue of their size or incidence if the financial statements are to give a true and fair view; examples are profits or losses on termination of an operation, costs of a fundamental reorganization and profits and losses on disposal of fixed assets
- **Expense**: a cost that is in the profit and loss (P&L) account of a year; it is the cost of operating a business, including capital, administrative and other operating expenditures
- **Exposure draft**: a document issue on a specific accounting topic for discussion
- **Extraordinary items**: material items possessing a high degree of abnormality that arise from events or transactions that fall outside the ordinary activities of the reporting entity and that are not expected to recur; they should be disclosed but are very rare
- **Factoring**: the sale of debtors to a factoring company to improve cash flow; factoring is a method of obtaining finance tailored to the amount of business done; factoring companies also offer services such as credit worthiness checks, sales and debtor recording, and debt collection
- **FICA:** Federal Insurance Contributions Act, commonly known as *Social Security*
- **FIFO (first in, first out)**: A method of recording and valuation of fungible assets, especially stocks, thatvalues items on the assumption that the oldest stock is used first; FIFO stocks are valued at most recent input prices
- **Finance lease**: a leasing contract that transfers substantially all the risks and rewards of ownership of an asset to the lessee; in effect the lessee is really buying the assets with the aid of a loan and the lease installments are really payments of interest and repayments of capital; they are accounted for as such in accordance with the accounting convention of substance over form
- **Financial leverage ratio**: provides information of the long-term solvency of the assisted living facility; dssimilar to liquidity ratios that focus on short-term assets and liabilities, financial leverage ratios measure the extent to which the assisted living community is utilizing its long-term debt; two primary financial leverage ratios are the debt ratioand the times interest earned ratio
- **Financial ratio analysis:** the analysis of quantitative indicators of the financial health of the organization; these ratios depict liquidity or the ability of the ALF to satisfy short-term obligations
- **Financial statements**: balance sheets, profit and loss account, income and expenditure accounts, cash flow statements, and other documents that formally convey information of a financial nature to interested parties concerning an enterprise; in companies, the financial statements are subject to audit opinion
- **Fixed assets**: business assets that have a useful life extending over more than 1 year; examples are land and buildings, plant and machinery, vehicles

- **Fixed cost**: a cost that in the short termremains the same at different levels of activity; examples are rent, real estate tax, and depreciation

- **Flexible budget**: a budget that is flexed to recognize the difference in behavior of fixed and variable costs in relation to levels of output; total budgeted costs are changed to accord with changed levels of activity

- **Floating charge**: an arrangement whereby a lender to a company has a floating charge over the assets generally of the company gives the lender priority of repayment from the proceeds of sale of the assets in the event of insolvency; banks frequently take a floating charge when lending

- **Format**: a specific layout for a financial statement; several alternatives are often prescribed by the prevailing governing authority or law of the country in which the enterprise operates or reports its financial performance

- **Functional classification**: the grouping of expenses according to the operating purposes (administrative, property, and related, etc.) for which costs are incurred; revenues are also classified functionally

- **Fund**: a self-containing accounting entity set up to account for a specific activity

- **Fund balance**: the excess of assets over liabilities (i.e., net equity); an excess of liabilities over assets is known as a *deficit in fund balance*

- **Funded debt**: also known as *long-term debt*

- **Funded depreciation**: the setting aside of a portion of retained earnings in a special account to be used for the purpose of new or replacement capital assets

- **Funds flow statement**: a financial statement that links balance sheets at the beginning and end of a period with the profit and loss (P&L) account for that period;replaced by the cash-flow statement

- **Gearing**: also known as *leverage*, the relationship between debt and equity in the financing structure of a company

- **General ledger**: a book that summarizes all journal entries for an accounting period in order to arrive at a trial balance

- **Generally accepted accounting principles (GAAP):** combination of authoritative standards (set by expert boards) and the commonly accepted ways of recording and reporting accounting information

- **Goal congruence**: the situation in which each individual, in satisfying his or her own interests, is also making the best possible contribution to the objectives of the enterprise

- **Going concern**: the accounting convention that assumes that the enterprise will continue in operational existence for the foreseeable future; this means in particular that the profit and loss (P&L) account and balance sheet assume no intention or necessity to liquidate or curtail significantly the scale of operation

- **Goodwill**: an intangible asset that appears on the balance sheet of some businesses; i is valued at (or below) the difference between the price paid for a whole business and the fair value of the net assets acquired

- **Gross**: usually means *before* or *without deductions,* for example, gross salary or gross profit

- **Gross income**: gross receipts of the assisted living facility before deductions or expenditures

- **Gross margin**: (or gross profit ratio), gross profit expressed as a percentage of sales

- **Gross profit**: sales revenue less cost of sales but before deduction of overhead expenses; in a manufacturing company, it is sales revenue less cost of sales but before deduction of nonmanufacturing overhead

- **Group**: a set of interrelated companies usually consisting of a holding company and its subsidiary and sub-subsidiary companies

- **Group accounts**: the financial statements of a group wherein the separate financial statements of the member companies of a group are combined into consolidated financial statements

- **Historical cost**: the accounting convention whereby goods, resources, and services are recorded at cost; cost is defined as the *exchange* or *transaction price*; under this convention, realizable values are generally ignored; inflation is also ignored; the almost universal adoption of this convention makes accounting harder to understand and lessens the credibility of financial statements

- **Hurdle**: a criterion that a proposed capital investment must pass before it is accepted; it may be a certain interest rate, a positive net present value (NPV), or a maximum payback period

- **Income and expenditure account**: the equivalent to profit and loss (P&L) accounts in nonprofit organizations such as clubs, societies, and charities

- **Indirect costs**: costs that cannot be traced to particular products; an example is rent or management salaries;these are usually shared by more than one product and are called *overhead*

- **Insolvency**: the state of being unable to pay debts as they fall due; also used to describe the activities of practitioners in the fields of bankruptcy, receivership, and liquidations

- **Intangible assets**: assets that have long-term value but no physical identity; examples are goodwill, patents, trademarks, and brands

- **Interim dividend**: a dividend paid during a financial year, generally after the issue of un-audited profit figures halfway through the year

- **Interim financial statements:** financial statements prepared at a date other than the end of the fiscal year (e.g., monthly/quarterly balance sheets and income statements)

- **Internal rate of return**: the rate of discount that will just discount the future cash flows of a proposed capital investment back to the initial outlay

- **Inventory**: a detailed list of things; used by accountants as another word for *stock*

- **Inventory turnover**: the cost of supplies used divided by the average inventory for the period

- **Invested capital:** equity capital that is supplied by the owner(s) or shareholders of the assisted living community

- **Investment appraisal**: the use of accounting and mathematical methods to determine the likely returns for a proposed investment or capital project

- **Invoice**: a document portraying the details of a sale

- **Journal:** the book of original entry

- **Labor-hour rate**: a method of absorption in which the costs of a cost center are shared amongproducts on the basis of the number of hours of direct labor used on each product

- **Lease:** a contract in which the lessee (user) pays the lessor (owner) for the use of an asset

- **Ledger:** the collection of all accounts used in the assisted living facility

- **Leverage**: another word for *gearing*

- **Lien**: a claim on particular property for payment of a debt or obligation

- **LIFO (last in, first out):** a valuation method for fungible items in which the newest items are assumed to be used first; this means stocks will be valued at old prices

- **Limited liability company (LLC):** a flexible form of enterprise that blends elements of partnership and corporate structures

- **Limited partnership:** similar to general partnership, but a framework for investors who do not want to be personally liable (as with the sole proprietorship or general partnership) for all activity of a business, but want to invest and be exposed only to the extent of their investment

- **Line of credit**: an arrangement whereby a financial institution commits itself to lend the assisted living facility a specified maximum amount for a specified period of time

- **Liquidation**: the procedure whereby a company is closed, its assets realized and the proceeds divided amongst the creditors and shareholders

- **Liquidity**: the ease with which funds can be raised by the sale of assets

- **Liquidity ratios**: ratios that purport to indicate the liquidity of a business; these ratios provide information about the assisted living facility's ability to meet its short-term financial obligations; they are of particular interest to those financial institutions extending short-term credit (i.e., bank loans) to the facility; two frequently used liquidity ratios are the current ratio (or working capital) ratio and the quick ratio

- **Long-term investments:** investments, generally in securities, that the assisted living facility intends to own for longer than 1 year or more from the balance sheet

- **Long-term liabilities:** debts and obligations of the assisted living facility not due for more than 1 year or more

- **Management accounting**: the provision and interpretation of information that assists management in planning, controlling, decision making, and appraising performance

- **Management by exception:** control and management of costs and revenues by concentrating on those instances where significant variances by actual from budgets have occurred

- **Margin of safety**: the excess of budgeted activity over break-even activity; usually expressed as a percentage of budgeted activity

- **Marginal cost**: the additional cost incurred by the production of one extra unit

- **Marginal costing**: a system of cost analysis that distinguishes fixed costs from variable costs

- **Marginal return**: the point at which income equals expenses; it is also referred to as the *break-even point*

- **Matching convention**: the idea that revenues and costs are accrued, matched with one another as far as possible so far as their relationship can be established or justifiably assumed, and dealt with in the profit and loss (P&L) account of the period in which they relate; an example is the matching of sales of a product with the development costs of that product; the appropriate periods would be when the sales occur

- **Master budgets**: the overall budgets of an enterprise comprising cash budget, forecast profit and loss (P&L) account and forecast balance sheet (BS); they are made from subsidiary budgets

- **Material management**: the integration of the processes of planning, acquiring, moving, and controlling materials

- **Materiality**: the accounting convention that recognizes that accounting is a summarizing process; some items and transactions are large (i.e., material) enough to merit separate disclosure rather than inclusion with others in a lump sum; examples are an exceptionally large bad debt or an exceptionally large loss on sale of a fixed asset

- **Minority interest**: the interests in the assets of a group relating to shares in group companies not held by the holding company or other members of the group

- **Modified accounts**: financial statements that are shortened versions of full accounts; small- and medium-sized companies can file these with the Registrar of Companies instead of full accounts

- **Money measurement**: the convention that requires that all assets, liabilities, revenues, and expenses shall be expressed in monetary terms

- **Mortgage**: a pledge of designated property as security for a loan (e.g., mortgage bonds)

- **National Investment Center for Senior Housing (NIC):** established in 1991 to enable access and choice in seniors housing and care by collecting data and providing analytics that investors and operators need to make informed decisions

- **Natural expense classification:** a method of classifying expenditures according to their natural classification such as salaries, utilities, and supplies

- **Net**: usually means *after deductions*

- **Net book value**: the valuation on the balance sheet of an asset; also known as the *carrying value* or *written down value*

- **Net income**: the excess of revenue over related expenses during an accounting period

- **Net present value**: the value obtained by discounting all cash inflows and outflows attributable to a proposed capital investment project by a selected discount rate

- **Net realizable value**: the actual or estimated selling price of an asset less all further costs to completion (e.g., cost of a repair if it needs to be repaired before sale) and all costs to be incurred before and on sale (e.g., commission)

- **New worth**: can be calculated by total assets minus total liabilities

- **Nominal value**: the face value of a share or debenture as stated in the official documents; usually will not be the same as the issue price, which may be at a premium and that will almost never correspond to actual value

- **Objectivity**: the convention of using reliable and verifiable facts (e.g., the input cost of an asset) rather than estimates of 'value' even if the latter is more realistic

- **Occupancy rate**: a key utilization measurement of success for assisted living facilities that is the ratio of actual number of resident days to the total possible resident days

- **OpCo/PropCo:** a common industry vernacular referring to the idea that owners will separate the property interest in a separate legal entity ("prop-co") from the ownership of the ongoing business operations ("op-co") for added liability protection

- **Operating budget:** includes anticipated incomes by source and anticipated expenses by category

- **Operating cycle**: the period of time it takes a firm to buy inputs, make or market a product and sell to and collect the cash from a customer

- **Operating ratio**: total operating expenses divided by total operating revenues

- **Opportunity cost**: the value of a benefit sacrificed in favor of an alternative course of action

- **Outsourcing**: the use of services (such as administration or computing) from separate outside firms instead of using the enterprise's own employees

- **Overheads**: indirect cost

- **Partnership:** when two or more persons (or entities) wish to work on a venture together and the profits and losses are shared proportionally

- **Payback**: the number of years that will elapse before the total incoming cash receipts of a proposed project are forecast to exceed the initial outlays

- **Periodicity**: the convention that financial statements are produced at regular intervals usually at least annually

- **Petty cash fund:** a small fund of cash maintained by the assisted living facility for the purpose of making minor disbursements (e.g., less than $25 or $50) for which the issuance of a bank check is impractical

- **Physical inventory**: the actual inventory as determined by physical count by auditors, usually at the end of a reporting period (usually annually)

- **Planning variance**: a variance arising because the budgeted cost is now seen as out of date; examples are wage or price rises

- **Pledging of receivables:** the use of resident account receivables as security or collateral for a bank loan

- **Position control plan**: a management tool for controlling the number of employees on the assisted living facility payroll and for assuring the utilization of each employee to the point of maximum effectiveness; also known as a *staffing plan*

- **Posting:** a transfer from the general journal to the ledger

- **Prepayments**: expenditure already made on goods or services but where the benefit will be felt after the balance sheet (BS) date; examples are rent or rates or insurances paid in advance

- **Price earnings ratio**: an investor ratio calculated asshare/earnings per share

- **Private company**: any company that is not a public company

- **Profit and loss (P&L) account**: a financial statement thatmeasures and reports the profit earned over a period of time

- **Profitability index**: in investment appraisal, the net present value of cash inflows/the initial outlays

- **Profitability ratios**: provides information on several different measures of success of the assisted living facility at generating profits; two key profitability ratios are the return on assets ratio and the return on equity ratio

- **Provision**: a charge in the profit and loss (P&L) account of a business for an expense that arose in the past but which will only give rise to a payment in the future; to be a provision the amount payable must be uncertain as to amount or as to payability or both; an example is possible damages awardable by a court in a future action over a past incident (e.g., a libel)

- **Prudence** (or **conservatism**): the convention whereby revenue and profits are not anticipated, but provision is made for all known liabilities (expenses and losses) whether the amount of these is known with certainty or is a best estimate;essentially: future profit, wait until it happensfuture loss, count it now

- **Publicly traded:** a company whose ownership is made up of shares of stock that are publicly traded on one of several stock exchanges or "over-the-counter" markets

- **Purchase order:** document issued by the assisted living community authorizing a vendor to deliver goods with payment to be made later

- **Qualified audit report**: an audit report including one or more qualifications or exceptions

- **Quantity discount:** a reduction in unit purchase cost received by those who acquire supplies in a quantity in excess of a specific amount

- **Quick ratio**: also known as *acid test ratio*, current assets (except stock)/current liabilities

- **Real estate investment trust (REIT):** a legal entity that will raise large amounts of funds for owning large portfolios of property and then lease large portions of their portfolios to various larger operating companies

- **Realizable value**: the amount that an asset can be sold for

- **Realization**: to sell an asset and hence turn it into cash

- **Realization convention**: the concept that a profit is accounted (or when a good is sold and not when the cash is received)

- **Receiver**: an insolvency practitioner who is appointed by a debenture holder with a fixed or floating charge when a company defaults

- **Reconciliation**: the procedure of checking bank accounts, deposits, and withdrawals against the bank statement

- **Redemption**: repayment of shares, debentures, or loans

- **Redemption yield**: the yield given by an investment expressed as a percentage and taking into account both income and capital gain or loss

- **Reducing balance**: a method of depreciation whereby the asset is expensed to the profit and loss (P&L) account over its useful life by applying a fixed percentage to the written-down value

- **Relevant costs**: costs that will only be incurred if a proposed course of action is actually taken; the only ones relevant to an actual decision

- **Relevant range**: the range of activity that is likely; within this range, variable costs are expected to be linearly variable with output and fixed costs are expected to be unchanged

- **Reporting**: the process whereby a company or other institution seeks to inform shareholders and other interested parties of the results and position of the entity by means of financial statements

- **Reserves**: a technical term indicating that a company has total assets which exceed in amount the sum of liabilities and share capital; this excess arises from retained profits or from revaluations of assets

- **Resource accounting and budgeting**: the use of normal accruals accounting and balance sheets in federal/government departments and agencies

- **Responsibility accounting**: a system of accounting which accumulates financial and statistical information according to the organizational units generating the revenues and responsible for incurring the expenses; the primary purpose is to obtain optimal financial management control

- **Retained profits**: also known as *retentions*, the excess of profits over dividends

- **Return on capital employed**: a profitability ratio being income expressed as a percentage of the capital that produced the income

- **Return on sales**: the ratio of profit to sales expressed as a percentage

- **Returns**: the income flowing from the ownership of assets; may include capital gains
- **Revenue**: amounts charged to customers for goods or services rendered
- **Revenue expenditure**: expenditure that benefits only the current period and which will therefore be charged in the profit and loss (P&L) account
- **ROP**: known as the *reorder point*; in inventory management, the point in time at which a new order should be placed for supplies and/or services
- **Safe harbor regulations**: federal regulations describing investment interest and other business transactions that are not violations of the Medicare and Medicaid antifraud and abuse laws
- **Salvage value**: also known as *residual value*, the amount estimated to be recoverable from the sale of a fixed asset at the end of its useful life
- **Secured liabilities**: liabilities secured by a fixed or floating charge or by other operation of law such as hire purchase commitments
- **Securities**: financial assets such as shares, debentures, and loan stocks
- **Shareholder**: individuals or entities that own shares of corporation's stock
- **Single asset entity**: a legal entity formed to hold a single asset, not multiple, such as when organizations hold the real estate and the operations together
- **Sinking fund**: funds required by external sources to be set aside to meet debt service charges and the retirement of indebtedness on plant assets
- **Sole proprietorship**: a business ownership form, usually for smaller concerns, with a single owner, in which the owner as an individual is not separate from the business
- **State of changes in financial position**: a financial statement summarizing the movement of funds (working capital) within the assisted living facility for a given period of time
- **Stockholder's equity**: the excess of assets over liabilities that consists mainly of invested capital and retained earnings
- **Subchapter S corporation**: a corporation that is taxed by the Internal Revenue Service as a private individual
- **Subsidiary ledger**: a group of accounts that is contained in a separate ledger that supports a single account (a control account) in the general ledger
- **Tangible asset**: an asset that has physical characteristics as equipment, land, and buildings
- **Third-party payer**: someone else paying for the ALC bill other than the resident; it could either be a commercial insurance company that offers long-term care insurance or state Medicaid; Medicare generally does not pay for assisted living facility's expenses
- **Trial balance**: a financial statement indicating name and balance of all ledger accounts arranged according to whether they are debts or credits; debits must equal credits
- **Turnover ratios**: financial indicators that measure the efficient management of assets by indicating the number of times assets (inventories, accounts receivables, etc.) are replaced during a period
- **Useful life**: an estimate of the number of years an item of plant and equipment will be used by the assisted living facility
- **Variable cost**: an operating cost that varies in direct proportion to change in volume; examples are salary costs, supplies, etc.

- **Variance analysis:** managerial control technique that identifies deviations from the original budget projections

- **Voucher system**: a system for the processing and control of cash disbursements

- **Weighted-average costing**: a method that determines the cost of supplies used and the valuation of inventory

- **Working capital:** available excess assets left over from subtracting current assets from current liabilities that the assisted living community can use in operations

- **Write off**: the removal of a bad debt from revenues that reduces its value to zero; an example is resident room and board charges that are written off because of nonpayment after failure of collection efforts by the ALC

- **Yield**: the actual rate of return on an investment as opposed to the nominal rate of return

INDEX

Printed in the United States
by Baker & Taylor Publisher Services